DIAGNOSIS IN SPEECH-LANGUAGE PATHOLOGY

Diagnosis in Speech-Language Pathology

EDITED BY

J. Bruce Tomblin, Ph.D.
Hughlett L. Morris, Ph.D.
D. C. Spriestersbach, Ph.D.

SINGULAR PUBLISHING GROUP, INC.
SAN DIEGO, CALIFORNIA

Singular Publishing Group, Inc.
4284 41st Street
San Diego, California 92105-1197

© **1994 by Singular Publishing Group, Inc.**

Typeset in 10/12 Garamond by CFW Graphics
Printed in the United States of America by BookCrafters

Library of Congress Cataloging-in-Publication Data

Diagnosis in speech-language pathology / J. Bruce Tomblin, Hughlett L.
   Morris, D. C. Spriestersbach, editor[s].
        p.   cm.
     Includes bibliographical references and index.
     1. Speech disorders — Diagnosis.   I. Tomblin, J. Bruce.
   II. Morris, Hughlett L.   III. Spriestersbach, D. C.
     [DNLM: 1. Speech Disorders — diagnosis.   2. Language Disorders —
   diagnosis.   3. Speech-Language Pathology.   WM 475 D5362 1994]
   RC423.D473   1994
   616.85′5075 — dc20
   DNLM/DLC
   for Library of Congress   93-23600
                                                                      CIP

CONTENTS

P R E F A C E

This book has had a long and, we trust, will have a venerable history. Its beginnings can be traced to the fall of 1939 when Frederic L. Darley and D. C. Spriestersbach were among the crop of new graduate students seeking master's degrees in the Department of Speech and Dramatic Art at the University of Iowa. One of the core courses required of all of them, regardless of their future major emphases, was the voice and phonetics course taught by a young, brilliant, dynamic professor, Grant Fairbanks. The course had the characteristics of all of Fairbanks' teaching: build on the meticulous attention to and mastery of the basic elements of the subject matter.

That year Fairbanks had distributed numerous handouts to each class member, providing drills designed to ensure proficiency in General American Speech. Each student was tested to make sure that she or he was able to speak within norms that Fairbanks and his assistant (an appointment eventually held by Spriestersbach) found acceptable. The class materials were soon published by Harper and Brothers in 1940 as *Voice and Articulation Drillbook*.

The experiences in that course and the exposure to the Fairbanks' teaching style left its mark on Darley and Spriestersbach. Some 10 years later found both of them on the faculty of the University of Iowa Department of Speech Pathology and Audiology (which had separated from the Department of Speech and Dramatic Art in 1956). Darley was teaching a course on the introduction to clinical practice and Spriestersbach was teaching a course on voice and articulation disorders, presumably with a "functional" origin. They found themselves teaching with approaches similar to those of Fairbanks, with emphasis on systematic and thoughtful observation of the client's communicative behavior. In the process, they generated many class exercises, which they put into a workbook with tear-out pages for students to use in making clinical observations. Wendell Johnson supported their plan and agreed to participate as well. The result was the publication of the *Diagnostic Manual in Speech Correction* by Harper and Row in 1952.

Understanding of normal and disordered communicative behavior grew. The exercise forms, preceded by cryptic "whereas" introductions, became increasingly unsatisfactory. Consequently *Diagnostic Methods in Speech Pathology* was published by Harper and Row in 1963. To be sure, some of the exercise forms were still in the new book as examples but arrangements were made with Interstate Printers and Publishers, Inc., of Danville, Illinois to supply the actual forms on a commercial basis.

The second edition of *Diagnostic Methods* was published by Harper and Row in 1978 by Darley and Spriestersbach, with contributions from Charles V. Anderson, Arnold E. Aronson, Margaret C. Byrne, Julia Davis, Hughlett L. Morris, and Dean E. Williams. The Preface includes the following:

> This is a textbook for students who are learning to be speech and language pathologists. It is designed to give them a philosophy for clinical practice, to teach them how to be efficient observers of oral communicative behavior and of the speech mechanism, and to help them develop skills for arriving at therapy decisions based on differentiations made among the possible etiological implications of the communicative behaviors they observe.

> The current edition represents yet another stage in our thinking about the most effective way to teach diagnosis and appraisal. The forms have largely disappeared and the substantive material has been further enlarged. The major change, however, relates to our recognition that the previous editions were concerned primarily with appraisal; little was said about diagnosis. In this edition a major section of the book concerns diagnosis.

We see the present book not as a revised edition, but as a continuation of the four earlier books. In the new book, we continue the philosophy for diagnosis in speech-language pathology of the earlier ones. That philosophy includes the importance of disciplined, comprehensive description of behavior using the best tools available, comparing that information with information about the normal population, and bringing these data together with clinical history information to arrive at hypotheses about diagnoses that can then be rationally tested through therapy in a problem-solving mode.

We focus on this philosophy because, in our opinion, a major hazard of diagnosis is the development by the clinician of preferences for specific diagnostic instruments and their continued use based, in large part, on familiarity with them. Any seasoned practitioner will recognize the potential for such practice. Here, we emphasize the need for the student to prefer a model of diagnosis that is more open-ended in nature. This philosophy leads the clinician to continually search for better descriptors to arrive at an overview of a given behavior, at the same time being mindful of the cost in doing so. The diagnostic goal we emphasize is to help clinicians arrive at defensible and workable diagnoses.

The book's chapters introduce you to the process of diagnosis in speech-language pathology. By design, the chapters are a mixed bag, containing different kinds of discussions from different perspectives. Some viewpoints are philosophic, intended to help you think about general issues of asking questions, making observations, and interpreting findings. The chapter on multicultural issues places the diagnostic process within societal influences.

Another group of chapters discuss "basic" parameters of oral communication: language, speech production, voice, and fluency. Obviously, material in these chapters has important generic use. That is, the information is relevant to a variety of complaints.

Another group of chapters covers specific disorders and demonstrates how we must adapt our general principles to fit the needs of the specific client. These discussions, as others, are not intended to be sufficiently comprehensive to qualify the reader for independent practice with the specific disorders. Rather, the material offers the beginning student some notion about questions to be asked and perspectives to be taken in approaching the task of diagnosis for each of the disorders.

Finally, several chapters illustrate differences in the clinical practice of speech-language pathology by setting: the classroom, the hospital, and clinic, and the private and public agency.

Note that the word we use to refer to the consumer of our service changes with setting. In general, a *patient* is examined in a health care setting, but a *client* is provided services in a free-standing speech pathology clinic or in a training clinic. The speech-language pathologist works with *students* or *children* in a school setting. One author (Kent-Udolf) reports even that, in programs where she works, services are offered to the *consumer*! We have no preference for any terminology, but instead urge the speech-language pathologist to follow the customs of individual work setting.

We've tried hard in our language use to indicate that some clients/patients/students/consumers are girls and women and some are boys and men, and that likewise some speech-language pathologists are women and some are men. We think our references to gender match are suitably done; forgive us if we missed one or two.

Finally, a word about the contributing authors. This is a University of Iowa book and all of the contributors have a connection with the university, either as alumni or present faculty. We're very proud to emphasize this Iowa connection. However, we are prouder still that all these Iowa-connected authors are accomplished and dedicated clinical speech-language pathologists who write about clinical diagnosis in practical terms and from extensive clinical experience. No ivory tower people here. Many thanks to them for agreeing to fit this assignment into their busy schedules.

A very big thanks to the Assistant to the Editors, Juanita L. Reckling. She kept us and the contributing authors on track with great efficiency and in good humor. As is usually the case for endeavors like this, we could never have managed without her good work. Thanks also to Linda Tomblin, who assisted greatly in the final stages of manuscript preparation.

We hope you find the book useful to your purpose and, better yet, that you find it interesting. Let us know if you have comments.

J. B. T.
H. L. M.
D. C. S.

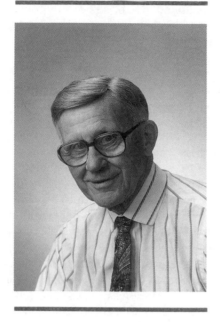

D. C. SPRIESTERSBACH, Ph.D.

M.A. 1940, The University of Iowa
Ph.D. 1948, The University of Iowa

Dr. Spriestersbach is Professor Emeritus at the University of Iowa.
He joined the faculty of the Department of Speech Pathology and
Audiology in 1948, and the faculty of the Department of Otolaryngology —
Head and Neck Surgery in 1957, was appointed Dean of the Graduate
College in 1965, Vice President for Educational Development and
Research in 1966, and served as Interim President of the University in
1981–1982. In speech-language pathology, his major interests are in
cleft palate and related disorders and in clinical outcome research. He
has served as President of the American Speech-Language-Hearing
Association and the American Cleft Palate-Craniofacial Association.
Currently, he is involved in the development of several for-profit
companies that are spinoffs of University research, an educational
software company, for which he now serves as a consultant.

Note: Identification for J. Bruce Tombline and Hughlett L. Morris is on pages
28 and 65.

CONTRIBUTORS

Frank M. Cirrin, Ph.D.
Special Education Service Center
Minneapolis Public Schools
Minneapolis, Minnesota

Jill L. Elfenbein, Ph.D.
Department of Speech Pathology and Audiology
Wendell Johnson Speech and Hearing Center
The University of Iowa
Iowa City, Iowa

Penelope K. Hall, M.A.
Department of Speech Pathology and Audiology
Wendell Johnson Speech and Hearing Center
The University of Iowa
Iowa City, Iowa

Linda S. Jordan, Ph.D.
Departments of Neurology and Speech
Pathology and Audiology
The University of Iowa
Iowa City, Iowa

Louise Kent-Udolf, Ph.D.
Private Practice
Houston, Texas

Hughlett L. Morris, Ph.D.
Department of Otolaryngology — Head and
    Neck Surgery
The University of Iowa Hospitals and Clinics
Iowa City, Iowa

Adrienne L. Perlman, Ph.D.
Department of Speech and Hearing Science
The University of Illinois at Urbana-Champaign
Champaign, Illinois

Sally J. Peterson-Falzone, Ph.D.
Center for Craniofacial Anomalies
The University of California
San Francisco, California

Donald A. Robin, Ph.D.
Department of Speech Pathology and Audiology
Wendell Johnson Speech and Hearing Center
The University of Iowa
Iowa City, Iowa

Shirley J. Salmon, Ph.D.
Veteran's Administration Medical Center
Kansas City, Missouri

Ann B. Smit, Ph.D.
Speech Pathology and Audiology Program
Kansas State University
Manhattan, Kansas

D. C. Spriestersbach, Ph.D.
Departments of Speech Pathology and
    Audiology and Otolaryngology — Head and
    Neck Surgery
The University of Iowa
Iowa City, Iowa

J. Bruce Tomblin, Ph.D.
Department of Speech Pathology and Audiology
Wendell Johnson Speech and Hearing Center
The University of Iowa
Iowa City, Iowa

Nancy A. Tye-Murray, Ph.D.
Department of Otolaryngology — Head and
    Neck Surgery
The University of Iowa Hospitals and Clinics
Iowa City, Iowa

Ann A. VanDemark, Ph.D.
Special Tree Rehabilitation System, Ltd.
Romulus, Michigan

Katherine Verdolini, Ph.D.
Department of Speech Pathology and Audiology
Wendell Johnson Speech and Hearing Center
The University of Iowa
Iowa City, Iowa

Amy L. Weiss, Ph.D.
Department of Speech Pathology and Audiology
Wendell Johnson Speech and Hearing Center
The University of Iowa
Iowa City, Iowa

Carol E. Westby, Ph.D.
University Affiliated Program
Albuquerque, New Mexico

Patricia Zebrowski, Ph.D.
Department of Speech Pathology and Audiology
Wendell Johnson Speech and Hearing Center
The University of Iowa
Iowa City, Iowa

CHAPTER

1

Perspectives on Diagnosis

J. Bruce Tomblin, Ph.D.

PERSPECTIVES ON DIAGNOSIS

If you are like most readers of this book, you are a student preparing for a career in speech-language pathology and/or audiology. For most students, the prospect of beginning work in a clinical field brings on mixed feelings. You are no doubt looking forward to clinical work because you will finally get to apply the information you have learned in the classroom. Furthermore, your practice may actually help someone else. Considerable apprehension may accompany this positive feeling, because speech-language pathology includes many roles and responsibilities that are unfamiliar to you. Few students have had the opportunity to receive services from a speech-language clinician and, unlike the professions of law and medicine, there are no television shows to inspire students and provide examples of the practice of speech-language pathology. You may have observed a speech-language clinician providing services and, if the clinician was skillful, you may have thought: "Will I be able to do that when I'm done with my professional education?" "Am I likely to have the talent to be able to provide clinical services?" And, worst of all, "what if I am no good at being a clinician or find that I don't like this type of work?"

It is very likely that these questions and other similar ones are going through your mind as you begin your professional education. Some of them cannot be addressed until you begin clinical work. Clinical work will require many things from you and only by actually doing the work will you begin to discover if this type of practice is satisfying to you. We anticipate, through the material in this book, that we can make at least one aspect of the clinical process more clear to you and reduce some of the uncertainty and mystery about the subject. This book provides you with information on how to perform one important aspect of clinical service — the assessment of speech and language disorders.

THE CLINICAL PROCESS

Speech-language clinicians engage in a variety of activities as they provide clinical services. Some of these activities are concerned with efforts to understand the client's communication problems. These activities are often referred to as diagnosis, or assessment. Other clinical activities include efforts to help modify, minimize, or resolve the communication problems and these are placed in the category called therapy, intervention, or treatment. Before we consider the assessment process, we need to consider what the clinical process is in general.

There are a variety of professions that, in one way or another, may be viewed as clinical. Certainly, physicians, dentists, clinical psychologists, and social workers perform clinical acts and their practices are characterized as clinical professions. What is it about the things these professionals do that lead us to refer to their activities as "clinical?" The most obvious commonality is that people go to these professionals to seek help for their personal problems. The clinical act, then, has as its basis a quality of "helping." In all human societies there are some who are given the role of providing assistance, in one way or another, to those individuals who are ill or suffering. In assuming this role, clinicians accept their client's trust that they will work in the client's best interest in relieving a problem. As a result, societies usually hold these "clinicians" in high esteem. The clinical process is, as a result, an act of helping and caring for others, while at the same time the clinician cannot become so emotionally involved as to be unable to exercise reasoned judgment. This aspect of the clinical process is one that most students in speech-language pathology and audiology understand and, in fact, it is what draws most of them to the profession.

A caring soul and a desire to help are not sufficient to produce a clinician. Part of the social contract between those who seek help and the clinicians who provide it is that the clinician actually has resources to help the client. The clinical process, then, also requires that the clinician have the ability to provide solutions to the client's problems. In the case of a tribal shaman, this may be the determination of the nature of the person's problem, the determination of the cause of the malady based on cultural lore, and the administration of an incantation or provision of herbs to remedy the problem. In such a case, the shaman is applying a body of knowledge to the problem being presented and, based on this knowledge, acting to help the affected person. Although we may view our clinical work as being much more sophisticated than the work of a native healer, the speech-language clinician also is expected to fulfill a similar role: as a thoughtful problem

Based on this definition, can you think of other professions that would also be clinical?

solver who brings current understanding of communication disorders to bear on the problems of the client.

Problem solving is a major part of the clinician's activities. The beginning student clinician often observes speech-language clinicians performing therapy or diagnostics, and what they see is the clinician doing things. It may be eliciting a speech sound from a child, instructing a person in better use of the voice, or administering a language test. Obviously, clinical work involves doing things and it is very logical for students to conclude that what they need to learn is how to do these things, and that if they learn about enough of these things they will also be capable clinicians. In fact, nearly all beginning clinicians, when assigned their first client, will ask themselves the question, "What am I going to do with this person?" Unfortunately, this is the wrong question, because it focuses your attention on doing something rather than the process of problem solving. Instead of asking what do I do, you must focus on the nature of the problem to be solved and the information you need to solve it. Once you have gotten to the point of knowing what information you need, the question of what you need to do will often become obvious. What you ultimately end up doing clinically should be, therefore, a logical part of the overall problem-solving process.

For the experienced clinician, the route between the problems presented by the client and the set of actions that need to be taken often requires little thought. Consequently, to the experienced clinician the problem-solving process may seem transparent or automatic. If you watch and even talk with an accomplished clinician, it may appear as though there is simply an obvious action for each clinical situation. For the beginning student or the experienced clinician with a difficult case, the problem-solving procedure is likely to be more difficult, requiring deliberate thought.

Let's examine this process by considering a situation in which a parent has come to you with a child whose speech is difficult to understand. How can we approach the problem-solving process in such a way that what we need to do becomes a product of our problem-solving process? We may start by beginning to frame a series of questions that we need to answer, such as "does the child have a communication disorder?" If so, "what aspects of communication are contributing to this problem?" Also, "are there factors that can be identified that are contributing to or complicating this problem?"

Having asked these questions, we can then begin to consider what information we need to answer them. For example, to answer the first question, "does the child have a communication problem," you need to know how old the child is — information you are likely to get by asking the child's mother. Obviously, we would interpret such a complaint differently if the child were 2 years old rather than 6 years old. In addition to the child's age, you will also want to hear the child speak. After obtaining the information you need to answer the initial questions, you will need to interpret the information using professional guidelines and standards to arrive at a conclusion.

The steps we just went through are depicted in Figure 1–1. We see that the first step is to determine what questions we should ask. Next, we establish what information is needed for us to answer the question. After

Good clinical work requires that you think about the problems you need to solve before you act.

Steps to Clinical Problem Solving

1. Establish the clinical question.

2. Determine the information needed to answer the question.

3. Determine how to obtain this information.

4. Gather the information.

5. Interpret the information using clinical standards.

6. Answer the question.

Figure 1-1. The clinical problem-solving process.

this, we can decide how to go about getting this information, that is, what we need to do. Notice that the question of what you are going to do becomes much easier to answer when it is placed in the framework of the general problem-solving process.

Once we have determined what we are going to do and, as a result, have gathered the information we needed, we are not done with this process. We still have to interpret the information in relation to the problem we were attempting to solve. This interpretation process is often the area where clinicians differ the most. As you develop as a clinician, you will acquire knowledge, beliefs, and attitudes that will determine your clinical interpretations of the information you have obtained. Therefore, these beliefs and attitudes will lead to your decision that a child is stuttering or that a teenager has a hoarse voice or that a person with aphasia should be seen for language therapy. I will term this collection of knowledge, beliefs, and attitudes *clinical standards*. Some believe this judgment process is the intangible quality that makes the clinical process an art and makes some clinicians better clinical artists than others.

Some believe that clinical arts cannot be taught, but only learned by extensive experience. If much of this is a definable judgment process, then it would seem that we should be able to teach it.

There is no doubt that, as one gains experience, this process of making clinical judgments becomes easier and probably more often correct. It is also true that, as our profession matures, these intangible notions contained in the mind of the master clinician can be made explicit and taught to beginning student clinicians. Much of what you will read in this book is just this sort of information. You will be reading about the kinds of decisions that confront the clinician in the diagnostic phase of clinical practice. Additionally, the kinds of information you need to obtain to address these questions are presented, as well as the ways in which you can gather this information. Finally, interpretation of the information gathered to answer these diagnostic questions will be covered.

I have just pointed out that the clinical process involves solving problems. That aspect of clinical work viewed as diagnosis addresses a set of common questions or problems with the objective of gaining an understanding of the client's communication disorder. Thus, *diagnosis is the clinical process concerned with understanding the client's communication disorder*.

This sounds rather simple, but actually understanding the client's communication problems involves multiple factors that go well beyond a characterization of a client's communication performance. Because of this complexity, a full understanding of a given communication problem is rarely attained; rather, this is a goal we work toward. Typically, this diagnostic process is the focal point of our clinical activities when we first begin to see a client. Obviously, any treatment efforts will be influenced by our understanding of the communication disorder. Rarely, is a full understanding of a problem arrived at before we initiate treatment. In fact, valuable information about the communication problem is often obtained during the treatment process, and therefore, we need to continually reassess the communication problem throughout treatment. Therefore, the diagnostic process is an ongoing aspect of the total clinical management process.

ASPECTS OF UNDERSTANDING A COMMUNICATION DISORDER

In other chapters you will be learning about what it is you need to know about specific types of communication disorders. In this section we will consider some basic questions that guide our diagnosis of most communication disorders.

Determination of the Complaint

The first question often confronting the clinician in the diagnostic process deals with determining what has led the person to be seen by the clinician. Unlike medicine or dentistry, few people seek out the speech-language clinician just to have a checkup to see that their communication skills are still fine. When people go to a speech-language clinician, they usually are seen because either they are concerned about their communication performance or someone else is concerned with their performance. The first question to be answered, therefore, often has to do with discovering what has caused the person to come to you for a diagnostic evaluation.

As a part of this question, we need to determine who is concerned about the person's communication performance and why they are concerned. In some instances, the client initiates the clinical contact and it must be determined what motivated the client to seek help. At other times the client is referred to the speech-language clinician by another professional, such as a physician or a teacher, because of concerns about the person's communication performance. The teacher may be concerned because a child is having difficulty with classroom learning activities and suspects that the child's language abilities are influencing the student's poor performance. The physician may be concerned because a patient has been having recurrent hoarseness and believes this results from the patient's vocal behavior. It is also common to have clients referred by family members — often parents or a spouse — because of concern about a child or spouse's communication.

In your clinical practice you will continually need to help teachers, physicians, and others know when and how to refer to you.

In such cases, we find ourselves having to address the concerns of the person who referred the client to us, as well as the concerns of the client, and we cannot always assume that these concerns are identical. An adolescent who stutters, referred to the speech-language clinician by a concerned teacher, may not view his stuttering as a problem. This certainly changes the nature of the problem we are dealing with and what it is that we need to understand. The key concept is that you must identify who is concerned and why they are concerned. It is very easy in a clinical setting to quickly focus on the issues that you think are important. Regardless of how important these issues are, if you do not address the concerns of the client and of those who have initiated the referral, your clinical efforts will fail because you haven't addressed the problem that originally brought the client to you.

Determining the Existence of a Communication Disorder

Whether the client is self-referred or referred by someone else, one of the questions we ask early in the diagnostic process is: "Does the client have a communication disorder and, if so, what aspects of communication are affected?" Usually, by the time we have addressed the first question concerning the complaint, we have some idea of the areas of communication that are likely to be contributing to the communication problem. If the complaint is linked to difficulties in being understood, we know that we need to obtain information about the person's speech sound production behavior. If the complaint is concerned with stuttering, we will look at the client's patterns of fluency and feelings about speech. Therefore, the complaint then directs our attention to obtaining sufficient information to determine if the person actually has a problem with that aspect of communication described in the complaint. Although we usually focus on those aspects of communication raised by the complaint, the cautious clinician will observe, at least informally, the person's competency across all domains of communication.

Earlier, we saw that information obtained in an evaluation needed to be interpreted by the clinician based on a set of clinical standards. In particular, in determining if a client has a communication disorder, we need to consider what our clinical standards are for the determination of a communication disorder. This seems like a straightforward problem and one that any speech-language pathologist should know how to handle.

Lee Edward Travis is viewed by many as the founder of American speech-language pathology. Van Riper was one of his most well known students.

Long ago Lee Edward Travis proposed that a "speech or voice defect may be defined as an unusually conspicuous deviation in the speech pattern of an individual which is incapable of bringing about an adequate social response and which by the same token constitutes a maladjustment to his environment" (Travis, 1931, p. 36). One of his students, Charles Van Riper, later stated that, "speech is defective when it is conspicuous, unintelligible or unpleasant" (Van Riper, 1963, p. 16). Although we have expanded the scope of our field to incorporate more aspects of communication than speech, these definitions provide a good starting point for considering what our standards for diagnosing a communication problem should be.

Each of these definitions recognizes that communication is a social tool. As such, a communication disorder will exist when a person's communication performance frequently fails to accomplish the social functions needed or the manner in which the person communicates is viewed negatively by either the speaker or the audience. In summary, the person's communication performance is either dysfunctional or displeasing. When you state that a person has a communication disorder, you are making a claim about the likelihood that the client will face difficulties because we all are required by society to accomplish various communication acts during our lives. A communication disorder, therefore, is not solely an attribute of the client, and it is not just the behavior of the client but rather *it is a relationship between the client and the person's current and future audiences*. The client is included as one of these audiences, because the client is often the individual most unhappy with his communication. Audiences have social values about communication and apply them to their communicative partners. As a clinician, you must develop an understanding of the uses of communication in a client's community and the values a given society places on communication. This will be easier if the client's social system is the same as yours. But if it is not, then you must try to understand the client's social system and make your clinical decisions in accord with the client's culture.

The ideas we have just discussed can be helpful in understanding the meaning of some terms used to refer to behavioral problems. You will also come across the terms "impairment," "disability," and "handicap" in some of the following chapters. These terms have been proposed to differentiate between different levels of an individual's communication disorder. *Impairment* refers to disruptions in the basic biological and psychological systems that are necessary for communication. The person who has difficulties with speech sound production because of a cleft palate has a speech problem because of an impairment in the palate. A *disability* is the inability to communicate because of the impairment. Therefore, the speech production difficulties arising from the cleft palate constitute a disability. The term *handicap* refers to the limitations in the fulfillment of social and cultural functions that result from impairments and disabilities.

> Cultures differ on how individual differences are viewed. For more information, see Chapter 2.

Here we see again that social values play a key role in determining when we say clients have a communication disorder. That is, when clients are handicapped by their communication skills we decide that they have a particular disability, namely, a communication disorder. We then attempt to explain why they have this communication disorder by looking for impairments in the basic systems involved in communication. The important thing to notice here is that when we say a person has a communication disorder we are making a statement about a relationship between the person's communication behavior and problems they may face in their life because of their communication skills.

The concepts we have discussed provide you with a general basis for developing your standards for the determination that a communication disorder exists. Once you have determined that a person presents a communication disorder, it will be necessary for you to begin to pose more questions to learn more about the client's communication disorder.

> Notice that I didn't give you a specific standard to use for the determination of a communication disorder. That's because the standards differ for different clients and different cultures.

Determining Client and Family Reactions and Attitudes to the Disorder

Communication is a fundamental aspect of being human. A limitation in this ability can lead to considerable social and emotional reactions by the client, the client's family, and friends of the client. These social and emotional responses often can be the most important aspect of the communication problem. Also, as you might expect, you will find that people respond differently to a communication disorder. For some clients, very subtle communication difficulties may provoke considerable concern in a parent or spouse; yet, in other cases, clients with rather striking difficulties may have relatives who are less concerned. Whether you view either response as under- or overreactions, it is very likely that any responses to your client's communication will influence the nature and success of your clinical management. Knowing about the variety of responses and including this information is necessary for a full understanding of a client's communication problem.

Identifying Associated Problems

Often, a communication problem occurs in the context of other problems. The child with a developmental disability such as cerebral palsy is very likely to have problems with feeding and ambulation, and the adult stroke patient may have problems with vision, as well as use of the right arm. Such concomitant problems can directly affect the way you will carry out your assessment and the way you will interpret some of the person's performance. For instance, a paralysis of the right arm of a person with aphasia may influence his performance on some assessment procedures requiring limb movement. So if this patient previously was right-handed, slow responses or even inaccurate responses may be due to the need to use the left hand rather than evidence of a language problem. Paralysis may be more troublesome for some patients than the communication problem that also resulted from the stroke. The relative importance of the communication impairment for such a person may be less than for a person who places high value on communication. Gathering such information is important in planning a program of rehabilitation combined with your judgment of the extent to which the communication problem handicaps the individual. This situation demonstrates that understanding the client's communication problem requires that you place the person's communication in the context of the client's needs.

See Chapter 7 for more on this topic in the context of acquired aphasia.

Determining Factors Causing or Exacerbating the Problem

Identifying the cause of something is usually considered an essential part of understanding it. Our ability to determine the cause of a communication disorder varies considerably across different types of disorders. You will also find that the importance of this decision in the clinical management of the client will vary.

A person with a chronic hoarse voice presents us with a situation in which determining the cause is very important. Often, an early sign of cancer of the larynx is hoarseness, so we must ensure that this causal factor can be determined and at least ruled out. If cancer is ruled out, as it often is, we may then hypothesize that vocal abuse may be the cause and use this causal hypothesis to guide our treatment.

There are other communication problems, such as developmental phonological problems, for which there are usually no known explanations. Even in dealing with these problems, however, it is important that you rule out the presence of hearing impairment, which could certainly cause a phonological problem. Once hearing impairment is ruled out, we are likely to proceed with a treatment approach that promotes phonological learning. In such a situation we don't know why the child has difficulty learning the sound system, but at least we can hypothesize that learning is at the root of the problem and that improved learning will remedy it.

These examples demonstrate that for all forms of communication disorder we will be concerned with determining the possible causes of the problem. In some instances, the cause of the problem can be treated, such as cancer of the larynx or hearing loss. In the best of cases treatment of causes will lead to a resolution of the communication problem as well. In other cases, such as a child with hearing impairment and a phonological problem, the treatment of the hearing impairment allows the phonological treatment to be more successful. In other instances, all we can do is rule out causal factors but even these negative findings are important. Often the client or family of the client will have developed beliefs about why the problem exists and such beliefs can generate unwarranted apprehension and, in some instances, blame. Addressing the causes and ruling out those that are groundless helps the client. Ruling out causal factors can also serve the clinician. As we will see in the next section, the course of the problem will frequently be different depending on the presence or absence of certain contributing factors.

Determining the Course of the Problem (Prognosis)

A basic property of humans is that we are always changing. You are capable of accomplishing different things today than you were a few years ago. It should come as no surprise that most communication problems change over time. For many, this change is toward improved communication skills. We often find this in children who, despite limited communication abilities, show gradual developmental growth. Likewise, the language skills of an aphasic will usually improve subsequent to the initial brain injury. Other communication problems may not be as predictable. The communication of a preschool child who stutters may improve or may become worse. As you study in this field, you will find that the prognosis for various types of communication disorders will depend on an array of factors, such as the client's age, the severity of the problem, and the cause(s) of the problem (to name some obvious considerations). You will also find that the crystal ball gazing required for developing prognoses is difficult but you won't be able to avoid this process. For the client and the family of the client this is *very* important. They usually know how the client is doing now. What they want to know is: "Will he get better?" If so, "How much better and how soon?"

Determining Treatment Alternatives

Earlier, I said that some clinical activities are focused on understanding the client's communication problem (diagnosis) and that other activities are concerned with efforts to modify the communication problem and that these two domains of clinical activity are closely related to each other.

A basic issue concerning treatment deals with whether or not initiating treatment or continuing treatment is warranted. Either can be one of the most difficult decisions you will face, and unfortunately, you will often lack a solid foundation for making such decisions. To make a decision to begin or continue treatment you will need to consider previous questions we have posed, that is, what is the prognosis for the problem and, in particular, will the outcome be improved if the person is provided with some form of treatment? Treatment can only be justified if the person will be better off for having had it. Likewise, treatment should only be continued for as long as you believe that the client will be better off for having received it. This leads us to want information about the client and the nature of the problem that will help us predict the client's future status when given a particular treatment, no treatment, or a different type of treatment.

In the later chapters you will be provided with information to help you determine treatment alternatives. At this point, I hope you have begun to see that diagnosis is, to a great degree, a thinking, problem-solving process. There are many questions that you will need to ask and with each question there are many procedures you may need to employ to address these questions. Your task at this point is to begin learning what questions you need to ask and what information you need to obtain to answer these questions.

Can you think of any ethical reasons why you might continue treatment when you have no reason to expect improvement?

MODELS OF DIAGNOSIS

The diagnostic process has been characterized as a decision-making process aimed at developing an understanding of the communication impairment. You will find that clinicians will vary on their views about what they think is required to understand a problem, and as a result, they conduct the decision-making process in different ways. Often, a given orientation will be influenced by the educational background of the clinician, as well as the work setting in which the person is employed. We will consider three different orientations to diagnosis that exemplify contrasting ways in which communication disorders can be understood through the diagnostic process.

The Medical Model

All of us at one time or another go to a physician because we are not feeling well. The doctor will ask some questions and make some observations, such as looking in our throat. After making these observations, we may be told that we have a particular illness, such as strep throat; and as a result, we are given a prescription for an antibiotic. This transaction exemplifies a medical approach to diagnosis. This orientation emphasizes the classification of symptoms into a disease category that often has a particular cause. Thus, the objective in medical diagnosis is on classification and explanation. Once the diagnosis is made, a physician can then turn to knowledge about the disease to make decisions about its course and treatment outcomes. In this orientation, the doctor is interested in the symptoms because they provide information about the type of the illness or disease which has a particular cause. It is assumed that the problems the patient presents with can be tied to one or more disease categories. Also, it is often assumed that the disease is something that is internal to the patient and that its nature and cause can be determined by examining the patient. Finally, notice that in this approach the treatment is often predicated on knowing the disease type, and, when possible, the treatment is focused on the cause of the disease. You should understand that I am describing this medical approach to diagnosis in its classic form. Often a physician treats the symptoms with a tentative treatment regimen, not fully understanding what is causing the symptoms, but this usually occurs because a traditional diagnosis cannot be made.

If you are working in a medical setting, you will find that your fellow health practitioners will assume that you are using this model. In many instances, however, the problems we are dealing with in speech-language pathology may not fit well into this framework. Some types of communication problems will not be the product of a disease process. In such cases, we may need to consider an orientation to the diagnostic process where categorization of problems and identification of causes are not considered to be very important.

Behavioral/Educational Model

Many clients with communication disorders are not being seen in a medical setting. Neither they, nor their families, view their problem as a sickness. The majority of clients who receive speech-language services are children or adolescents in school or preschool settings. The problems they have may be viewed as learning or developmental problems and, in many instances, we don't know why they are having these problems or, if we do know, there is little that can be done to resolve the cause. Because of the educational nature of the service setting and the developmental nature of the problems confronted in these settings, those working in educational settings tend to employ an orientation to assessment that is often referred to as a behavioral, or educational, approach.

Within the behavioral approach, the primary interest is in characterizing the client's performance in tasks that are viewed as important for educational or social success. The focus of this approach is on describing the child's performance on relevant tasks, rather than on identifying certain behaviors that are suggestive of a particular disease. Because the causes of these problems are usually difficult to determine and even more difficult to change, this approach focuses on conditions that may lead to improved communication performance even if these factors were not involved in the cause of the problem. For instance, a clinician may decide that a 4-year-old child with a language problem will be helped if the parents spend more time reading bedtime stories, even though the clinician does not believe that the absence of bedtime stories contributed to the child's language problem. Thus, we see that the clinician using this approach is interested in finding ways to change the child's behavior, often by using educational or behavioral models to encourage change.

Systems Model

The two models we have considered so far assume that to learn about a problem we must look carefully at the client and learn about the person's behavior and possibly factors within the person that led to the communication problem. In contrast, some argue that an adequate account of a communication problem requires that we look at the familial and cultural context within which the person lives. This view leads the clinician to include the parents, spouse, and/or teacher of the client in the diagnostic process to learn about the dynamics of the communication problem. Also, those using this approach often observe the client in a natural context. Accordingly, rather than performing the assessment in the clinician's office or examination room, the clinician will observe the client at home or in the classroom. Furthermore, the clinician will seek to learn which contexts and interactions seem to promote better communication and which seem to impede communication success. The communication problem, in this case, is seen as a mismatch between the client and the environment.

The three models presented are not the only approaches you will encounter in your career, but these three show us that as clinicians we adopt general philosophies about what we think is important in our attempt to understand the nature of a communication problem. It is difficult to argue that one of these models is better than the others. Each provides a different view of the problem, and if you are going to be a thoughtful clinician, you should be able to adopt all or part of each model, depending on the needs of particular clients. For instance, the acceptance of a behavioral orientation should not lead you to assume that you can simply ignore assessment questions that are associated more with the medical approach, such as etiology and prognosis. Likewise, the clinician using the medical model will sometimes deviate from the standard medical model and treat the symptoms in a way that is similar to the behavioral model. All clinicians should be able to move from one model to another and sometimes combine approaches. In this way our understanding of the communication disorder is enriched, and hopefully, we are provided with more insight into the problem.

METHODS FOR OBTAINING INFORMATION

It should be very clear by now that the assessment of communication disorders requires the clinician to obtain a variety of types of information and that this information gathering is conducted for a variety of purposes. The clinician has a wide range of methods of assessment from which to choose to obtain information. The most prominent of these assessment methods are discussed in following chapters, and you will see that these methods fall into one of the following five categories.

Interviews

See Chapter 3 for an in-depth discussion of interviewing.

A very common diagnostic method is by some form of interview. In an interview the clinician usually poses questions to an informant. The questions are designed to obtain information to help make some of the basic diagnostic decisions. The informant is often the client with a communication problem; however, it is also common for us to interview parents, spouses, teachers, or even employers. No doubt, the most common type of information obtained by means of interview has to do with the basic complaint. That is, early in the diagnostic process you need to hear why the client is coming to you. Along with this, you will probably obtain a basic description of the communication problem through an interview.

Some interviews are unstructured in that the questions asked are generated by the clinician "on the spot" and are driven by the clinician's problem-solving goals. In other instances, the clinician may administer a structured interview by following a script and, therefore, systematically gathering information regardless of the particular client and clinical situation. It is not at all uncommon for clinicians to develop their own structured interview tool, particularly to collect information on the history of the communication problem.

Written Questionnaires

The use of a written questionnaire is another method that is similar to the structured interview. There is a wide variety of questionnaires. Many are generated by clinicians for their own use; others are available from commercial sources. The items in these questionnaires may require that the informant respond to yes-no type questions and others may ask for open-ended responses which allow the client to provide input. The information obtained from questionnaires often covers background information on the client and the history of the client's problem, but the forms may also allow for information gathering on the client's feelings about the communication disorder and/or the communication settings that are most troubling to the client. The informant may also be someone other than the client. Parents can provide developmental history through questionnaires, teachers can provide systematic information on children's school performance, and nurses and other caregivers can provide insight into how a patient is communicating.

You can see that questionnaires are handy tools. They can provide you with useful information that may be difficult to obtain in other ways. Also, you can use them to obtain information efficiently and inexpensively because you don't need to be involved in the information collection. Efficiency is important because, as a professional clinician, your time has to be paid for by someone. As you consider your diagnostic procedures, you will have to consider the cost involved in obtaining the information you seek and try to find ways to reduce it.

Standardized Tests

The standardized test is one of the most common assessment tools used by clinicians. A standardized test is usually designed to measure a client's performance in one or more domains of performance, such as phonological ability or sentence comprehension. Some tests are developed to measure some presumed individual trait such as intelligence. Usually the authors of such tests assume that the *trait* being measured is an enduring characteristic of the person similar to hair color. Traits of communication may include the client's ability to understand words and sentences or the client's word retrieval ability. These trait-oriented tests, therefore, test some hypothetical enduring property of the client.

Some other examples of traits measured by tests are aptitude measures for music or college performance.

In contrast to trait-oriented tests, there are tests designed to characterize or describe a person's speech and language behavior, such as the rate of certain types of speech disfluencies. These tests are designed to tell the clinician if and how much the client does of something and, thus, provide information on the characteristics of the client's communicative performance. Usually no effort is made to use these measures as evidence of some underlying trait.

The important point to be understood here is that tests are designed for different purposes. The people who develop the tests should be very clear about a test's purposes and provide you with evidence that the tests measure what they are purported to measure. Later we will see that this property of a test is called its validity. As a clinician, you must determine if the test will provide you with appropriate information to help you address the clinical problem confronting you.

I said earlier that there is a variety of types of tests. For a test to be considered a *standardized* test, it must be constructed to ensure that whatever is being measured is not influenced by the person administering and interpreting the test. That is, we want the measurement procedure to be uniform across examiners. Written directions must clearly outline what the examiner says and does during the testing, including "scripts" for the instructions to the client. Also, the stimuli used to elicit the client's behavior must be given and, finally, explicit rules for scoring the client's responses must be provided. By standardizing the method of a test, it should be possible to compare the results of one test administration with another. As I show you later, this allows us to compare a client's test performance either with the same client's earlier performance, with the performance of some normative group, or with some established standards for performance on a given test. Standardization allows us to assume that differences in performance are based on differences in the client's ability or trait status rather than differences in the test circumstances.

The value of standardized tests as tools for the assessment of communication performance has been debated for many years. Often, clinicians believe that, by being so structured, standardized tests destroy the fundamental social-interactive quality of communication. Many of the tests available to us attempt to isolate and measure particular aspects of communication such as expressive grammatical ability, but in so doing strip away the pragmatic and semantic dimensions of language that naturally interact with the grammatic skill in which we are interested. As a result, the standardized tests of communication are usually less natural. Better and more thoughtful test construction may solve some of these problems; nevertheless, we also must recognize that the price to be paid for replicable and objective measures is a restriction on some of the things that the clinician can measure. Standardized tests are likely to be valuable tools for you to use, but they need not be the only tools you use. As I have been saying throughout this chapter, your decision to use a standardized test should be dictated by the clinical problem you are trying to solve. In many instances the criticisms of standardized tests have more to do with the inappropriate use of tests than with the inadequacy of standardized testing per se.

In quantum physics, it has been found that the act of observing atomic particles changes their character. Likewise, it seems difficult to measure communication performance precisely without disrupting it in some way.

Observation

The standardized testing method of assessment attempts to measure a person's performance on explicitly defined tasks. The advantage of this assessment method is that the measures should be replicable. The disadvantage is that the things being measured are in an unnatural context and, therefore, we are often left wondering how the person performs in the "real world," or at least in settings that are like the real world. In some assessment situations, the clinician may want to change a task to see how the variation influences the client's performance — something you are not supposed to do within strict standardized testing situations.

To meet the needs for naturalness and flexibility, the clinician often turns to observation. The clinician may observe the characteristics of a person's voice, fluency, or language during a conversation. During such an activity the clinician may notice a relationship between her speaking rate and the rate of disfluencies by the client. Having noted this, she could be in a position of manipulating her rate systematically while continuing to track the client's disfluencies.

The observation of communication performance is certainly a vital and useful assessment method. However, for this method to be useful the clinician must know what to observe. To do this you need to have developed a general framework for describing the various dimensions of communication. You have already begun to do this by learning about the nature of normal and disordered communication. As you gain experience, you will refine this scheme. In other chapters you will also be given some protocols to provide you with schemes to observe systematically a variety of the client's characteristics, including such things as the client's oral mechanism, various aspects of his language, as well as properties of his voice and fluency.

Instrumented Observation

A number of aspects of speech and swallowing are difficult to observe without the aid of instruments. For these circumstances, technological advances have provided the clinician with an ever-increasing array of tools to aid in observation and measurement of these physical systems. The acoustic properties of voice and speech can be obtained from a computer equipped to analyze acoustic data. Also, through the use of a fiberoptic tube, clinicians can look directly at the vocal folds. Also, in association with a radiologist, the clinician can use x-ray images to observe the actions of the oral mechanism during swallowing. With such technology, the clinician can make very detailed observations and measurements. Whereas clinicians were denied such precision in the past, now you will be faced with having to determine which of the measures will be useful in your clinical problem solving. Otherwise, you will spend a great deal of your time and the client's time and money gathering information of limited use. As in all fields, as we obtain new technology we have to learn to use it appropriately.

BASIC CONCEPTS OF CLINICAL MEASUREMENT

So far we have talked about the various ways we can obtain diagnostic information, that is, the different measurement methods. You can see that a wide variety of tools is available to you and you must learn to select the measurement methods that will be accurate and meaningful, because your clinical decisions depend on the data obtained from them. To make selections wisely, you will need to know how to interpret the accuracy and meaningfulness of a clinical measure. But before we discuss this, we need to talk briefly about the categories of measurement scales used, because the type of measurement scale will influence how we can describe the accuracy and meaningfulness of our measure.

Measurement Scales

A nominal scale employs categories that have names as values. Thus, "stuttered" and "fluent" are nominal values in a scale of speech fluency.

Sometimes the measure you use allows you to represent your observation in terms of a category, or name, such as hoarseness, and therefore, a category measure can be represented as either being present or absent. This type of measurement scale is a *nominal scale*. At other times, the measure may be in the form of a scale having to do with more or less of something such as with a judgment of the severity of stuttering. With such a scale you might have possible values ranging from 1 to 7, in which a value of 4 would be viewed as greater than 2, but we may not be able to justify saying that a severity of 4 is twice as severe as a severity of 2. This form of measurement is termed *ordinal* because order or ranking information is contained in the measure. Finally, we also have measures that employ numbers in their ordinary sense in that the numbers represent counts of the number or magnitude of something. For example, we may measure the rate a person can repeat a syllable over the span of 10 seconds. The person who produces 30 syllables is speaking twice as fast as the person who only produces 15 syllables. This type of measurement scale is usually referred to as a *ratio scale*. You can see that there are various ways in which the measures you make can be represented, ranging from a nominal system to one that involves true counting. Now we can turn to the ways in which we can describe the accuracy and meaningfulness of our measures.

Reliability

Regardless of the method of measurement you employ, there will always be error associated with the measure. One type of measurement error reflects variability between repeated administrations of a test or observation. Even when we use the same test and give the test under apparently identical circumstances, we will usually obtain somewhat different results. The property of a test or measure having to do with its replicability is termed *reliability*, and it is important for a clinician to know something about the reliability of the measures obtained. If a test is not very reliable, the clinician needs to be cautious about interpreting the results.

The reliability of a measure can be influenced by several factors. Some portion of the error can be a product of the behavior of the client. On one administration the examinee may have been more attentive or less fatigued than during another examination session. Also, measurement error can be introduced by the examiner or person doing the measurement. For instance, a clinician may be interested in the fundamental frequency of a speaker's voice and use electronic equipment to obtain this information. If a different microphone is used for separate sessions, there may be a slight variation in the fundamental frequency even though the speaker may have actually produced the same acoustic signal during both sessions.

Many of the factors that influence the reliability of a measure are random or at least not systematically associated with the measurement process. Sometimes error will cause a measure to be too small; at other times the error will cause the measure to be too large. This points to a way to improve the reliability of a measure. If you repeat the measure several times, the errors will tend to cancel each other out. As you can see, the more measures you take, the more stable your overall measure will be. Therefore, if you are interested in a child's grammatical ability and you measure this by means of the average number of words in the child's utterances, you will have a more reliable measure if you compute this measure of grammatical ability on 100 utterances than if you compute it on 50 utterances. Likewise, all other things being equal, longer tests are more reliable than shorter tests. It is also true that longer tests and repeated administrations of a measure take more time than shorter tests and single administrations. For the clinician, this often means balancing the need for greater reliability against the cost of conducting additional measures.

Ways of Describing Reliability

The reliability of a clinical measure is often provided to you by those who have developed the tool. Many of the clinical measures you will be using are commercial products that cost quite a bit of money. Part of the publisher's or manufacturer's justification for the price of the tool is the cost associated with determining its reliability. As an educated consumer, you need to require that the supplier and developer of a tool provide information concerning its reliability. You will need to be able to read the manual and understand and evaluate the information provided on reliability.

You will find that there are different types of reliability indices reported for particular instruments. Remember that earlier I talked about the fact

Often the reliability of our clinical measures is based on normal speakers. Do you think this creates a problem when we use the tools on speakers with communication disorders?

that we could measure things with different measurement scales. Such information is used in describing reliability. The type of measurement scale employed influences the way the test developer reports reliability.

Agreement

If the instrument uses a nominal scale for measuring aspects such as the presence or absence of a moment of stuttering, then the reliability of the measure is in the form of a measure of agreement. Let's assume that a clinician reviews a video tape and tallies the occurrences of stuttering and then repeats this observation of this video tape again the next day. Table 1-1 displays the results of our hypothetical clinician. Notice that the clinician wasn't always consistent in these judgments. This inconsistency can be represented by rate of agreement. There are several ways that this agreement can be computed. The generally accepted method uses the formula in Figure 1-2. Using this method, our clinician achieved a 71% agreement. As both sets of observations were performed by the same clinician, this is an *intrajudge agreement* measure. If, in our example, the second set of observations had been performed by another observer, this measure would have been a measure of *interjudge agreement*.

Reliability

In many measurement situations the scale used will involve a test score or a physical measure, such as a person's fundamental frequency. Earlier, we described this type of scaling as a ratio scale. In this case the reliability measure should reflect the *stability* of the measure or score. Let's assume that we administered a vocabulary test to a group of children twice. This would allow us to determine the *test-retest* reliability of the measure. We could look at the stability of the scores by plotting each child's scores. Data like these are contained in Figure 1-3. Each child's score on the first administration is plotted on the horizontal axis, and the second score is plotted on the vertical axis. Given perfect reliability, the scores should line up on the diagonal. You can see that they don't. The extent to which the scores deviate from the diagonal reflects the unreliability of the test. If you have had a basic course in statistics, you know that we can measure the correspondence between two such sets of measures, by calculating a correlation coefficient. A common correlation coefficient used for this purpose is the

Table 1-1. Decisions made by a clinician regarding instances of stuttering during two different listening sessions of a video tape.

Listening Session	Word 1	Word 2	Word 3	Word 4	Word 5	Word 6	Word 7
1	Yes	No	No	Yes	No	Yes	No
2	Yes	Yes	No	Yes	No	No	No
	Agree	Disagree	Agree	Agree	Agree	Disagree	Agree

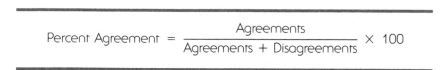

$$\text{Percent Agreement} = \frac{\text{Agreements}}{\text{Agreements} + \text{Disagreements}} \times 100$$

Figure 1-2. Formula for computing percent agreement.

Pearson Product Moment (r). In our example the test-retest reliability co-efficient is .93. Some believe that a test should have a test-retest reliability coefficient of .90 or greater (Salvia & Yessldyke, 1991) for it to be used with confidence.

So far we have considered test-retest reliability. In many cases, a score will consist of several items combined to measure a trait such as vocabulary level. The test developer can obtain a measure of reliability by comparing the scores obtained on one half of the test, for instance the odd items, with those obtained on the other half, that is the even items. This type of reliabil-

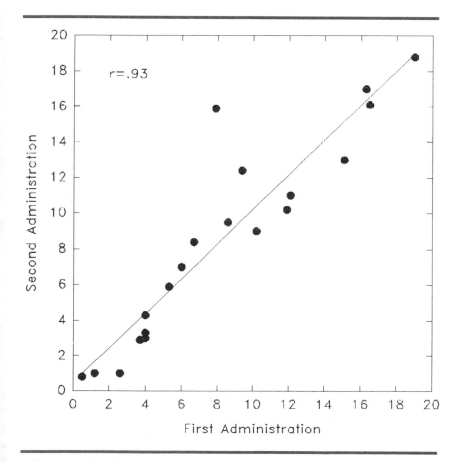

Figure 1-3. These data are hypothetical scores from two administrations of a test to the same individuals. Notice that the scores don't change much and thus the correlation (.93) shown by the straight line is high.

ity is called *split-half reliability* and reflects the internal consistency of the test in contrast with the test's stability reflected in the test-retest reliability.

Validity

The validity of a measure refers to how accurately the measurement tool measures the characteristic in which we are interested. Validity provides us with information about what the measurement means and, therefore, what conclusions can be made from the measure. In a sense then, validity is concerned with the truthfulness of the measure. For instance, there may be several ways to obtain a measure of a speaker's fundamental frequency. If these measures provide conflicting results, which do you believe, which is the most truthful index of fundamental frequency?

It shouldn't surprise you that a concept dealing with meaning and truth is not clear-cut. Although some people will make a blanket claim that a certain clinical measure is valid, in fact, it is always necessary to specify the measurement purpose when discussing validity. A given measure can have strong validity for some purposes and poor validity for other purposes. The *Peabody Picture Vocabulary Test — R* (PPVT-R) originally was designed to be used as an intelligence measure. Over the years, psychologists have found that it is not a particularly good measure of intelligence, because it depends on only one skill. Hence, it is not regarded as a valid intelligence measure. In contrast, the PPVT-R is viewed as a valid measure of receptive vocabulary. This demonstrates that, as a clinician, you are responsible for learning about the issues of validity associated with the measures you use.

To evaluate the validity of a new measure, we must have some external standard of truth. Then we can compare our new measure with this standard. There are three common types of external standards used by test developers to establish validity, resulting therefore, in three types of validity indicies. The first type of validity is *concurrent validity*. To establish this type of validity a new or untested measure is compared with another measure that is widely regarded as accurately measuring the same property. The *Stanford-Binet Intelligence Test* has served as a standard against which many newer intelligence tests have been validated and thus shown to have concurrent validity with the Stanford-Binet.

In other situations, a test developer may want to show that the measure can be used to make predictions about a person's likely performance in some other place or time or maybe on another type of task. This type of validity is called *predictive validity*. A speech-language pathologist may develop a listening task that will predict how well a child will understand classroom instructions. This requires a predictive validity type of interpretation, and therefore, the measure needs to be compared with an acceptable measure of classroom comprehension to determine its predictive validity.

There is one other common form of validity. Often our measures have to do with some hypothetical trait or attribute that we believe underlies a person's performance. In our clinical practice we may use many hypothetical constructs such as short-term memory, anxiety, or linguistic competence. These are usually things about a person that can't be directly observed, and it is possible that the thing being measured may not actually

Validity is dependent on the reliability of a measure. Why do you think this is so?

exist. When we think we are measuring such a construct, our measurement instruments need to demonstrate *construct validity*. An example may help you get a sense of what construct validity involves. Let's assume that we want to develop a measure of English grammatical competence. First we need a theory about the nature of grammatical knowledge, therefore, we need a grammatical theory. Next, based on our theory we will need to make some predictions about how people may differ with respect to this knowledge and who is likely to show these differences. Thus, we may expect children to have a different knowledge than adults. Also, the theory needs to predict how this construct should be displayed in a person's grammatical performance. Therefore, we may expect to see evidence of grammatical knowledge in listening, speaking, and maybe judgments about the grammaticality of sentences. With this theory in mind we must develop tasks that will measure this construct in the most straightforward manner so that differences in people's performance are likely to be due to differences in their grammatical knowledge and not other extraneous factors. Finally, research will be needed to show that our test of grammar does appear to be consistent with the predictions of the theory and that persons who are likely to have differences in grammatical knowledge do indeed differ on our test. Moreover, we would expect that their performance on our test correlates well with other indices of their grammatical knowledge.

As you can see, construct validity is most difficult to achieve. First, it requires that your measurements be based on a theory. Then the test must be developed in a way that is consistent with the theory. Finally, there must be considerable supporting reasearch demonstrating that the test does conform to the predictions of the theory. Because of the complexity of this process, the construct validity of a test may gradually be documented over time.

Diagnostic Accuracy

Our attention so far has been directed toward the measurement tools we use in the assessment process. These clinical tools that provide us with measures of speech, language, or swallowing do not make decisions; that is what the clinician does. In order to do this, recall that the clinician must bring a set of interpretive standards to bear on the information gathered in making decisions. The measures used by the clinician might be highly reliable and very valid, but if the standards used to interpret these measures are poor, the clinical decision will be poor. Therefore, not only is it possible for us to evaluate the accuracy of the measurement process, it is also possible to evaluate the accuracy of the whole diagnostic process involving both the instruments and the diagnostic standards used by a clinician to arrive at a final decision.

The notion of diagnostic accuracy is very similar to that of measurement validity, in that it deals with the correctness of the clinical decision. Just as we needed some standard of truth for establishing validity, we also need one for diagnostic accuracy. This standard is referred to as the "gold standard" because, whatever it is, it is assumed to be the truth against which clinical decisions are measured. In medicine, a gold standard can often be a laboratory test or an autopsy performed by a pathologist. The results of such extensive examinations are then compared with the clinical diagnosis made by a physician. We must realize that gold standards often are not perfect, but rather represent the best that can be done at a given time.

Once a gold standard has been established, we can compare clinical decisions with the gold standard to judge how accurate these decisions are. Let's assume we screen by observation for hoarseness in a group of children and then perform a more in-depth examination that determines their true hoarseness status. The results of such a hypothetical clinical study are displayed in Figure 1–4. We can see that the screening decisions did not always agree with the gold standard of the in-depth study. Of those children who were thought to be hoarse from the initial screening, 20 (25%) turned out to have normal voices, meaning the screening decision had a *false positive rate* of 25%. Also, there were 9 children (3%) who were thought to have normal voices but were found to be hoarse. Accordingly, the screening test had a *false negative rate* of 3%. The terms "positive" and "negative" are a little confusing here. A positive decision is one that says the person has the clinical condition, thus positive usually means bad because it indicates a clinical condition. A negative decision, on the other hand, is construed to be good, because it represents an absence of the clinical condition. Clinicians want to have low false positive and false negative rates. No one likes making mistakes, but how can you reduce your mistakes? One way you can lower both of these error rates is by using better measurement tools. But if you can't change your measurement instruments, the only thing you can change is the diagnostic standard you are using.

In the voice diagnosis example we have been talking about, you might believe that you are diagnosing too many children with normal voices as having hoarse voices. In such a case, you will want to reduce your false positive rate. The way you can do this is by becoming more reluctant to say a

		Gold Standard		
		Hoarse	Normal	
Diagnostic Test	Hoarse	20	60	False Positive .25
	Normal	9	291	False Negative .03

Figure 1-4. Diagnostic accuracy of hoarseness.

child has a hoarse voice. As a result, some of those cases that were marginal, but considered to be hoarse during the earlier screening example, now will be judged as normal. Unfortunately, this change in your standard will also probably have an impact on your false negative rate, and it won't be a good change. By becoming more stringent in your determination of hoarseness, you will have a greater tendency to say a child has a normal voice and therefore you will increase your false negative rate — saying a child is normal when actually the child is hoarse. That is, when you change your diagnostic standard to reduce one type of error, you will usually increase the other type of error.

When making clinical decisions we have to decide what kind of error is the worst to make — saying someone is okay when they are not, or saying they have a problem when they don't have one.

The major point is that the accuracy of our clinical decisions can be evaluated. By studying our decisions we can begin to learn where errors are coming from and we can discover ways to reduce errors. Remember, the way to become better clinicians is by making better, more accurate decisions. As our measures improve and our standards for making decisions improve, our clinical effectiveness will improve.

APPROACHES TO MEASUREMENT INTERPRETATION

So far, what we have talked about are rather abstract ideas that affect the quality of our clinical measures. How do clinicians actually interpret the data they obtain from their clinical observations to arrive at conclusions about the performance of their clients?

The specific approaches and standards used to make diagnostic decisions will be detailed in subsequent chapters. You will find that most of the approaches for interpretation of clinical information can be placed in three general categories: (1) norm-referenced interpretations, (2) criterion-referenced interpretations, and (3) client-referenced interpretations.

Norm-referenced Interpretation

One common way that we can interpret measures we obtain is by comparing the client's performance to some other group of individuals, sometimes called the normative group. Often the normative group is a representative sample of individuals who are of the same age and possibly same sex as the client. There are two ways we can compare a client's performance to a normative group — standard scores and equivalent scores.

Standard Scores

For norm-referenced measures, the standard score approach evaluates the client's placement within the normative group. To understand this, we need to review some basic characteristics of the *normal distribution*. Figure 1–5 depicts such a distribution. You can see that there is a concentration of people toward the middle and then a rapid decrease in the number of individuals as you move away from the middle of the distribution. If we divide the group up into the upper half of the distribution and the lower half, the dividing line represents the *median* score for the group. This would also be

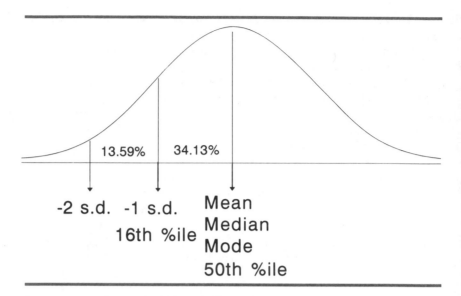

Figure 1-5. The normal curve and the terms used to identify the location of a score on this curve.

the 50th percentile. We can also compute the average score for the group. This *mean* value will also be near the center of the distribution and, for truly normally distributed data, the median and the mean will be the same. The extent to which scores deviate away from the mean is represented by the *standard deviation*. For scores with a normal distribution, 34.13% of the scores will fall within 1 standard deviation above the mean and 34.13% will fall within 1 standard deviation below the mean. These statistical descriptors for characterizing the middle of the distribution and then the location of a score's distance from the middle of the distribution allow us to describe where our client stands in this distribution, using scales based on the normal distribution.

A very common scale, based on the normal distribution is the percentile scale. Percentile should not be confused with the percentage correct on a test. Your client could get 65% of the items on a test correct and yet be at the 10th percentile. The client's percentile score will depend on how the person performs in relation to her comparison group. The 10th percentile means that 90% of the comparison group received higher values on the measure than the client. You can see in Figure 1-5 that the 50th percentile is equivalent to the median and the mean. People who have scores placing them 1 standard deviation below the mean will be slightly below the 16th percentile. If the person's score is 2 standard deviations below the mean, the person will be close to the 2nd percentile. Notice that changes in percentile and changes in standard deviation are not consistent with each other. The change from the mean (0 standard deviations) to −1 standard deviation involves 34 percentile points whereas the change from −1 to −2 only represents 14 percentile points.

You can see that we can describe how a person has performed on a norm-referenced test by converting the actual test score, which might be the number of correct responses, into standard deviation units. Standard deviation units are a little awkward because they may involve negative values and decimals. Because of this, most norm-referenced measures allow you to convert the test score, also called the raw score, into a *standard score* that does not have a negative number or decimals. The intelligence quotient (IQ) is an example of a standard score. When a test is developed, a number is established that will represent the mean. In the case of IQ, the number representing the mean is 100. Also, a value is given to represent the standard deviation for the standard scores, which in the case of most IQ tests is 15. The test publisher will usually provide you with tables that allow you to convert the raw score into standard score units. Further, there are likely to be different tables for different age groups, which allow you to select the group that best matches your client. Once you know what the standard score equivalent is for your client's raw score, you can use your knowledge about what the mean and standard deviation is for this standard score to determine where on the normal distribution the client's score will fall.

Another standard score system is used with the SAT and GREs. For these tests, the mean is 500 and the standard deviation is 100.

Equivalent Scores

We have been talking about interpreting measures by comparing an individual to a group of individuals by describing where in the normal distribution the person falls. It is also possible to interpret the score by identifying the group of individuals that are most likely to achieve a given score. Let's assume that a client obtains a score of 25 on a vocabulary test. Because children's vocabulary improves with age, we could then ask what age group is most likely to obtain this score. Our client may be 4 years old, but we may find that the obtained score is typical of 3-year-old children. Therefore, we might put in a diagnostic report that the child's vocabulary age is 3 years. This is an example of an age-equivalent score, but you will also find grade-equivalent scores. Parents find age- and grade-equivalent scores easy to understand, and because of this, many clinicians employ equivalence scoring. We have to be cautious about how we interpret the equivalent scores, however. With these scores, we have no idea whether differences in equivalent scores are unusual or common in the general population, and uncommonly low performance often is taken as a sign of a problem. For instance, returning to our example, although we know our 4-year-old obtained a vocabulary score similar to the typical 3-year-old, we don't know how unusual this is. It may turn out that our vocabulary score of 25 places the child at the 40th percentile for 4-year-olds, and therefore, this score is not particularly discrepant for all 4-year-olds. On the other hand, this score could place the child -2 standard deviations below the mean and therefore be unusual for a 4-year-old. It is because of this problem with equivalent scores that clinicians are being discouraged from using them.

Criterion-referenced Interpretation

Norm-referenced interpretation of measurement information makes the measurement interpretation meaningful by comparing the client's performance with that of some group of other individuals. There are some decisions, nevertheless, that don't call for this type of interpretation. For instance, you may be working with a patient who has a swallowing disorder that results in the aspiration of material into the lungs during swallowing. It is not important how this person's swallowing behavior compares with a group of adults. Instead, you are interested in whether there is significant aspiration. In such a case you need a standard defining unacceptable aspiration which may be based on data about the likelihood of respiratory complications. Clinical standards such as these are sometimes referred to as criterion-referenced standards. That is, there is some level of performance that can be viewed as minimal for acceptable performance. What is acceptable may be determined by a group of experts or, as in the case of our swallowing problem, be evidence that undesirable outcomes become common below or above some level of performance. You should be able to see that criterion-referenced interpretation often involves a qualitative evaluation of the performance having to do with "good-bad" or at least "acceptable-unacceptable," whereas, a norm-referenced interpretation brings with it more of a quantitative meaning having to do with "common-uncommon," "typical-unusual," or "high-average-low." The two can be combined in some instances because "unusual," "low" levels of performance may often also be associated with unacceptable or undesirable outcomes.

Client-referenced Interpretation

So far we have talked about ways of interpreting a client's performance by comparing the measures we have obtained with similar measures obtained on another group of individuals or against some criterion-based standard of performance. There are times that neither of these two approaches serve the decisions we need to make. Instead, we may be more interested in comparing some clients' performance to themselves. In fact this type of comparison may be the most common form of clinical interpretation. We frequently do this as we track the client's progress in therapy by comparing levels of performance at different points in time. In many settings it is necessary to document that, in association with clinical intervention, there is improvement and this requires that we obtain repeated measures of the same or very similar behavior from the client across the treatment period.

Sometimes the questions we are addressing call for comparing the client's results on two or more different tasks or different types of behavior. When evaluating young children with speech sound production difficulties, we often need to determine the likelihood that the child will make improvements in speech sound production without therapy. That is, we need to predict future developmental change in the child's communication. We can make this prediction by observing the children's speech sound production in spontaneous speaking tasks such as picture naming, and comparing this performance to the child's spontaneous performance when given auditory and sometimes visual models of how to produce the sound. Improvement when going from spontaneous productions to modeled production is a positive sign for future improvement in sound production. Client-referenced interpretations that involve either the same type of measures at different times or different types of measures obtained during the same examining session will be covered in other chapters.

SUMMARY

In this chapter you have been introduced to the process of diagnosis. We have seen that it is a problem-solving task requiring the clinician to set up the problem, gather data, interpret the data, and arrive at conclusions. The objective of the diagnostic process is to develop an understanding of the multiple dimensions of a client's problem. In so doing, the clinician employs a wide range of skills and knowledge having to do with ways of evaluating measurement methods, as well as the interpretation of the information obtained from these methods. Thus, although the diagnostic process does involve actions that we have described as measurement, these actions all must serve the specific problem-solving purposes you require to best help your client.

REFERENCES

Travis, L. E. (1931). *Speech pathology*. New York: Appleton-Century.
Van Riper, C. (1963). *Speech correction*. Englewood Cliffs, NJ: Prentice-Hall.
Salvia, J., & Yessldyke, J. (1991). *Assessment*. Boston: Houghton Mifflin.

RECOMMENDED READINGS

Bellack, A., & Hersen, M. (Eds.). (1988). *Behavioral assessment: A practical handbook*. Boston: Allyn & Bacon.
McCauley, R. J., & Swisher, L. (1984). Use and misuse of norm-referenced tests in clinical assessment: A hypothetical case. *The Journal of Speech and Hearing Disorders, 49*, 338–348.
Nunnally, J. (1972). *Educational measurement and evaluation*. New York: McGraw-Hill.

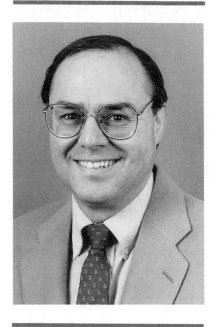

J. BRUCE TOMBLIN

M.A. 1967, The University of Redlands
Ph.D. 1970, The University of Wisconsin at Madison

Dr. Tomblin is a Professor in the Department of Speech Pathology and Audiology at the University of Iowa. He was previously at Syracuse University. His special interests are in language development and disorders of children, including possible genetic influences on specific language impairment.

CHAPTER

2

Multicultural Issues

Carol E. Westby, Ph.D.

A man's home is his castle. (English)
Mi casa, su casa. (Spanish)

The squeaky wheel gets the grease. (American)
The duck that quacks loudest gets shot. (Chinese)

Take care of #1. (American)
The group always comes first. (many traditional cultures)

Appropriate assessment and treatment of culturally/linguistically diverse clients requires an understanding of their culture. What does it mean to understand a culture? Numerous misconceptions of culture exist. It is often equated with art, music, food, and holiday celebrations or with the language one speaks. Such a view of culture results in the belief that understanding another culture can be accomplished simply by participating in its celebrations and learning the language. But culture involves more than the things people make and use. It also includes how people interact with one another and their belief and value systems. The statements at the beginning of this chapter represent contrasting values that can affect persons' interactions.

Being bilingual is often equated with being bicultural, but a bilingual person is not necessarily bicultural. Being bilingual will not ensure effective communication, if you do not recognize a person's values, beliefs, and patterns of interaction. In fact, some of our most serious miscommunications may occur when we are speaking the same language.

Describe your family's culture. How does your family's culture differ from the family culture of some of your friends?

Gary Larson, author of the Far Side cartoons, mistakenly assumed that being bilingual results in effective communication. In one cartoon he depicts a man attempting to talk with a duck. The man tries, "Sprechen sie deutsch?" and gets no response. Next he tries, "Habla español?" and still he receives no response. He then tries, "Parlez vous francais?" The duck continues to stare at him. Finally the man looks at the duck and says, "quack?" The duck responds with "Quack!" and the man and the duck continue their conversation. The byline reads "It's nice to have someone who understands me."

Now, I have a pet duck, Mocha, and I have learned that speaking quack is not sufficient for effective communication with a duck. I speak quack. I know that a loud, prolonged "muck muck muck" means, "You've left me outside, and I want in." I know that a soft, short, quick series of "muck, muck, muck" means, "I've just seen a big, black New Mexican cockroach." — which are the chocolate chips of the duck world. Despite being bilingual in English and Quack, I have not been able to avoid miscommunication problems with Mocha.

We bought Mocha shortly after he hatched from his egg at the feed store. He quickly imprinted on my husband and for several months followed him everywhere. Eventually, he began to show an interest in me. He would nibble at my ankles and stretch and bob his neck. Because he looked uncomfortable as he did this, I thought that he had a sore throat or something in his throat. I took him to the vet. It cost me $15 to learn that this duck was a drake, he was going through his second imprinting, and his head bobbing meant he was propositioning me to be his wife.

You can see that an adequate evaluation of Mocha's behavior requires an understanding of duck culture. I cannot assume that what I know to be true of humans is true for ducks. Otherwise, I might treat Mocha's normal behaviors as pathological and seek unnecessary and inappropriate treatment.

THE NEED FOR UNDERSTANDING CULTURAL/LINGUISTIC DIVERSITY

I do not believe that Mocha has suffered from my lack of knowledge of duck culture. Inadequate understanding of human cultural/linguistic diversity can, however, harm persons. Culturally/linguistically different clients frequently have been inappropriately placed in special education classes; treatment approaches have been used that violate their values and beliefs; and true speech, language, and hearing problems have sometimes not been identified.

Demographic changes are resulting in significant changes in the types of clients being served by speech-language pathologists and audiologists. According to the 1990 U.S. Census, which admittedly undercounted people of color, the minority population of the United States exceeds 60 million persons. One American in 4 already is self-defined as Hispanic, African

---

Not counting Native American languages, school districts in the United States have identified more than 100 languages from more than 120 countries.

Can you think of a situation in which you experienced a miscommunication with someone with whom you were speaking even though the two of you were speaking the same language?

It is estimated that in certain categories of special education individuals from culturally/linguistically different populations are overrepresented as much as 60–80%.

American (Black), Asian American, Pacific Islander, or Native American. If current trends in immigration and birth rate continue through the end of the 20th century, the Hispanic population will have further increased by an estimated 21%, the Asian population by about 22%, Blacks by almost 12%, and Europeans by a little more than 2%. Several states already have a third or more of their populations from nondominant cultural groups, who combined, are now more than 50% of many large cities. Following current demographic trends, by 2010, one third of the American people will be people of color and by 2056, caucasians will be a minority group. The implication is that, whether you identify yourself with the Euro-American culture or with a minority culture, many of your clients will come from a culture different from your own. The American Speech-Language-Hearing Association estimates that 10% of the population in the United States has a disorder of speech, hearing, or language. If the prevalence of communication disorders among minority groups in this country is consistent with that for the general population, it is estimated that 2.9 million African Americans, 190,000 Native Americans, 720,000 Asian Americans, and 2.2 million Hispanic Americans have communication disorders (Battle, 1993).

> Presently, less than 5% of members of the American Speech-Language-Hearing Association are from Asian, Hispanic, African American, or Native American backgrounds.

This chapter familiarizes you with the issues and considerations you will encounter in assessing individuals from culturally and linguistically diverse backgrounds. Other chapters will provide you with specific means of assessing a client's speech and language abilities. In this chapter I give you few specifics of what to do. Instead, I focus on why it is difficult to conduct valid and reliable speech and language assessments of culturally/linguistically diverse clients. In assessing the speech and language abilities of culturally/linguistically diverse clients you must possess the information provided in all the other chapters of this book, plus have an understanding of:

1. The development of communication in different cultures;

2. The causes and effects of communication disorders in various racial/ ethnic populations;

3. The effects of culture and second language acquisition on the process of testing and test interpretation;

4. Dialect differences versus speech-language disorders; and

5. Alternative assessment approaches for culturally/linguistically different clients.

> Information necessary to work with clients from culturally diverse backgrounds can be gained from fields such as anthropology, linguistics, sociology, and teaching English as a second language.

Speech-Language-Hearing Disorders in Diverse Ethnic/Racial Groups

As a speech-language pathologist or audiologist, you need to be alert to risk factors for communication disorders in different populations. Although persons from nonmainstream American backgrounds generally have the same types of communication disorders as those in the dominant culture, the frequency and causes of particular conditions may vary. Native American populations have a higher incidence of otitis media, or middle ear infections, than other racial/ethnic groups (Downs, 1985). These infections occur earlier and more frequently than in the general population. Otitis media is associated with mild, intermittent hearing loss and, in some circumstances, may result in delayed speech and language skills. White adults are more likely to experience significant hearing loss associated with aging than are Black adults (Post, 1964). Native American and Asian populations exhibit a higher incidence of orofacial anomalies such as cleft lip and palate (Vanderas, 1987). There are distinct differences in frequency of occurrence of cleft lip and palate among skin color groups, with clefts less frequent in darkly pigmented skin colors and more frequent in lightly pigmented skin colors (McWilliams, Morris, & Shelton, 1990). African-American populations are at greater risk for high blood pressure, which increases their risk for strokes that can affect their speech and language (Spector, 1985). Persons of African and Mediterranean descent are more likely than other populations to carry a gene for sickle cell anemia. This genetic condition causes the red blood cells to be abnormally curved. These malformed cells tend to clump together, blocking blood vessels and causing, among other difficulties, strokes. Strokes can occur in all parts of the body, including the blood vessels in the inner ear and brain, thus causing hearing loss and speech, language, and cognitive disabilities (Scott, 1985).

Knowledge about racial/ethnic differences is critical in counseling families about possible causes of communication disorders and risk of communication disorders in other family members.

Lead poisoning is also known especially for young children to cause decreased cognitive abilities and associated speech and language delays. Individuals from low socioeconomic urban environments are at greater risk for lead poisoning than middle class individuals from suburban or rural areas because of unreplaced lead plumbing and lead-based paints in old buildings or exposure to lead fumes from vehicle exhaust or factories. Even when socioeconomic levels and environment are held constant, persons of color appear to have a higher incidence of lead poisoning than White persons (Mayfield, 1985).

Cultural Attitudes Toward Disabilities

What people do about speech, language, and hearing disorders is related to their beliefs about what is a disability. Professionals from mainstream American culture families generally regard hearing loss and speech-language delays and disorders as potential and significant disabilities. Consequently, they are likely to seek medical treatment for otitis media, hearing aids for sensorineural hearing loss, and therapy for speech-language delays and disorders. In taciturn cultures and cultures where children learn by watching and not questioning, families may not recognize the hearing or speech-language disorders that concern mainstream professionals. Mainstream culture places a high value on communication skills. Adults encourage children to ask and answer questions and tell stories. Once a child walks, parents focus on a child's talking. If a mainstream child is not talking by age 18 months or 2 years, parents express concern. In contrast, many nonmainstream cultures do not place a high value on verbal children. Crago (1988), in a study of Inuit children, reports being intrigued with a young Inuit child who was more verbal than other children. Crago viewed the child as highly capable. When Crago questioned adults about this child, however, she gained a different perspective. They reported that they too were concerned about the child — because he didn't know when to keep quiet!

To understand peoples' responses to communicative disorders, you must understand what they value. Figure 2–1 summarizes the dimensions of cultural value-orientation systems (Sue & Sue, 1990). Persons in the mainstream American culture tend to look toward the future. They focus on being active and demonstrating their accomplishments. Who they are and what they are worth are dependent on what they do. Children are socialized to be independent. They are rewarded for accomplishments they achieve on their own. People are viewed as having power over nature. As adults, the value is that persons be responsible for mastering circumstances that arise. With this value system, mainstream families tend to think about the significance of a disability in terms of the future. They may ask, "When will she learn to talk?" " Will therapy correct the problem?" or "When can he return to his teaching position?" They express concern regarding what persons cannot do, what they will be able to do, and when they will be able to do it. Parents, spouses, or clients take responsibility for alleviating the disability. Persons with these mainstream values seek treatment for speech-language-hearing disabilities and are active co-participants in their therapy.

Many nonmainstream American cultures focus on the present and value the past. Persons are valued simply for their existence or being, not for what they can do. Persons are interdependent, not independent. Families may consist not only of children and parents, but also of grandparents, aunts, uncles, cousins, and even nonrelated friends. People believe that they cannot affect nature and what happens to them; they may attempt to live in harmony with events or the world as it is, or they may believe there is nothing they can do about their circumstances. In such nonmainstream

Think about your family. What are your value orientations with respect to time, human activity, social relations, and relationship with nature?

In nonmainstream families, older siblings are primary socializers who may be candidates for training to carry out therapeutic activities with a younger brother or sister.

Dimensions	Value Orientation		
1. *Time Focus* What is the temporary focus of human life?	*Past* The past is important. Learn from history.	*Present* The present moment is everything. Don't worry about tomorrow.	*Future* Plan for the future: Sacrifice today for a better tomorrow.
2. *Human Activity* What is the modality of human activity?	*Being* It's enough to just be.	*Being & In-Becoming* Our purpose in life is develop our inner self.	*Doing* Be active. Work hard and your efforts will be rewarded.
3. *Social Relations* How are human relationships defined?	*Lineal* Relationships are vertical. There are leaders and followers in this world.	*Collateral* We should consult with friends/families when problems arise.	*Individualistic* Individual autonomy is important. We control our own destiny.
4. *People/Nature Relationship* What is the relationship of people to nature?	*Subjugation to Nature* Life is largely determined by external forces (God, fate, genetics, etc.)	*Harmony with Nature* People and nature co-exist in harmony.	*Mastery over Nature* Our challenge is to conquer and control nature.

Figure 2-1. Value-orientation model. From Sue, D. W. & Sue, D. (1990). *Counseling the culturally different: Theory & practice,* p. 139. New York: John Wiley, with permission.

cultures, people generally have a greater tolerance for variation; they may feel less need to "fix things" and focus, instead, on learning how to accept and cope with their circumstances. Families may recognize that a family member is different, but accept that difference as being a natural aspect of who the person is. As a Hispanic mother said when enrolling her non-speaking child in kindergarten, "Luis is my quiet one." She was aware that Luis did not talk much, but she accepted his quietness as just being Luis. Because of such outlooks, persons from cultures with nonmainstream values may be less likely to seek out evaluation and treatment services. When they do become involved, it is important to include the extended family in decisions.

Even when a speech, language, or hearing problem is recognized, nonmainstream families may not approach treatment in the expected way. Mainstream professionals generally believe that a physician or certified therapist should be immediately consulted to perform necessary surgery or treatment when a handicapping condition is diagnosed. In contrast, Native American families may first need to consult a tribal healer before having their child treated for otitis media. Hispanics may employ the services of a *curandero* (healer) before or while they are receiving mainstream therapies.

NO SUCH THING AS CULTURE-FREE TESTING

When you work with nonmainstream American cultures you may need to spend time laying the groundwork for referral for evaluation and intervention services. Evaluation may involve:

1. Testing of clients' abilities through the use of published standardized, normed tests.

2. Testing of clients' abilities through the presentation of activities structured by the evaluator. The evaluator may present the tasks in a standardized format and use developmental information to interpret clients' performance, but no normative data may be available. Narrative language sampling is a form of this type of testing.

3. Assessment of clients' abilities through observation in naturalistic environments. Clients are not required to perform a particular activity. Instead, the evaluator observes the client performing familiar activities in familiar settings and makes an assessment of how adequately the client performs.

Once the clients do come for evaluation, other issues arise. Traditional evaluation often emphasizes administration of tests: standardized tests, normed tests, and test-like activities. Professionals who evaluate bilingual and culturally different clients frequently ask me, "What tests should I use?" Or they tell me, "As long as I test in the client's dominant language or use nonverbal tests, then the client's language background is not an issue." Such questions and statements reflect the fallacious assumption that there are valid tests for culturally different persons. You need to understand why there are no valid tests for culturally/linguistically diverse populations.

Because the act of testing is itself culturally biased, testing in the native language or using nonverbal tests are not adequate solutions to the problems of assessing culturally different individuals with limited English proficiency. Testing involves the presentation of decontextualized tasks and structured professional-client interactions that are unfamiliar to persons from many cultures. Therefore, because the decontextualized tasks and the communicative interaction patterns of the testing situation are unique, there can be no valid tests for culturally different clients, regardless of the content and language of the tests. To understand the issues in assessing culturally different clients, you must understand how the behavioral interactions and language requirements of the testing culture differ from the culture of the clients being assessed.

Persons raised in societies with square houses are more likely than persons raised in societies with round or octagonal houses to perceive the top figure as longer than the bottom figure.

$$\longleftrightarrow$$

$$\mathrel{\rule[0.5ex]{3em}{0.4pt}}$$

Nonverbal Aspects of the Testing Culture

Perception and Use of Time

We are apt to view testing as a time-bound activity. Testing is scheduled: for instance Tuesday, September 2, 10 A.M.–noon. Subtests within the assessment are also time bound. One activity is completed before moving on to the next. There is no going back, even if the client later realizes the answer to an earlier question. Time is of the essence — the faster the better. To appear intelligent, clients must perform quickly within the given time limits. Native American, Latin, and Middle Eastern cultures are less bound to this view of time (Hall, 1984). In such cultures, activities are done "when the time is right" and need not be started and completed within a specified time frame. Culturally different persons may not respond to efforts to have them complete a task as quickly as possible, either because they do not view speed as critical or because they have not previously had to manage time in the way demanded by testing.

In mainstream society, time is monochronic — things are accomplished one-at-a-time in a linear fashion. In many nonmainstream societies, time is polychronic — many activities take place simultaneously and schedules are invisible.

Learning and Displaying Learning

Beliefs about how learning occurs vary in different cultures. In mainstream American culture, adults assume that for learning to occur children must be explicitly taught with words. In many African American, Hispanic, and Native American cultures, learning more often occurs by observing others. Children are encouraged by adults to "watch me." Adults may seldom give verbal explanations. Children watch until they can do the task. They may watch for many months or years before they are expected to do the task, and they may not attempt the task until they are certain they have mastered it. Children from nonmainstream cultures may expect you to show them how to do the tasks, and few standardized tests permit this. Clients who are used to having tasks demonstrated for them may lack strategies for trial-and-error learning. They may be hesitant to attempt unfamiliar tasks of the type that you present in testing situations, even if they understand the words of the language and the instructions of the test.

Watching approaches to learning tend to result in field dependent learners who are good at global perception and sensitive to the social environment.

Group Versus Individual Orientation

Mainstream American culture values and encourages individual achievement (Stewart, 1972). From infancy, children are encouraged to display their abilities and the child who displays the best skills is publicly rewarded. In contrast, in a number of cultures, a high value is placed on being part of the group and not appearing better than others in the group. In these cultures, showing how well one can do, as required by tests, is socially inappropriate, and persons may be hesitant to perform if they feel their performance will separate them from their peers. Also in such cultures, children may not be expected to perform a new, unfamiliar task alone. Children expect assistance from peers and readily give assistance to peers.

How could you encourage and reinforce good performance in children from a group oriented culture?

Verbal Aspects of the Testing Culture

Language differences complicate any testing, and differences involve not only the dialect or language that is spoken but also the functions of language, the content of the language, and the way the language is organized for the various functions and content in the test situation.

Asking "What's that?" may get children to label, while asking them "What's that like?" may get them to give an analogy.

Language Function

Testing often involves questioning. Cultures vary in terms of who asks questions, the types of questions that are asked, and the reasons they are asked. In all cultures people generally ask genuine questions when they need information. Adults from mainstream American culture, however, also engage in much pseudoquestioning (asking questions to which they know the answers). They do this from the time children begin to talk. They ask "What's this?" while looking at a picture book. Mainstream children know that the adults asking the questions know the answers and they recognize these pseudoquestions as requests to perform.

Some cultural groups rarely ask pseudoquestions. Native American children are unlikely to answer a question if they think the adult should know the answer. To do so would be insulting because it would suggest that the adult does not know. Heath (1982) noted that members of a Black community in the Carolina Piedmont seldom asked pseudoquestions. When pseudoquestions were asked, they were usually asked by an adult following some transgression by the child ("Who ate the last piece of cake?"). A pseudoquestion signaled to children that they were in trouble. They could either leave the scene quickly, they could produce a highly creative response/excuse that might distract the adult from punishing them for the transgression, or they could claim no responsibility for the act. At a workshop I conducted in Mississippi, a psychologist commented that she frequently received the response, "I didn't do it!" or "Not me!" when she asked the question, "Who discovered America?" on the Wechsler Intelligence Scale. These students believed they were being accused of a bad deed.

Questioning is inherent in the testing process. If clients are not familiar with the ways questions are used in testing, any test you give will be culturally biased regardless of the language you use and the specific content of the items.

Language Content — Where Is the Meaning?

In everyday conversation, speakers and listeners rely heavily on the context to communicate the meaning of a message. Much testing, however, presents tasks without any context. Persons are expected to follow instructions in which there are no contextual cues as to the appropriate response (e.g., "Touch the blue square to the yellow circle after you pick up the red circle."). They are expected to be able to reason from the words, even if they are unfamiliar with the content. Clients who expect to look to the context for meaning and not the words alone will not perform well on decontextualized test items. Many will attempt to make sense of the items by personalizing them or searching the environment for cues. This results in responses such as "I got one at home" or "Where is it?" when you ask them to define words such as coat or bird or they give responses based on their own experiences that are judged as associative or illogical.

Language Organization Structure

Conversational discourse is symmetrical. Anyone can talk at any time and participants can assist one another in carrying on the conversation by helping each other find necessary words and clarify ideas. Testing involves asymmetrical communicative interaction; one person asks and the other answers. Asymmetrical communications require more language organizational skills, because speakers are responsible for organizing the entire discourse in a manner that will be understandable to the listeners, and because they cannot rely on assistance from the listeners. Speakers must constantly remember the topic and make certain that each statement is related to the topic and to preceding and following statements. Speakers from both the mainstream and culturally/linguistically varied communities may exhibit apparently similar difficulties in producing cohesive and coherent asymmetrical discourse, but for different reasons. Mainstream speakers with intrinsic, neurologically based language problems may have difficulty with asymmetrical discourse because they cannot simultaneously keep the topic and the individual statements in mind. Clients from nonmainstream may experience problems because they have never been assisted in producing this type of discourse. Consequently, tasks such as telling a story may be overwhelming. The performance of a nonmainstream culture client may appear disorganized like that of the client with language-learning disabilities.

Formal testing generally cannot be used to determine if clients from nonmainstream cultures are language-learning disabled. Testing shows only if they are familiar with the culture of testing. Poor performance on testing may predict a client's performance in a school or work setting that requires skills similar to those on the tests, but it does not tell us if a client has an intrinsic language disability. We can make adequate evaluations of the speech and language of clients from other than mainstream culture only over time by identifying their language-learning needs in different situations, provid-

> Asymmetrical communication is organized differently in different cultures. Mainstream English speakers use a sequential linear organization. Spanish speakers use frequent topic-associated digressions. A Navajo educator has suggested that Navajo thought is like frybread — "an idea bubbles up here, and another idea bubbles up over there."

ing appropriate programming, and observing how quickly they learn what is taught.

EVALUATION OF CULTURALLY NONMAINSTREAM OR POTENTIALLY ENGLISH PROFICIENT CLIENTS

We must understand dialect variations and the process of second language learning if we are to provide appropriate assessment of individuals who do not speak the mainstream or standard variant of English and those whose first language is not English.

Dialect Variations

Some clients speak only English, but the English they speak is not the type that is heard on the 6 P.M. news. Not all English speakers use the same phonological, morphological, syntactic, semantic, and pragmatic rules. The variations in a language used by a racial, ethnic, geographical, or socioeconomic group are called **dialects**. Every dialect represents the phonological and grammatical rules used by persons in a speech community. A dialect should not be considered deviant or deficient because it differs from the dialect of Standard American English. Consequently, persons with dialect differences should not be treated as though they have a speech disorder. To assess a client who speaks a nonmainstream dialect of English we must know the characteristics of the client's dialect. We must be able to differentiate the elements of clients' language production that are characteristic of their dialect and those that may indicate a speech and language delay or disorder. Two major racial/ethnic dialects in the United States are Black English and Spanish-influenced English. Figure 2–2 shows some common characteristics of Black English and Spanish-influenced English. Saying "baf" for "bath" in Black English may represent a dialect difference; although saying "ba" for "bath" may represent a speech disorder because Black English dialect would not omit the final sound in "bath."

> Some dialects have more social prestige than others. What dialects are considered prestigious in the United States and what dialects are not considered prestigious?

Language Dominance/Language Proficiency

We sometimes refer to individuals who are learning English as a second language as limited-English proficient (LEP) or as potentially English proficient (PEP). When we evaluate PEP clients, we must assess their **language proficiency** and their **language dominance**. Language proficiency refers to a client's ability to comprehend and produce language. Language dominance refers to the language in which a person is most fluent and proficient.

Commercial, standardized tests are available that reportedly assess language dominance. Such tests generally evaluate a person's vocabulary and syntactic knowledge in two languages by having the person select a picture that best represents a word or sentence. Language dominance is not, however, a stable phenomena. It is dependent on the situation and the people being spoken to. A client may be Spanish-dominant at home, but

> A balanced bilingual is equally proficient in both languages. Being a balanced bilingual, however, is not necessarily indicative of a high level of language proficiency.

Black English	Spanish-influenced English
Phonological	
Consonant cluster reduction: *hol/hold;*	Substitutions because many Spanish dialects have no /ı/, /sh/, /dʒ/, /z/: *confuse sheep/ship; choose/shoes; yellow/jello; sue/zoo*
Substitutions: *f/θ (baf/bath); v/ð (brover/brother); skr/str (skreet/street)*	Devoicing final consonants *k/g, f/v, t/d, p/b, s/z*
Consonant omissions: *r (ca/car; sto'y/story; potect/protect); l (too/tool)*	One sound for /b/ and /v/
	Addition of /e/ for /s/ initial words *estudy/study*
Devoicing final consonants *p/b, t/d, k/g*	
Syntactic	
Nonobligatory plural markers on count nouns *(two dog)*	Adjectives follow nouns *house white/white house ball of tennis/tennis ball*
Nonobligatory possessive markers *(John cousin)*	No set word order for questions and no auxiliaries *When Mary came?*
Omission of copula and auxiliary be *(He a big dog. That your dog?)*	No auxiliaries in negative sentences *I no understand*
Multiple negation *(I don't got none/I don't have any)*	Double negatives *I not saw nobody*
Regularize third person *(he swim/he swims)*	Simple present used to refer to future *I see her next week*
Regularize plural copula/auxiliary *(I was, you was, he was, we was, they was)*	Possessives expressed with prepositional phrases *the book of Rosa*

Figure 2-2. Common phonological and syntactic dialect variations.

English-dominant at school or work. Clients may not have English words for items and events talked about at home; and they may not have Spanish words for items and events talked about at school or work. Hence, we cannot determine a client's language dominance by only administering a test. We must also interview clients regarding the language they use in different situations and with different people. We need to be aware that a client may be dominant, but not proficient, in a language. This frequently is true of students who are English-dominant at school, but speak another language at home. We must determine not only the client's language dominance, but also the client's degree of proficiency in the dominant language.

Contexts for language use are different for clients of different ages. What language contexts might you consider for a preschool child, a school-age child, and an adult?

Language Loss

Evaluating speech and language skills in bilingual clients is complicated by the fact that clients, especially children, may be losing their first language while acquiring their second language. In such circumstances, many children do not have age-level proficiency in any language. Figure 2–3 displays this situation. If children are monolingual, they generally exhibit a steady increase in language skills over time. If a child is introduced to a second language, the degree of concurrent exposure to the first language may be reduced. In such a case, the rate of language learning in the first language is slowed; and, in some cases, first language learning stops and the child loses some or all of that language. As this is occurring, the child is not yet proficient in the second language. Consequently, such children are likely to appear delayed in both languages.

Children may also experience language loss because they elect not to speak their first language because they want to fit in.

Types of Language Proficiency

In evaluating a client's language proficiency, we must consider the person's language proficiency in everyday familiar communication contexts as well as in academic or work contexts. The language used in familiar social interactions is termed basic interpersonal communication skills (BICS). The type of language necessary in school settings is called cognitive academic language proficiency (CALP). Persons with BICS proficiency have sufficient vocabulary and skill in morphology and syntax to make their

Children who have CALP proficiency in a first language develop CALP proficiency in a second language more easily than children who have only a BICS proficiency in a first language.

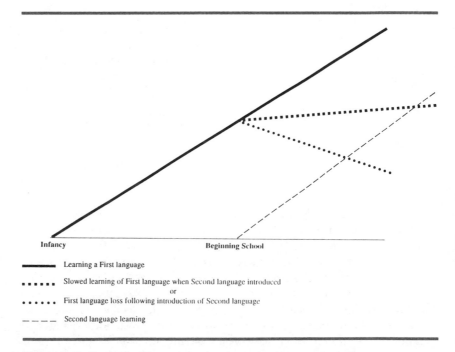

Infancy   Beginning School

———— Learning a First language

• • • • • Slowed learning of First language when Second language introduced
                    or
• • • • • First language loss following introduction of Second language

– – – – Second language learning

Figure 2-3. Patterns of language development.

needs known, share familiar experiences, and repeat and paraphrase information. CALP language involves the ability to use language to talk about language and to analyze, synthesize, and evaluate information. These language skills are particularly needed in social studies, science, and literature classes. Because clients can sound fluent in BICS language, deficits in CALP language often go unrecognized. In a supportive environment, it takes approximately 2–3 years to achieve proficiency in BICS and 5–7 years to achieve proficiency in CALP (Cummins, 1984).

When assessing language proficiency, we must consider two components or dimensions: (1) the cognitively familiar, undemanding/cognitively unfamiliar, demanding dimension, and (2) the context-embedded/context-reduced dimension. Figure 2–4 shows evaluation activities that can be used to assess these aspects of language proficiency.

The cognitively familiar, undemanding tasks or activities are ones the client has mastered and thus require little need for active thinking. Unfamiliar, demanding tasks and activities require more active processing by the client. What might be a familiar task for one person may be an unfamiliar task for another person. For example, arroyos, cactus, and volcanos are familiar to persons living in Albuquerque, New Mexico, but not to persons living in Cedar Rapids, Iowa. Both dimensions need to be probed through a variety of assessment activities. We want to see how clients perform on activities that they have been specifically taught or should be familiar with and how they approach unfamiliar activities that should be manageable for their developmental level. We will need to interview the client and family members or the client's teachers to determine what may be familiar and unfamiliar materials and activities for any one person.

The context-embedded versus context-reduced dimension deals with the range of contextual support available for understanding and performing an activity. In a context-embedded activity, persons can rely on people and objects in the environment to provide them clues about meaning and feelings about how well they are doing. Contextually reduced activities require reliance primarily on verbal instructions alone. Understanding these two continua helps us understand why a child's performance on formal assessments may differ from parental reports of children's abilities at home or a teacher's estimate of children's proficiency based on the language the child uses on the playground and in the cafeteria. Home, playground, and cafeteria activities are familiar and context-embedded; many classroom activities and assessment tasks are unfamiliar and context-reduced.

> Review some tests that are commonly used. What items may be unfamiliar to a client? For example, have children ever seen a squirrel or used a taxi?

Problems With Common Suggestions for Evaluation of PEP Clients

Schools, clients, and hospitals often require that speech-language clinicians use standardized test procedures to document a client's disability and justify treatment. Formal tests can be useful if you want to determine if an individual has the speech and language skills expected of mainstream individuals in a particular situation. The reasons for poor performance of a person from a cultural minority on such testing, however, is not easily interpretable. Without other information we cannot know if the person has

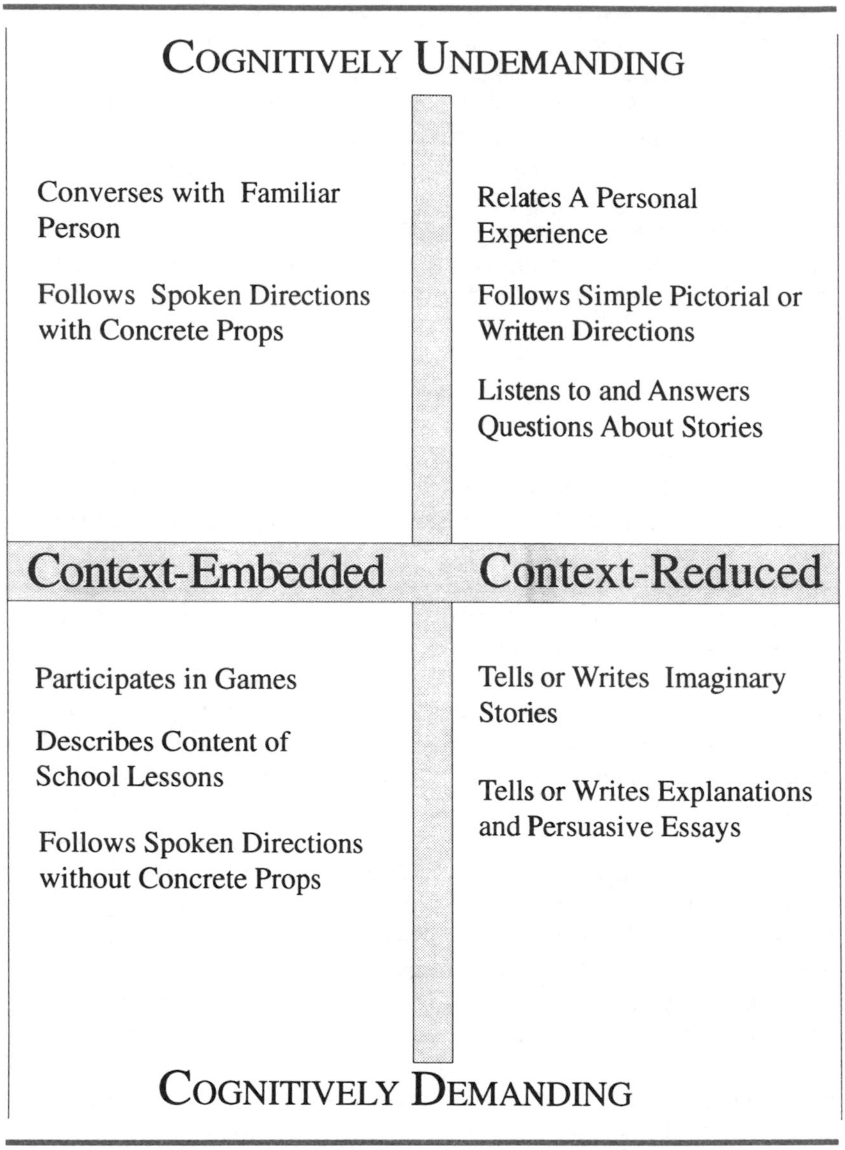

COGNITIVELY UNDEMANDING

Context-Embedded	Context-Reduced
Converses with Familiar Person	Relates A Personal Experience
Follows Spoken Directions with Concrete Props	Follows Simple Pictorial or Written Directions
	Listens to and Answers Questions About Stories
Participates in Games	Tells or Writes Imaginary Stories
Describes Content of School Lessons	Tells or Writes Explanations and Persuasive Essays
Follows Spoken Directions without Concrete Props	

COGNITIVELY DEMANDING

Figure 2-4. Framework for language assessment.

done poorly because of an intrinsic, neurologically based language-learning disability, or if the poor performance stems from unfamiliarity with the test items and the testing interaction patterns. Several methods have been suggested to modify tests to make them more useful; however, none seem wholly satisfactory (Damico, 1991; VaughnCooke, 1983). As speech-language pathologists or audiologists we must be able to discuss effectively and convincingly the problems associated with such test modifications when administrators or supervisors suggest that we use these methods to evaluate culturally/linguistically varied clients. That is, we must be able to explain why modifications currently suggested do not successfully deal with the problem of validity.

1. *Translate the test.* Some concepts don't have a direct translation. For example, there is no single word in Navajo that can be translated for the word *construction*. The concept is translated as "there is a man hitting a board with a hammer." Clearly, this sentence is not as complex as the word *construction*. Many aspects of English morphology and syntax do not have counterparts in other languages. For example, many Native American languages do not have gender pronouns; Vietnamese does not have plural and possessive markers. Even if test items can be translated from one language to another, the order in which concepts are learned may vary among cultures. When testing hearing of English speakers, audiologists use single syllable words and spondee words such as *baseball* and *hot dog* to assess speech reception. An equivalent Spanish test is not possible because the Spanish language has very few single syllable words and no spondee words.

2. *Standardize existing tests on minority populations.* Ethnic norms are potentially dangerous because they provide a basis for invidious comparisons between racial/ethnic groups. Standardized tests are based on mainstream culture. Consequently, nonmainstream individuals who are unfamiliar with the concepts on the tests will usually score lower than mainstream individuals. There is a tendency to assume that lower scores are indicative of lower innate potential.

3. *Use tests that include a small percentage of minorities in the standardization sample when developing tests.* This is a common practice of commercial standardized tests. The problem with this approach is that the norms represent no one. The mean scores are below the mean for mainstream students and still above the mean for students from nondominant cultural groups.

4. *Modify existing tests to make them appropriate for clients from other cultures.* This is easier said than done. It is difficult to maintain similar complexity of content. We must have sufficient knowledge of the culture and be able to modify the tests in a way that the revisions provide the possibility of equal credit.

5. *Use a language sample and other observations.* Presently, we do not have adequate developmental information on nondominant cultural groups and non-English speakers. Without normative data we cannot evaluate the quality of a language sample or make a diagnosis regarding the normalcy of a client's language.

6. *Use criterion-referenced measures.* What should the criterion be and who establishes it? How do we know what the order of progression should be in the criterion? More data are needed about developmental sequences in children from nondominant cultural groups if we are to develop criterion-referenced measures.

When asked to explain the term "learning disability" to Navajo parents so they would sign permission for special education, a Navajo interpreter reported that she told the family, "Your child can't do white people things in school. Sign the paper and they'll teach him to do white people things."

Alternative Assessment Approaches

If formal tests are generally inadequate for assessing nonmainstream populations, what is appropriate? Three general approaches are available: (1) ethnographic interviews, (2) observational inventories, and (3) dynamic assessment procedures.

Ethnographic Interviews

Ethnographic interviews enable us to attempt to see the world through the eyes of the clients and their families. Ethnographic interviewing techniques provide a means for assessing the client's strengths and needs in an ecological (naturalistic) framework and from the client's and family's perspective. In traditional interviews, professionals predetermine the questions that are to be asked; and in some cases they predetermine the range of responses that can be given. In ethnographic interviewing, both questions and answers must be discovered from the people being interviewed. Different information is collected from different clients because the values, beliefs, strengths, and needs of each client varies.

All ethnographic interviews have the goal of helping the interviewer understand the social situations in which the clients live and how the clients and their families perceive, feel about, and understand situations. This understanding is especially critical when the clients' cultural values and beliefs are different from the interviewers. We can gain a great deal of information by asking clients or family members to describe their typical day. As they discuss their typical day, you will note what is important to them — their concerns, what they like and do not like, what they do and how they do it, and so on. Depending on the reason for the referral, you can ask about specific activities or events. Types of information that are important for making speech and language assessment decisions may include:

> You should approach the ethnographic interview with the attitude, "I don't know much about this person's point of view so I've got to encourage him or her to set the agenda for this interview."

The language skills expected of children at different ages;

Who talks to children and who children talk with;

How people talk with children;

The topics of conversation for boys, girls, men, women;

The beliefs about how children learn to talk;

Reasons for talking (giving directions, asking questions, telling stories, joking, etc.);

Roles of boys, girls, men, women in the culture; and

How the culture defines and views a "handicap."

We want to know if other members of the client's culture view the child or adult as having speech and language differences or disorder. If they believe that a little girl, for example, has a speech and language disorder, it is likely that she does have an intrinsic speech or language disorder. If they do not regard her as having a speech or language disorder, then according to the standards of her culture, she does not have a disorder in situations that are common to her cultural community. She may, however, have an actual intrinsic disorder that is not recognized by members of her culture. This is particularly possible for language disorders that affect academic performance, because schools require structures and functions of language not required in other settings. If family members have not had much experience with the formal educational system, they may not recognize the reasons a child may be having difficulty.

Inventories and Work Sample Analysis

Inventories and work sample analysis involve observing clients in naturalistic environments. The observer considers the demands of the situation and the behavior and use of speech and language by others in the setting. We may observe the purposes for which the client uses language in a setting, such as:

Greeting,

Requesting,

Describing objects and events,

Reporting past experiences,

Directing self or others,

Reasoning,

Predicting what will happen, and

Projecting into the thoughts and feelings of others;

or how the client participates in conversation such as:

Initiating topics,

Taking turns appropriately,

Maintaining topic,

Giving off-topic responses,

Elaborating on topics already established, and

Repairing communication breakdowns.

When employing this observational assessment strategy, we should note the frequency of these language functions (in categories of frequently, occasionally, not observed) and identify specific examples for each category and how the frequency compares to the frequency of the functions' use by others in the setting.

For school-age students, we need to evaluate the student's ability to comprehend the content of the school curriculum and to complete necessary written work. We can do this by observing the student, asking the student's teacher to describe her concerns, and exploring the student's ability in activities such as:

Understanding elements of stories

Causes of events and characters' feelings in stories

The problem and solution in stories

Telling coherent stories of personal experience

Telling imaginary stories

Comprehending complex sentence patterns

Comprehending assigned texts

Writing coherent and cohesive texts

You may choose to be a passive observer watching, but not interacting with the client in the situation, or an active observer participating in the activities with the client being observed.

Dynamic Assessment

An adequate evaluation of persons from nondominant cultural groups can be done only over time. The purpose of a single evaluation of a culturally/linguistically different client should not be to determine if a client is delayed or disordered and "qualifies" for services. Rather, the purpose of an evaluation should be to determine how the client learns and how easily the individual learns. Feuernstein (1979) proposed the concept of dynamic assessment. Dynamic assessment focuses on the **process** of how people learn in contrast to traditional assessment that focuses on the **product** or what has been learned. When a client does poorly on a traditional assessment, we have little information regarding the reasons for the difficulty or of the person's ability to learn. The intent of dynamic assessment is to improve understanding of the learner.

Figure 2–5 shows the process of dynamic assessment. A person is surrounded by other people (humans) who filter information that the person receives. At a point in time, an evaluation is conducted; and based on that evaluation, an appropriate educational/therapeutic program is developed for the client. When we use dynamic assessment we consider the referral questions and concerns and design an evaluation to assess the client's ability to learn skills related to the area of concern (i.e., language in social interactions with family members, classmates, or co-workers; reading and writing skills; etc.). We need to know the skills that are expected of others in these environments. Based on this evaluation, we design a therapeutic program in which you mediate the client's learning by explaining expectations and by modeling and prompting how to do the task. Persons who respond well to mediation can be expected to make steady, significant progress in treatment (Figure 2–5, line A) and it is unlikely they have intrinsic, biologically based delays and/or disorders. Their apparent language problems on the initial assessment most likely were caused by cultural differences. Persons who do not respond to mediation are likely to make very little or very slow progress compared to other individuals from a similar background. They most likely do have intrinsic learning problems that can-

Feuerstein referred to a person's ability to learn as "cognitive modifiability."

Feuerstein developed a structured intervention program called "instrumental enrichment" to teach students to use language to mediate their problem solving.

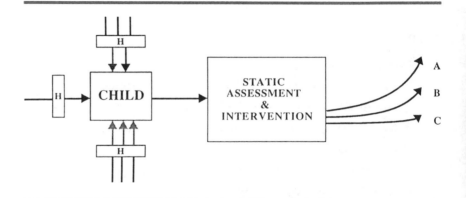

Figure 2–5. Issue of assessment is can child learn?

not be accounted for by cultural differences (line C). One can assume that persons who are slow to respond to mediation will make an intermediate degree of progress over time. They may have mild, intrinsic learning disabilities or may simply be persons who demonstrate normal variations in learning rates (line B).

Evaluation of culturally/linguistically different clients should determine how easily their learning can be modified (Lidz, 1991). Cuong and Tueyen were two fifth grade Vietnamese boys in an Albuquerque school who were experiencing difficulty in language arts. They were no longer eligible for English as second language (ESL) classes because they had passed an oral language proficiency test. Their teacher, however, was concerned because Cuong and Tueyen could not tell or write a coherent story and could not comprehend the stories they read. The speech-language pathologist conducted a dynamic assessment to determine how modifiable the boys were for narrative skills. For the pretest she had the boys tell stories about two poster pictures. She then planned a series of lessons over a 2-week period in which she and the boys read short stories and identified the parts of the stories. Together she and the boys constructed a story with all the parts. After these activities were completed, she asked the boys to tell stories about two more poster pictures. Modifiability was determined from the students' responsiveness to mediation, the effort required by the speech-language pathologist to induce changes in the students, and evidence of the students transferring the narrative skills to their language arts class. Figure 2-6 shows the results of mediation for Cuong and Tueyen. Cuong exhibited greater modifiability than Tueyen. He was more attentive to the tasks, retained the information better, and was better at self-monitoring.

Strategy	Cuong	Tueyen
Attention	Attentive to all activities; rarely required reminders to pay attention	Lost interest part-way through lessons; required frequent reminders from the examiner to look at what they were doing
Style	Reflective; waited for instructions before beginning tasks	Impulsive; tried doing activities before examiner gave all the instructions; examiner had to keep materials out of his reach until they were ready to begin
Memory	Could tell the examiner what was done in a previous lesson	Examiner needed to give clues for student to remember previous lesson
Monitoring	Self-corrected omissions in his stories	Examiner had to remind him of the parts to include
Transfer	Recognized character goals in story read in language arts	Could relate beginning and ends of stories, but could not answer questions about the goals in stories

Figure 2-6. Dynamic assessment results.

INTERPRETING ASSESSMENT INFORMATION FOR OTHERS

The gender, age, life experiences, race/ethnicity, language skills, and education of the person conducting the interpretive session can make a difference in what clients hear and how they hear it.

Interpreting evaluation data to clients and their families is as important as conducting the evaluation. Severai factors are particularly important to consider when interpreting assessment data with culturally/linguistically different clients and their families.

Include the Extended Family

Always include family members when assessing a child. Inform the parents that they can bring any other family members or friends they would like to have with them at the interpretive session. In some cultures the parents do not make the decisions for the child's care. Grandparents, godparents, aunts, uncles, or tribal elders may determine if, when, and how medical, thera-peutic, or educational services are sought and accepted. Consequently, it is important to have individuals who are involved in the decision-making process at the interpretive session.

Cultural Interplay

Be aware that miscommunication may arise because of differences in val-ues, beliefs, and communication patterns. In some traditional cultures, men are reluctant to accept information given by a woman. A mother may not accept suggestions given by a clinician who does not have a child of her own. Different cultures use different rates of speaking and different pat-terns in taking turns in a conversation. These differing speaking rates and turn-taking patterns may affect the client's or family's ability to participate in a discussion with you.

Rudeness Bias

Mainstream professionals like to ask questions. These questions may ap-pear rude and overly personal to some clients and families. Some topics may not be permissible topics for strangers to raise. When you must ask questions, explain why the questions are important (e.g., "The answer to this next question will help me know how to work with your child").

Courtesy Bias

Most clients and families do not wish to cause problems or create friction. They wish to be polite or to "save face." They may not believe what you are saying and they may disagree with your recommendations, but often they will not tell you so. Instead, during the meeting they may agree to anything, although they have no intention of following your suggestions.

Racial Difference Bias

If families have had a history of negative experiences with individuals from your ethnic/racial group, they may not trust you or may not feel comfortable with you. If families have negative self-esteem for their own racial ethnic group, they may not trust a professional from their own group. They may think that the professional is no longer part of the group, or they may think that the person is a token professional and does not really have the skills necessary to do the job.

SUMMARY

Speech, language, and hearing evaluation of culturally/linguistically diverse clients is a complex task. It requires not only knowledge about development and disorders in mainstream populations, but also knowledge about cultural variations in the development and use of language, causes and manifestations of speech and language disorders, and values and beliefs associated with disabilities and intervention. Valid evaluations for all clients require sensitivity to their cultures. As a mother of a child with developmental disabilities (Poyadue, 1979) stated:

> Don't put the other fellow in your shoes — wear his. Tis true, if "I were you" I could use the logic that you espouse to solve my problem. But, since I am me, we must find a solution that fits well into the scheme of my mold. We must cloak the solutions of my problems in garments wrinkled by my needs and desires, otherwise, what you are saying to me is not, "If I were you," but "If you were me;" and since I am not, your answers help me little.

REFERENCES

Battle, D. E. (1993). Introduction. *Communication disorders in multicultural populations* (pp. xv–xxiv). Boston: Andover.

Crago, M. B. (1988). *Cultural context in communicative interaction of young Inuit children.* Unpublished doctoral thesis, McGill University, Montreal.

Cummins, J. (1984). *Bilingualism and special education.* San Diego: College-Hill Press.

Damico, J. S. (1991). Descriptive assessment of communicative ability in limited English proficient students. In E. V. Hamayan & J. S. Damico (Eds.), *Limiting bias in the assessment of bilingual students* (pp. 157–217). Austin, TX: Pro-Ed.

Downs, M. (1985). Language disorders from hearing losses in multicultural populations. In L. Cole & V. Deal (Eds.), *Communication disorders in multicultural populations.* Washington, DC: American Speech-Language-Hearing Association.

Feuernstein, R. (1979). *Dynamic assessment of retarded performance.* Baltimore: University Park Press.

Hall, E. T. (1984). *The dance of life: The other dimension of time.* Garden City, NY: Doubleday.

Heath, S. B. (1982). Questions at home and school. In G. Spindler (Ed.), *Doing the ethnography of schooling.* New York: Holt, Rinehart and Winston.

Lidz, C. S. (1991). *Practitioner's guide to dynamic assessment.* New York: Guilford.

Mayfield, S. A. (1985). Excess lead absorption and language disorders in Black children. In L. Cole & V. Deal (Eds.), *Communication disorders in multicultural populations.* Washington, DC: American Speech-Language-Hearing Association.

McWilliams, B. J., Morris, H. L., & Shelton, R. L. (1990). *Cleft palate speech.* Philadelphia: B.C. Decker.

Post, R. H. (1964). Hearing acuity among Negroes and whites. *Eugen Quarterly, 11,* 65–81.

Poyadue, F. M. (1979). Visiting parents: Peer counseling training manual. San Jose, CA: Parents Helping Parents (535 Race St., Suite 220).

Scott, D. (1985). Hearing loss and sickle cell anemia. In L. Cole & V. Deal (Eds.), *Communication disorders in multicultural populations.* Washington, DC: American Speech-Language-Hearing Association.

Spector, R. E. (1985). *Cultural diversity in health and illness.* Norwalk, CT: Appleton-Century-Crofts.

Stewart, E. C. (1972). *American cultural patterns: A cross-cultural perspective.* Yarmouth, ME: Intercultural Press.

Sue, D. W., & Sue, D. (1990). *Counseling the culturally different: Theory & practice.* New York: John Wiley.

Vanderas, A. O. (1987). Incidence of cleft lip, cleft palate, and cleft lip and palate among races: A review. *Cleft Palate Journal, 24,* 216–225.

Vaughn-Cooke, F. B. (1983). Improving language assessment in minority children. *Asha, 25,* 29–34.

RECOMMENDED READINGS

Adler, S. (1993). *Multicultural communication skills in the classroom.* Boston: Allyn & Bacon.

Hamayan, E. V., & Damico, J. S. (Eds.). (1991). *Limiting bias in the assessment of bilingual students* (pp. 157–217). Austin, TX: Pro-Ed.

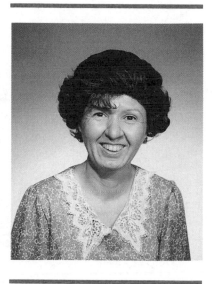

CAROL WESTBY, Ph.D.

M.A. 1968, University of Iowa
Ph.D. 1971, University of Iowa

Dr. Westby is a senior research associate with the New Mexico
University Affiliated Program, Albuquerque. Among her special
interests are the development of culturally appropriate assessment and
intervention programs, infancy through young adulthood; play and
narrative development; language/literacy connections; ethnographic
interviewing, and cultural variations in narration and adult-child
interactions.

CHAPTER

3

The Clinical History

Hughlett L. Morris, Ph.D., and
Penelope K. Hall, M.A.

Our purpose here is to provide guidance in acquiring the skill of taking a clinical history. The term *clinical history* is used to refer to background information about the communication disorder so that we can better understand its nature and can assist in its treatment. In other words, we need to know what has come before, before we can proceed!

Common sense tells us that the "history" of a speech and language disorder varies with its individual nature and, therefore, the process of history taking must certainly be tailored to the disorder and the patient at hand. For example, the questions asked of an adult with a voice problem of recent onset obviously will be different from those asked a parent of a child who shows evidence of problems in language acquisition. In the first case, the informant is the woman or man with the problem and information about childhood development is probably not relevant (although vocal use patterns during adolescence may be!). In the second case, the informant is the parent or the responsible adult and detailed information about development will probably be crucial to the clinical purpose. Health status, family, school/work status, and personal reaction to the problem will be important for both.

Even so, it seems reasonable that the beginning speech-language pathologist is well advised to focus on several aspects of the clinical history interview common to all or the majority of patients with speech and language complaints. That is the objective of this chapter. Details of the history relevant to specific disorders are discussed in other chapters.

Finally, as have other contributors to this text, we have taken some shortcuts in our language use for reading ease. Sometimes we use the feminine gender and sometimes the masculine gender pronoun. We use *patient* throughout, but in some settings *client* would be preferred. In the context of history taking, we describe discussions with the *patient* but obviously, if the patient is a child, these discussions will be held with a parent or responsible adult.

With these thoughts in mind, we proceed.

WHY DO WE NEED TO KNOW THE CLINICAL HISTORY?

The clinical history tells us a lot about the problem under consideration, as well as the patient with the problem. It gives us ideas about what we can do to help. And, it saves time. Without the clinical history, we approach the clinical problem blindly and in a vacuum. Good history taking is the hallmark of a good clinician.

WHEN DO WE TAKE THE INFORMATION?

The clinical history usually begins even before meeting the patient. That an examination has been arranged tells us that there is a concern about some aspect of communication. It further tells us that the concern is important enough to seek our professional advice as a speech-language pathologist.

The setting in which we work may provide some automatic clues about the nature of the suspected disorder. The speech-language pathologist who practices in a school setting quite naturally expects prospective patients to be children; she who practices in a rehabilitation center expects patients who have chronic disorders that are frequently debilitating; he who conducts a wide range private practice can expect almost anything!

The age of the patient provides some clues, as well. The referral of a young child is likely to indicate a problem in development, a congenital disorder, or a pediatric disease. An older adult more likely has chronic disease, a neurologic disorder or disease, or deterioration of previous functional abilities.

Spouses, chidren, and other relatives may be helpful in providing such information when the medical problems of some adults limit their participation in gathering the clinical history.

Information available from the request for appointment or from the referral may be useful in identifying the possible problem, depending on the level of sophistication with which the request or referral is made. Although the public and our colleagues from other disciplines are generally on-target about whether there *is* a problem (after all, the public is the final authority about the matter), they frequently are poorly equipped to describe with any precision the *nature* of the "speech" problem. Frequently, the report is that the child or adult "can't talk plainly," "has trouble saying certain words," "repeats," "can't get the words out," "can't think of the right words," "doesn't talk much," "can't talk," "talks too slowly," "talks through her nose," "nobody can understand him," "her teacher can't hear her," "I don't sound like I used to," "I lose my voice a lot," "on the phone, people mistake me for a man (woman)," and so forth.

The experienced speech-language pathologist can probably identify the general nature of the disorder from such information. On the other hand, all or most of this type of information can be misleading about the "real" problem. Therefore, the speech-language pathologist must be alert to avoid a bias of expectation that interferes with her ability to make observations.

What we typically regard as the taking of clinical history takes place when we begin our interview with the patient and family. We use this occasion to get acquainted with the patient and to learn as much as possible, or as much as needed, or both, about the problem and the patient to add to our previous knowledge. Actually, we continue this process of learning throughout all our encounters with the patient, but this initial interview is the starting place.

FROM WHAT SOURCES DOES A CLINICAL HISTORY COME?

Usually we begin a clinical interview with background information in hand, noting particularly what we know thus far about why and how this initial appointment was made. We will also be familiar with any available reports from colleagues, including those from other disciplines. These reports will be in the clinical file, along with information about previous examinations or treatment the patient has received in this clinic. Sometimes the patient will bring reports from other facilities to the interview.

Be sure to have clients sign appropriate forms so that you can request relevant information from other facilities.

In most cases, the heart of the clinical history is taken during the initial portion of the examination period. The main strategy is to ask questions of the patient and family to gain information about the problem and to form an impression about the needs, restrictions, and motivations that seem relevant to the clinical problem.

HOW SHALL WE INTERVIEW THE PATIENT AND THE FAMILY?

Certainly we want to conduct the interview so that, when finished, we will have the information we need. That calls for considerable attention to *what* you want to ask. Before we consider the *what*, let's think about the *how*, the manner with which we talk to the patient and family about the problem.

Let's begin by agreeing that there's no one right way to do this. The patient has come for help and is anxious, if not always able, to tell you what she knows or suspects about the problem and how it affects her life. The patient also may not be aware of the extent of the problem. In the same way, by virtue of our interest in speech-language pathology, we proclaim a strong interest in people and an uncommon skill in talking with them. So, the objective is to bring these two motivations together as well as possible for the benefit of the patient. Following are several questions that we must think about as we strive to accomplish that objective.

1. *Can our manner during an interview be both friendly and professional?* It may be difficult to describe in writing what constitutes a friendly manner, but most of us know one when we see it! Certainly, as described in Chapter 2, there may be variations among cultures in what constitutes "a friendly manner." In general, in the majority North American culture, it includes smiles and handshakes. A professional manner is even more difficult to describe but, again, we know it when we see it! It includes discussion focused on the problem in clear and direct language. It reflects a nonjudgmental attitude that makes it possible for the patient and family to answer questions, to confide, to relate feelings, and to ask questions without undue embarrassment. It assures the patient that all clinical information will be confidential within the appropriate clinical setting. It demonstrates interest and concern about the problem and the patient. It conveys the ability to discuss good news and bad news with equal clarity and compassion.

2. *What can we do to foster a professional manner?* We can seek to work in a physical environment that is adequate in size, comfortable, attractive but not distracting, and easily accessible to all. We can present a physical appearance that is pleasing and consistent with the standards of the community and work setting. That includes choice of clothing and personal grooming. We can make arrangements about payment for our services (if there is an exchange of money) that are convenient, comfortable, and easily understood.

3. *Can we use both technical and everyday language?* Yes. Not only can we, but we must. Everyday language is needed to put the patient at ease and to help him feel confident of his ability to talk with you about the problem. Questions put in everyday language will lead to dependable, honest answers that will be useful for your purpose. At the same time, we also use technical language in our discussions. Frequently, technical language is more precise and more descriptive than everyday language: *phonological disorder* tells us more than *doesn't talk clearly*, although, for many pur-

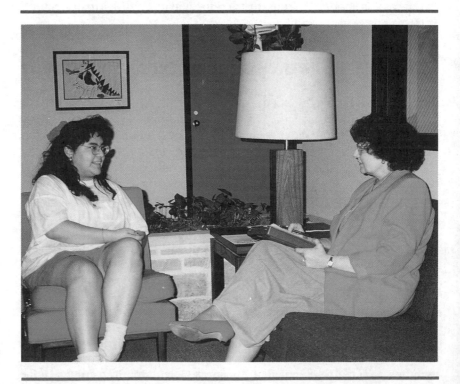

poses, the two terms may be used interchangeably. When we use technical language, we must be certain that the patient knows what the words mean, how to say them, and how they are written. (Parents are sometimes embarrassed when they learn that *pharyngeal* does not begin with an *f*!) Acquainting the patient and the family members with technical language gives them more confidence in their ability to understand the problem and, certainly, to ask better questions in the future.

Don't lose your patients by using professional jargon.

4. *Can we structure the interview for the sake of efficiency and yet make it possible, even easy, for the informant to volunteer information that may be useful?* The question indicates the two competing objectives. In most circumstances, the time available for history taking is limited and so the discussion must be carefully focused to obtain the desired information. Yet it is crucial to pace the interview so that the patient has the easy opportunity to volunteer comments that, from her perspective, are relevant. If comments are relevant, we must be prepared with follow-up. If they are not, we must be able, in a friendly manner, to move on with the interview.

5. *How can we be sensitive to cultural differences that are important to observe in interviewing?* Obviously, there's no easy answer here. North American peoples encompass such a large number of cultures that it would be impossible here to consider them all in this regard. The key word, of course, is *sensitive*. That includes clear acknowledgment of the possibility and probability of important cultural differences among us, our genuine efforts to learn about these differences and how they influence our professional practices as speech-language pathologists, and our best attempts to incorporate these understandings into our daily dealings with patients and families. Although sensitivity to these "ethnographic issues" is important during all of our clinical activities, it is especially crucial in our first interviews, because initial relationships set the stage for all that follows. Useful discussions of these ethnographic issues are provided in Chapter 2 and by Battle (1993), Christensen and Delgado (1993), Taylor (in preparation), and Westby (1990).

6. *What about confidentiality?* The speech-language pathologist, as all professional workers who deal with human problems, is pledged to keep all information about the patient and her problems in confidence. That means that we maintain privacy of what we know about her and her problems, to be discussed or shared only with her and with whomever else she names in written consent for that specific release of information. Otherwise, we are ethically obliged to restrict our discussions of her problem to our colleagues within the institutional setting where we work.

In the same way, we require her consent to obtain information about her and her problem gathered as a result of professional services from any other clinician. One way to do this is to simply ask her to request that the information be sent to us. Another is to make the request ourselves, including with our query her written permission for release of information for this purpose.

7. *How can we continue to improve our interviewing skills?* We can improve by practice, by reflection, by observing others, by increasing our sensitivity, and by learning more about disorders we treat.

Some additional discussions of interviewing techniques are provided by Evans, Hearn, Uhlemann, and Ivey (1989) and Shipley (1992).

Sometimes the clinical
history is also called a case
history.

HOW DO WE ASK QUESTIONS
WHILE TAKING A CASE HISTORY?

We all recognize that the way in which questions are asked can influence the amount, quality, and specificity of the answers. Some types of questions elicit factual information; others lead to clarifying information or allowing the informant to voice feelings about the problem. As we collect background information, we must be aware of the different types of questions and use them appropriately.

Some questions are requests for general information and can be regarded as *open* questions. Some examples are: "What are your concerns about your daughter?" "What do you do when you can't understand your son?" "Tell me about your husband's job," or "Describe your daughter's academic program." Although we control the general background areas being explored, we do not control the range of responses we receive. Nor do we control how extensively an informant responds. However, open questions often allow us to help the informant expand on issues that need further exploration. These types of questions can even help an informant clarify her own thinking about an issue. Open questions allow the informant to be an active participant in the information-gathering process.

Other questions that the informant can answer with very few words can be regarded as *closed* questions. Closed questions have a legitimate place in obtaining background information. For instance, closed questions help us get correct factual information about the patient, such as "What is your son's birthdate?" "Who was the speech-language pathologist who evaluated your wife after her stroke?" and "How old was your daughter when she began receiving remediation?"

Another example of closed questions are those that can be answered "yes" or "no." Yes/no questions can be useful, particularly when very specific information is needed to clarify what areas may need to be discussed further. Examples are: "Does your husband wear a hearing aid?" or "Is your son receiving physical therapy now?" On the other hand, yes/no questions are not likely to stimulate further discussion and should be used sparingly in most interview situations.

Another example of closed questions is one in which we provide several possible answers. This type of question can help the informant recall specific information, such as "Did your daughter take her first steps around the time she celebrated her first birthday, or did she do this at a later age?" or "Did a speech-language pathologist talk with your husband before he had his laryngectomy, or was it after the surgery?" After the specific information is recalled, use of other types of questions will help the informant give further expanded information about the situation.

Finally, we need to consider the limitations of an interview that consists solely of question-answer discourse. For many purposes and with many patients and families, the question-answer format needs seasoning with strategies that include "supportive" comments by the interviewer, encouraging the patient to spontaneously continue the discussion of the topic at hand or change the topic to one not previously included in the interview. The ability to keep the interview on track, yet permit or even encourage such excursions from the routine questions, is the prime example of interviewing skill.

WHAT DO WE WANT TO KNOW?

We begin by asking what the problem is and we listen carefully to the answer. Most often the first answer is consistent with our expectations, but sometimes not. In either case, we continue to discuss the problem until we have a satisfactory understanding. Sometimes we need also to ask to whom is this a problem. The answer tells us about social, educational, and occupational perspectives of the problem.

Next we ask when the problem began and how it has developed. Information about onset provides valuable clues about causes of a number of speech and language disorders and hence appropriate treatments. We also ask how the disorder has developed, seeking to understand whether the severity of the disorder is stable, improving, or worsening.

We also want to ask about how troublesome the disorder is, and in what ways it interferes with patterns of living (school, work, social interactions, health, etc.)

For many communication disorders, asking about variability of the problem has special significance for planning treatment, so these questions merit careful consideration. If the answers indicate that the disorder varies, we need to ask specifically about when is it better and when worse. Of equal importance is the question of whether, today, the disorder is "typical" (or better than usual, or worse than usual). If not typical, and especially if better than usual, we need to find ways to find out about the usual severity of the disorder.

Information about previous treatment or previous efforts to seek treatment is vitally important in setting the stage for our examination and treatment planning. We learn what the patient has previously done about the problem and whether she thinks it helped. Did she understand the previous examination and the recommendations? Did she follow the recommendations? If not, why? Did conditions improve? Sometimes we ask why she came to us rather than continuing with the previous clinical program.

Sometimes we ask the patient and family what they think has caused the problem. The answer provides insight into what the patient understands about the disorder in general and specifically in his case. The answers will reflect whether his understanding is a reasonable explanation or whether it is based on misconception. Frequently we refer back to this discussion at the end of the examination when we are reporting our findings and our recommendations.

Another important group of questions are asked to understand family-social-school-work history and the interactions between the communication disorder and that history. For example, whether the patient is an adult or child, we want to estimate family and social relationships and the extent to which the interactions are influenced by the disorder. For some disorders, especially those that have genetic implications, we ask whether other members of the family have this or other disorders of communication. If so, what are the disorders and what is the relationship? Also, has the problem been resolved?

We need information about daily life. We ask the child and his family about school activities. What grade level is he placed in? How is he doing in his academic work? What kind of problems is he having? How are they being dealt with? If the child is of preschool age, we want to know about child care or preschool arrangements. To what extent are the communication problems causing him problems? We ask the adult about daily life and activities. Again, how is his life influenced by the disorder?

For some speech and language disorders, information is needed about general and specific aspects of health. We ask about a child's developmental patterns, illnesses, disorders, treatment, and medication. We ask the adult about general health, whether there have been diseases and treatment, including surgery. Does the informant see any connection between any health problem and this disorder that led to this examination? Who is providing health care, and is there progress in any treatment? We limit these questions about health to areas that are directly or indirectly relevant to the disorder under consideration. Further, we must be able to easily defend, in everyday language, the relevance of the information asked for to the disorder.

Our major focus in these questions about health is on matters directly relevant to the communication disorder. However, sometimes we need to know about health problems that have indirect relevance. Does she have visual or reading problems that will interfere with our examination? How might his treatment program for dialysis influence a language therapy program for aphasia? Sometimes such factors become clearly apparent during the interview; other times we find out about them later.

WHAT IF THE INFORMANT DOESN'T HAVE THE INFORMATION YOU NEED, OR SEEMS RELUCTANT TO GIVE IT?

In many instances, the informant doesn't have the information needed. Neither she nor her family can tell you much about her medical status or what medical or surgical treatment is planned. He is unclear when he became hoarse and whether the medical doctor who examined him was in general practice or was an otolaryngologist and what the findings were. She is an adopted child, placed, at age 4, and not much is known about her early development or her biologic parents. He can't remember much about recommendations or treatment provided by a previous speech-language pathologist. If the information is crucial to the diagnosis, every attempt should be made to get it. Usually that requires action by the patient: "Please ask (the local speech pathologist, the special education resource teacher, the school psychologist, the pediatrician, the neurologist, the otolaryngologist, etc.) to send me a report about her findings and your plans for management." Sometimes we offer to make the request, especially if we want to ask for specific information. If we do, we must obtain proper written consent from the adult patient or the parent/legal guardian to be included with our written request. In all matters of seeking or giving information about a patient, we must carefully follow procedures of informed consent and confidentiality. These procedures are necessary to ensure trust that our information about the patient is obtained and will be kept in confidence. These procedures are always in writing, properly dated, and kept on record.

What if the informant seems hesitant to respond to questions or appears hostile? On occasion the patient or family have mixed feelings about the clinical appointment and show their uncertainty by appearing uncooperative or even antagonistic during the interview. Or their demeanor indicates such feelings, even if that's not their intention. The interviewer must be prepared to carry on in the face of such apparent reluctance to cooperate, taking care to explain why certain information is needed. If the perception of noncooperation continues, we must offer to terminate the interview and the clinical examination. In our experience, some offers are refused, with disclaimers that the perception is true and the interview is continued with more success. Some offers to discontinue are accepted, with obvious relief. When that happens, we must offer another appointment, or if the patient is inclined, other assistance in a way that the offer can be accepted without loss of face.

HOW CAN WE TELL IF THE INFORMATION GIVEN IS DEPENDABLE?

Our expectation is that the history information we are provided is dependable. After all, the patient came or was brought to us for assistance and presumably wants to cooperate. Sometimes, however, during the course of the interview we notice sufficient inconsistency among various details that we must repeat questions or ask for further clarification. Usually that clarifies the confusion. If not, we proceed as best we can, including our concerns about reliability in our written report of the interview.

Remember to specify in the written report of the interview who provided the information, such as "Mr. Hernandez *stated* that his daughter walked at 24 months of age."

WHEN AND HOW DO WE CONLCUDE THE HISTORY?

As indicated earlier, we strive for a balance between a conservative use of time and a need to be comprehensive. We make a judgment call about when we have the information necessary to proceed with the examination. Sometimes the transition between history and examination is indicated verbally. Sometimes we ask: "Is there anything else that you think we should talk about before we proceed?" In other circumstances, the transition is hardly apparent. Certainly, we all agree that the history-taking process continues throughout this and subsequent interviews with the patient, as we learn more and more about the disorder and the patient.

SHALL WE USE A PREVIOUSLY PREPARED OUTLINE AS WE ASK OUR QUESTIONS AND WHEN WE WRITE OUR REPORT?

Many practitioners prefer to use a preprepared outline to assist them in remembering to ask relevant questions and to use time efficiently. An example of such an outline developed by Darley and Spriestersbach (1978) is presented in Figure 3-1. Others have been developed by Haynes, et al. (1992), Meitus and Weinberg (1983), and Shipley (1992).

Other practitioners find it effective to have several leading questions in mind when the interview begins but to allow the informant considerable freedom in determining the direction of the discussion and the interrelationships among the various aspects of the problem. Probably most of us seek a moderate path between the two extremes.

Basic Case History Outline

Name: _____

Birthdate: _____

Address: _____

Date history taken: _____

Interviewer: _____

Informant(s): (Full name and relationship to speaker)

_____

Complaint:

State in informant's own words, if possible. Is this the only problem?

Referral:

Full name of individual or agency making referral. Indicate relationship.

History of Speech Problem:

Age of patient when first regarded as having a speech problem? Who first so regarded him or her? Under what circumstances? What sort of treatment has been attempted? By whom? Have parents made any effort to correct problem at home? What have they done? What results from treatment? Has patient made any effort to improve his or her speech? If so, what has he or she done? What results? What has been the general course of the problem — has it become better or worse? Parents' estimate of present severity. Patient's own estimate of present severity. What things have seemed to affect the severity of the problem? Anyone else in family or among friends with similar problem or other speech problem? Did problem cause any adverse comment from relatives and others? Were such comments made in patient's presence?

   Patient's attitude toward speech problem. Has he or she withdrawn from speech or other situations because of it? Attitude of parents, siblings, and other relatives. Variations in attitude with different situations.

   (If the problem has been present from the time the child would normally have started to talk, complete the supplementary case history on language development and its disorders. If the problem developed after language was partially established, complete those sections of that supplementary case history that are appropriate for the age of the patient or the general level or functioning.)

Developmental History

Birth weight. Unusual birth circumstances? Any feeding difficulties? Ages of sitting up, first steps, bowel and bladder control. Toilet training techniques. Handedness, manual dexterity, bodily coordination.

Medical History

Illnesses — age of patient at each significant illness, degree of severity, duration, amount of fever, any complications or sequelae. Care provided when ill. Were parents overly concerned or solicitous or matter of fact? Same for all injuries and operations. Condition of tonsils and adenoids. History of mouth breathing? Ever worn glasses? If so, why? Parents' or patient's own estimate of hearing and vision.

School History

Age when entered school. Ever failed or skipped a grade? Present grade placement. Kind of grades child makes. Any special difficulties with school subjects? How has patient gotten along with teachers and schoolmates? Amount of education completed. If patient is a child, parents' estimate of his or her intelligence.

Social History

Estimate of family socioeconomic status, based upon parents' occupations, amount of education, source of income, house size and type. Leisure-time activities of family and of patient, community activity participation. Parental, parent-child, and sibling relationships. Discipline practices of parents when patient was a child; present relationship between patient and parents. Personality characteristics of patient. Behavior abnormalities as a child — thumb sucking, temper tantrums, destructiveness, hyperactivity, nail biting, et cetera; present adjustment problems. Age of patient's associates, especially in childhood. If patient is an adult, include work history and estimate of his or her own socioeconomic status.

Family History

Age and health of parents and siblings. Any family health problems? Speech abilities and disabilities in the family background, and family reactions to them.

Comments on Interview

Development of rapport, nature of informant's language behavior, expressive movements, emotional reactions, insight, evidence of rationalization, of unconscious projection. Any other important observations.

Figure 3-1. An example of a history outline. From *Diagnostic Methods in Speech Pathology* (2nd ed., pp. 58–59) by F. L. Darley and D. C. Spriestersbach, 1978, New York: Harper & Row. Copyright 1978 by Harper & Row. Reprinted by permission.

An outline is very helpful to refer to in writing the report, particularly if there is considerable similarity between one patient and another. In such cases, a checklist may even be sufficient. If there are differences among patients in the sort of information needed, each report must be tailor-made or nearly so. In some work settings, reports are written from an outline. Again, it seems probable that most practitioners choose a moderate path between the extremes.

WHAT ELSE DO WE LEARN ABOUT THE PATIENT AND THE PROBLEM IN ADDITION TO THE "FACTS"?

The history-taking interview gives us, usually, our first impression of the patient as a speaker. We can judge for ourselves her conversational skills, what disorders are apparent, and their severity. We also can make observations about how easy or how difficult it is for her to discuss the problem and any influences it has on her life. We also get an impression of her personal and social interactions in such a situation. These observations and impressions, so much a part of our clinical science and art, help us connect what we learn about the communication problem to the person(s) who lives with the problem and who deals with it as best possible on a daily basis.

HOW CAN WE USE THE HISTORY-TAKING PROCESS TO MAKE THE ENTIRE CLINICAL RELATIONSHIP EFFECTIVE AND EFFICIENT?

By many standards, this initial interview during which we take history sets the stage for all that follows. We want to show our genuine concern about the patient and her problem so we can be effective. We want to create an atmosphere in which she can easily express her concerns, impressions, and questions. We want to identify as quickly as possible aspects of the disorder that need further examination so time will be well spent. And we want to achieve both these goals as well as possible.

SUMMARY

The clinical history is our personal introduction to the patient. During the history interview, we hear the patient tell us about the problem and how it influences her life. We ask about onset, variability, and previous treatment. We identify her purposes in asking for our assistance. We structure the interview so that our discussion will yield useful information. We also set the pace so that she can ask questions or volunteer comments. During the interview we make our own judgments about the disorder and its severity. During the discussion, we observe the patient for indications about attitudes and feelings relevant to our purpose. At the conclusion of the history-taking interview, we can expect to have considerable information to use as our basis for the clinical examination. Further, we should expect to have formed a comfortable relationship with the patient to enhance effective evaluation.

ACKNOWLEDGMENT

Our thanks for assistance from Kenneth Tom, Margie Crawford, Harry Seymour, and Orlando Taylor.

REFERENCES

Ethnographic Issues

Battle, D. E. (Ed.). (1993). *Communication disorders in multicultural populations.* Boston: Andover Medical Publishers.

Christensen, K. M., & Delgado, G. L. (1993). *Multicultural issues in deafness.* White Plains, NY: Longman.

Taylor, O. L. (in preparation). Clinical practice as a social occasion: An ethnographic model.

Westby, C. E. (1990). Ethnographic interviewing: Asking the right questions to the right people in the right ways. *Journal of Childhood Communication Disorders, 13,* 101–111.

Interviewing Techniques

Evans, D. R., Hearn, M. T., Uhlemann, M. A., & Ivey, A. E. (1989). *Essential interviewing: A programmed approach to effective communication* (3rd ed). Pacific Grove, CA: Brooks/Cole.

Shipley, K. G. (1992). *Interviewing and counseling in communication disorders: Principles and procedures.* New York: Merrill.

Case History Forms

Darley, F. L., & Spriestersbach, D. C. (1978). *Diagnostic methods in speech pathology* (2nd ed., pp. 58–59). New York: Harper & Row.

Haynes, W. O., Pindzola, R. H., & Emerick, L. L. (1992). *Diagnosis and evaluation in speech pathology* (4th ed., pp. 373–376). Englewood Cliffs, NJ: Prentice-Hall.

Meitus, I. J., & Weinberg, B. (1983). *Diagnosis in speech-language pathology* (pp. 60–70). Austin, TX: Pro-Ed.

Shipley, K. G. (1992). *Interviewing and counseling in communication disorders: Principles and procedures* (pp. 24–32). New York: Merrill.

RECOMMENDED READINGS

Emrick, L. L., & Haynes, W. O. (1986). *Diagnosis and evaluation in speech pathology* (2nd ed., Chapter 2). Englewood Cliffs, NJ: Prentice-Hall.

Haynes, W. O, Pindzola, R. H., & Emerick, L. L. (1992). *Diagnosis and evaluation in speech pathology* (4th ed., Chapter 2). Englewood Cliffs, NJ: Prentice-Hall.

Meitus, I. J., & Weinberg, B. (1983). *Diagnosis in speech-language pathology* (pp. 60–70). Austin TX: Pro-Ed.

Nation, J. E., & Aram, D. M. (1984). *Diagnosis of speech and language disorders* (2nd ed., Chapter 4). San Diego: College-Hill Press.

Peterson, H. A., & Marquardt, T. P. (1990). *Appraisal and diagnosis of speech and language* (2nd ed., Chapter 2). Englewood Cliffs, NJ: Prentice-Hall.

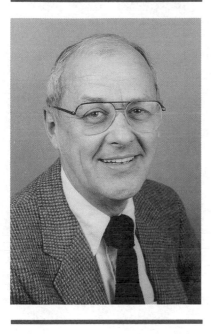

HUGHLETT L. MORRIS, Ph.D.

M.A. 1957, The University of Iowa
Ph.D. 1960, The University of Iowa

Dr. Morris is Professor Emeritus, Department of Speech Pathology and Audiology and of the Department of Otolaryngology-Head and Neck Surgery, The University of Iowa. His special interests are in cleft palate and related disorders, voice disorders, and speech and voice disorders associated with head and neck cancer.

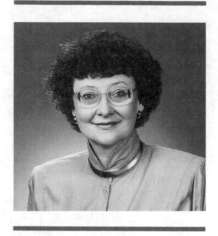

PENELOPE K. HALL, M.A.

M.A. 1967, The University of Iowa

Penelope K. Hall is Associate Professor, Department of Speech Pathology and Audiology, The University of Iowa. Her teaching, clinical, and research interests are in the areas of assessment and remediation of speech sound disorders and developmental language disorders, including developmental apraxia of speech.

The Oral Mechanism

Penelope K. Hall, M.A.

As you know by now, the clinical process is one of asking questions with the goal of solving problems. Questions that must be asked for each and every client or patient include: "Are there any problems with the mouth that might be the cause of, or contribute to, the communication disorder?" and "If there are problems with the mouth, what specific communication disorders might we suspect?"

The answers to these important questions are obtained by developing subquestions about specific parts of the mouth and related structures. Then, the questions are put to the test by conducting a physical examination, which consists of a collection of specific procedures. The physical examination of the speech producing mechanism goes by various names, including the "speech mechanism examination," "oral mechanism examination," "peripheral speech mechanism examination," "oral peripheral examination," and "orofacial examination."

WHY DO WE WANT TO ASSESS THE SPEECH MECHANISM?

In the minds of many people, "speech" is the most readily apparent part of the communication process. And, if there are problems with "speech," the problem must be related to how the mouth works, because "speech" is produced by the mouth. Further, the "speech" problem might be solved by "fixing" the part of the mouth that is "broken" or "not working well." Even though this is not the case for most speech and language problems, it is true for some communication disorders. As a result, the speech-language pathologist must be skillful in estimating the degree to which the oral structures and functioning are normal. Thus, the purpose of the speech mechanism examination is to evaluate how well the parts of the mouth, or articulators, and to some extent, the face and oral cavity, function in the production of speech. When conducting an examination of the speech mechanism we evaluate the face, lips, tongue, teeth, hard palate, soft palate, and pharynx.

WHAT DO WE WANT TO LEARN ABOUT THE SPEECH MECHANISM?

We examine the oral mechanism to answer our questions about how adequate each structure of the mechanism is for the production of speech, and how well each structure functions for the production of speech. To determine adequacy for speech production, each physical structure within the mechanism and its function must be evaluated individually and then, again, as part of the entire mechanism. From these observations, we can make estimates about the speech mechanism's structural and functional adequacy, each of which must be considered separately, as they are very different aspects.

Structural adequacy deals with the normalcy of the structures and the normalcy of the structures in relationship to each other. Some questions to ask about structural adequacy include: Is the tongue normal in size and appearance? Is there an unrepaired cleft palate? Are any front teeth missing? As well, assessment of the structural adequacy of the speech mechanism looks at whether any problems of the physical structures might interfere with speech production. *Functional adequacy* is concerned with how well these structures, regardless of intactness and relationships to each other, move and perform during speech production. The following questions may give you information about the functional adequacy of the speech mechanism: Does the tongue move normally? Is there the ability to open and close the velopharyngeal port rapidly?

Attempting to understand the difference between structural and functional adequacy is fundamental to the evaluation of the peripheral speech mechanism. Also, it is important to understand that problems with structures of the mechanism may, or may not, be related to the functional use of the mechanism for speech. For example, one client's mechanism may exhibit many structural "problems," but function adequately for speech. In contrast, another patient's mechanism may be structurally "perfect," but may not have adequate function during speech.

Some structural abnormalities are present from birth and are known as congenital problems. An example is cleft lip and/or palate. Structural abnormalities also may be acquired through accidents or diseases, such as traumatic injuries to the mouth or surgical removal of parts of the oral structures because of cancer.

Frequently, assessment of the functional adequacy of the oral mechanism is more difficult than assessing the structural adequacy. In arriving at judgments, the speech-language pathologist looks at the *rate* at which speech productions, or movements, are performed, as well as the *accuracy* of the productions. As with structural abnormalities, difficulties with the functional adequacy of the speech mechanism may be the result of developmental problems, problems acquired as a result of trauma or disease, or simply be unknown. We may find problems with the functional adequacy of the speech mechanism in patients exhibiting cerebral palsy and those who have had neurological insults as the result of stokes, traumatic accidents, and neurological system cancers. These functional problems sometimes may be more narrowly specified dysarthria or apraxia. For other clients, such as children with developmental apraxia of speech, problems in functional adequacy may be apparent even though the basis for the problem is not clear. With still other clients and patients you will find problems in the function of the speech mechanism during speech, but will be unable to describe it as a specific type of disorder; the mouth just doesn't seem to "work" very well during speech.

See Chapter 14 for more information on cleft lip and palate and Chapter 12 for additional information on head and neck cancer.

Discussions about dysarthria and apraxia are continued in Chapters 8 and 9.

HOW DO WE LEARN ABOUT THE SPEECH MECHANISM?

With the majority of your clients, the evaluation of the speech mechanism will be a clinical procedure that relies heavily on observations, estimates, and clinical judgments. There are a few direct measurements that can be made, such as the dimensions of a cleft palate and the measurements of dental occlusion and dental relationships. However, the relationships between these measurements and the production of speech are unclear. Further, the equipment to perform these measurements is often not readily available to most speech-language pathologists nor have most speech-language pathologists been trained to make the measurements.

Clinical judgments are often required when conducting a speech mechanism examination.

There are some tasks that have been standardized through "norm-referenced" information that will help you in interpreting a patient's performance on a task. These norms compare a given client's performance of a specific task to the performance of a group of persons with "normal" speech doing the same task. "Norm-referenced" information is available for some tasks used to assess the speech mechanism, such as some diadochokinetic rates. Such norm-referenced information may be helpful in understanding the functional adequacy of a client's mechanism. The norms can also be used to obtain "client-referenced" information, as when we compare a particular patient's performance on assessment tasks conducted across time. Client-referenced information can be particularly helpful in determining if there has been a change in the client's performance over a period of time. These changes may indicate that such aspects as remediation, maturation, or spontaneous recovery have or have not helped the patient use the speech mechanism with improved rate and accuracy during specific tasks.

However, mouths and oral structures come in a variety of shapes and sizes and with different degrees of mobility. Thus, clinical judgment, gained from your clinical experiences, will form the basis for many of the interpretations you will need to make when evaluating structural and functional adequacy of a patient's oral mechanism.

There are a few pieces of equipment you will need when conducting an examination of the peripheral oral mechanism. A flashlight is essential for observation of the structures and movements at the back of the mouth. Other equipment you will need includes sterile, individually wrapped tongue depressors, a stop watch, and a small mirror that will fit comfortably under a patient's nostril, sometimes known as a "nasal mirror." The use of examination gloves is required when doing a physical examination of the oral cavity as a precaution against bloodborne pathogens.

HOW DO WE ASSESS THE SPEECH MECHANISM AND WHAT MIGHT OUR FINDINGS MEAN?

There are a number of formats that can be used as the basis of your assessment of the speech mechanism. Some of these forms providing an outline for recording results are commercially available; others were developed by clinicians working to solve their own professional assessment needs. Some forms are very general, such as the one provided by Spriestersbach, Morris, and Darley (1978) and presented in Appendix 4-A. Others are developed for very specific populations of clients with communication disorders. A list of forms is included at the end of the chapter.

Speech mechanism examination forms should be thought of as "guides" to help you organize your assessment and observations, ensuring that your evaluation is comprehensive. Although the organization of the assessment forms will vary and the suggested tasks may differ, they all usually address the structural and functional adequacy of the various parts of the face, mouth, and oral cavity.

Patients often are asked to attempt diadochokinetic tasks to evaluate the functional adequacy of the oral mechanism. These tasks call for the rapid repetition of either a speech or nonspeech task. The purpose is to assess how *consistently*, *accurately*, and *rapidly* the patient is able to make the repeated movements. Diadochokinetic tasks place "stress" on the speech mechanism, because we rarely (if ever) use our most rapid possible rate of speech. But when the maximal movement or speech rate is attempted, you have the opportunity to observe how well the entire mechanism works as a whole and to assess how well the individual articulators function in the task.

There are two ways in which diadochokinetic tasks are performed. In the first method, the client produces the speech or nonspeech task for a specified period, often 5 seconds, which is then repeated for a total of three or more trials. The average number of productions *per second* is then calculated. The second method involves having the patient produce a specified number of productions or movements, with the speech-language pathologist timing the trial to determine how much time the client needs to complete the entire task.

Diadochokinetic tasks involve repetitive movements or speech sounds, such as repeating the syllable "tuh" or opening and closing the lips as fast as possible.

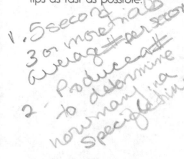

Norms are available for some of these diadochokinetic tasks, although there are two reasons why the norms should be used with caution. First, much of the research that includes diadochokinetic information was conducted with small subject groups. Second, the age groups for which the norms were developed are sometimes very narrow or, in other cases, are not precisely specified. Available research findings also indicate that diadochokinetic rates increase with age, starting at age 2 years, 6 months. However, when norms are available for a task, an "average" performance range, summarized from the research literature, will be reported in the margin notes in this chapter. It is hoped this placement will help you quickly find the information when needed. However, you may find it helpful to memorize these average rates, which can assist you in evaluating the function of the mechanism. At the end of the chapter is a reference list that contains the sources of these diadochokinetic norms.

Getting Started

It is best to establish a degree of rapport with the patient before conducting the oral peripheral examination because some clients are hesitant to have you look into their mouths. Before you begin the actual examination, briefly explain what you will be doing and why it is an important part of the total diagnostic evaluation. Remember that for some clients the things we are asking them to do may be new to them or they may feel uncomfortable in performing them. Some young children may even refuse to do the tasks or will do so only after you go to considerable efforts to make a series of "games" or "challenges" out of the tasks. Explanations and encouragement help assure the patient that you respect them and their dignity.

WHAT KINDS OF OBSERVATIONS AND EVALUATIONS DO WE MAKE?

The Face

The face is a part of the speech mechanism evaluation because of the important role facial expression plays in nonverbal communication. The examination will give you clues about muscle weakness and possible problems with the innervation of the face and mouth, which can be associated with problems of speech production as well as facial expression. Such problems need to be documented and may also give us hints that other parts of the speech mechanism, such as the tongue, might demonstrate similar problems.

Part of the assessment of the face can be done by observing the client during conversation, perhaps as part of rapport-building or as you obtain background information. Look at the general symmetry of the face when it is at rest. Is there a drooping of the corner of the mouth? Is an eyelid partially or completely closed? Is the mandible, or jaw, drooping on one side?

The symmetry of the face also can be assessed by asking the patient to make specific movements. Ask him to open his mouth as far as possible. Does the jaw move, or deviate, to one side or the other? Can he raise both of the eyebrows? Can he close both eyes tightly?

Summary of Procedures

To assess the structural adequacy of the face you can ask the client to do the following after having observed the general symmetry with the face at rest:

1. Open mouth as far as possible.

2. Raise both eyebrows.

3. Close both eyes tightly.

Lip Structure

The lips are very important in the production of speech; they are used to impound the air for the plosives /p/ and /b/, to restrict air flow for the fricatives /f/ and /v/, and to help shape the oral cavity in the production of vowels. The ability to seal the lips so that they remain closed is important in the swallowing process by holding food or liquids within the mouth. Deviations in the structure of the lips may interfere with these roles. We must also recognize that the entire oral mechanism has a great capacity to compensate for and overcome structural problems.

There are several observations you need to make of the lips when they are at rest. Look for symmetry, general contour, or shape, and the condition of the lips. A lack of symmetry may indicate the presence of a neuro-motor problem and may be apparent as you look at general facial symmetry. Does there seem to be an adequate amount of tissue in the lips? Can the lips be closed? Do you observe drooling? Does the lip tissue appear healthy or are there indications of inflammation, infection, or growths that might need medical attention?

You also may see a cleft lip, which may be a unilateral (on one side only) or a bilateral cleft. The cleft may not have yet been repaired, particularly in infants and very young children. For most patients, however, look for a scar line that may indicate a cleft lip repair. Remember that not all scars in the lipline are the result of a cleft lip repair. If present, note the shape of the scar(s) and how tight the tissue appears to be.

Lips are usually very mobile and, as stated previously, are used to compensate for many structural deviations. Thus, the explosion of air needed to produce the /p/ or /b/ sounds can usually be achieved even if either the upper or lower lip is very short or thin. Clinical and research findings tell us that, except in extreme cases, even an unrepaired cleft lip does not cause significant problems with speech sound production. However, you must look at the "total client" and question the possible negative impact of a scarred and uneven upper lip on the person's self-concept and personal adjustment.

Summary of Procedures

To assess the structural adequacy of the lips, you can make a number of observations.

1. At rest, observe the lips for symmetry, contour, condition, and an adequate amount of tissue.

2. Observe any presence of scar tissue.

Lip Function

The function of many of the oral structures is assessed using several different types of tasks: tasks that involve nonspeech movements and tasks that involve speech movements. Comparing the performance of the various parts of the mechanism for these varying tasks will help you to determine if there are problems with the mechanism and, if so, of what type. However, there is disagreement about the degree to which information about non-speech movements is predictive of speech movements. Even if they are not predictive, the use of nonspeech tasks in your speech mechanism examination will give you some idea of how well the structure can function in various ways. This includes the range of movement, the duration of movement, and the strength of movement. The range of movement indicates how far a structure, such as the tongue, is able to move. The duration of movement indicates how long a single or repeated movement can be maintained or sustained. The strength of movement indicates how well a structure can achieve and maintain a position when an external force is applied.

Nonspeech Movements

There are a number of nonspeech tasks that you may use to assess lip function. You may begin by asking the client to make static movements, or movements that are made and then "held in place." Examples are the unilateral retraction of the lips to each side of the face and the bilateral retraction of the lips. Remember, this is not a "smile," so requesting a smile for this movement is an inappropriate prompt.

The adequacy of lip function also needs to be assessed with non-speech diadochokinetic tasks that require the lips to move, as opposed to remaining in "static" positions. A task often-used for this assessment is to have the patient alternatively protrude and retract the lips by giving her the direction to "pucker, then smile, pucker, then smile," and so on. This is an example of a "reciprocal" movement task where the lips alternately make series of backward and forward movements. Another task is to ask the patient to approximate, or open and close, the upper and lower lips without making any speech sounds. While the client is performing these series of movements, be sure to look for the symmetry of the movement, how easily the movement seems to be made, how rapidly the movements are made, and how long the client is able to continue making the movement series.

Clients who have problems accomplishing these nonspeech movements with their lips may have neuromotor deficits, which, in turn, require further evaluation and may result in referrals for medical examination. Or, the client may have a history that indicates neurological problems, so the problems the client has in making nonspeech movements may not be a sur-

[handwritten margin note: reciprocal mvmt task pucker/smile]

The normal adult is able to open and close the lips without sound 5–6 times per second.

prise to you. However, when you observe patients having problems with nonspeech movements, you should not automatically assume that these are caused by underlying neurological problems. Perhaps the requests seemed "silly" and unnecessary to the client. Perhaps they are movements that the patient has seldom made and are, therefore, "unpracticed." Should you suspect the latter, the client's performance may improve in subsequent trials with the tasks.

You may find that "prompts" (things that clinicians can do to help clients' achieve success with the requested movement or speech act), using the patient's auditory, visual, and tactile-kinesthetic sensory modalities, are necessary to help her achieve the best performance she is capable of giving on nonspeech tasks. These sensory prompts often are used in a hierarchy, so that at first only verbal requests are made by the speech-language pathologist. If the client has problems performing the task after receiving only auditory cues, you can provide visual cues by modeling the movements yourself and/or using a mirror for the patient to visually self-monitor after watching you. If the visual clues do not result in successfully made movements, you can provide tactile cues by lightly touching the part of the face that is to make the movement.

Summary of Procedures

Nonspeech tasks that may help you assess the functional adequacy of the lips are:

1. Unilateral retraction of the lips to each side of the face.

2. Bilateral retraction of the lips.

3. Series of "pucker, smile."

4. Series of upper and lower lip approximations.

Speech Movements

A reciprocal speech movement task that can be used to help assess the functional adequacy of the lips and that is diadochokinetic in nature, involves asking the client to make a series of the vowels /u/ and /i/ (e.g., /uiuiuiui/, etc.). Remember that this task is different from the nonspeech task of completing a "pucker, smile" series. There are no known norms for this task, so you need to observe accuracy, smoothness, and the rate during the task. Another diadochokinetic speech task used to assess the functional adequacy of the lips is the repetition of the monosyllable /pʌ/ ("puh").

The normal diadochokinetic rate for /pʌ/ is 3–6 per second for children, and 6–7 per second for adults.

Summary of Procedures

The functional adequacy of the lips during speech can be assessed by:

1. Repetitions of /uiuiui/.

2. Repetitions of /pʌ/.

Lip Strength

The strength of the labial seal can be assessed by asking the patient to puff out each, and then both, cheeks, sealing the air by tightly closing the lips. Then, you gently press on each cheek, and both cheeks, with the flat of your hand to see if the labial seal is broken with the air escaping out the mouth.

Summary of Procedures

The strength of the lip seal can be evaluated by the procedure:

1. Request that the patient puff out the cheeks and seal the air, then gently push against each cheek, and both cheeks.

Teeth

Teeth are involved in the production of a number of consonant sounds by channeling the airstream. These phonemes are the labiodentals (/f/, /v/), the linguadentals (/θ/, /ð/), and the fricatives (/s/, /z/, /ʃ/, /ʒ/). Because the teeth are easily observable, dental deviations often are identified as the cause of a speech sound disorder. In fact, this may or may not be correct. We need to be very aware that most speakers are able to make major compensations for dental deviations, such as children who continue to produce correct /s/ and /z/ sounds despite the loss of deciduous ("baby") central incisors and the gradual growth of new, larger permanent teeth. But, it is important to be able to identify clients whose dentition actually may be a factor in their communication problems.

You need to learn the names of teeth and the typical ages when the permanent teeth emerge. This information is important because you will be dealing with children who are in the process of losing their deciduous teeth and gaining their permanent ones, as shown in Table 4-1.

You also must assess the dental "occlusion," which is the relationship of the upper and lower dental arches and the alignment of the teeth when the jaw is closed. This is done by telling the client to "bite down" on the back teeth and then to spread the lips or to "show the gums," which prevents the client from thrusting the jaw forward. This allows you to see the first upper and lower molars easily, which is crucial to the determination of occlusion.

Many dentists use the Angle classification system to describe occlusion and malocclusion, and you also will find this adaptation of it helpful.

Table 4–1. Eruption of dentition.

Primary Dentition		Permanent Dentition	
Teeth	**Age of Eruption**	**Teeth**	**Age of Eruption**
Maxillary		Maxillary	
Central incisor	7.5 months	Central incisor	7–8 years
Lateral incisor	9 months	Lateral incisor	8–9 years
Cuspid	18 months	Cuspid	11–12 years
First molar	14 months	First bicuspid	10–11 years
Second molar	24 months	Second bicuspid	10–12 years
		First molar	6–7 years
Mandibular		Second molar	12–13 years
Central incisor	6 months	Third molar	17–21 years
Lateral incisor	7 months		
Cuspid	16 months	Mandibular	
First molar	12 months	Central incisor	6–7 years
Second molar	20 months	Lateral incisor	7–8 years
		Cuspid	9–10 years
		First bicuspid	10–12 years
		Second bicuspid	11–12 years
		First molar	6–7 years
		Second molar	11–13 years
		Third molar	17–21 years

Source: Adapted from *Pediatric Dentistry: Infancy Through Adolescence* by Pinkham, J. R., Casa-massimo, P. S., Fields, H. W., McTigue, D. J., and Nowak, A. J., Philadelphia: W. B. Saunders Company. 1988.

The four occlusions with which you need to be familiar are:

1. *Normal occlusion*
   The cusps, or points, of the first upper molar should fit into the "groove" between the two anterior and posterior cusps of the lower molar. A handy way to think of normal occlusion is that the mandibular (lower) first molar is "half a tooth ahead" or in front of the maxillary (upper) first molar, as shown in Figure 4–1. It is important to keep in mind that a normal occlusion is not the "average" occlusion. Very few individuals have an occlusion that is "normal" in every way.
   You will need to modify this evaluation for young children who do not have permanent first molars. For these youngsters, you can examine the most posterior teeth that are in place. Then, line them up the same way you would when viewing the first permanent molars.

2. *Neutroclusion (or Angle's class I)*
   The upper and lower dental arches are in correct occlusion, when a person presents with a neutroclusion, but individual teeth are misaligned. For instance, a tooth, or teeth, may be rotated or teeth may be jumbled.

3. *Distoclusion (or Angle's class II)*
   A distoclusion occurs when the lower dental arch is "too far back" in relation to the upper dental arch. This is apparent when you align the up-

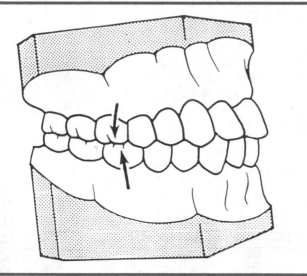

Figure 4-1. Normal occlusion. The arrows indicate the normal occlusion relation ship of the first molars. From Bloomer, H. H. "Speech Defects Associated with Dental Malocclusions and Related Abnormalities." In Travis, L. E. (Ed.), *Handbook of Speech Pathology and Audiology.* Englewood Cliffs, NJ: Prentice-Hall, Inc., 1971. Reprinted with permission.

per and lower first molars, as illustrated in Figure 4-2. It often also is apparent when the individual has closed the mouth because the chin looks as if it is receding.

4. *Mesioclusion (or Angle's class III)*
Mesioclusion exists when the mandible is "too far forward" in relation to the maxilla. Thus, the lower dental arch overlaps the upper dental arch, which can be observed when you align the first molars, and as seen in Figure 4-2.

You also will need to be familiar with several other aspects of dentition as you conduct your speech mechanism examination. One involves the relative positions of the front (anterior) parts of the upper and lower arches. These terms and explanations are:

Openbite is the lack of contact between the upper and lower anterior teeth (incisors, cuspids, and bicuspids) when the first molars are in normal occlusion (See Figure 4-3).

Overbite, or *closebite,* is the excessive vertical overlapping of the lower anterior teeth by the upper anterior teeth, as shown in Figure 4-3, with occlusion by the first molars. The upper central incisors normally cover one-half to one-third of the lower central incisors.

Crossbite is a lateral, rather than a parallel, overlapping of the upper and lower dental arches. When a crossbite occurs, it appears as if the lower jaw is located either to the right or left of a normal, central position relative to the upper jaw.

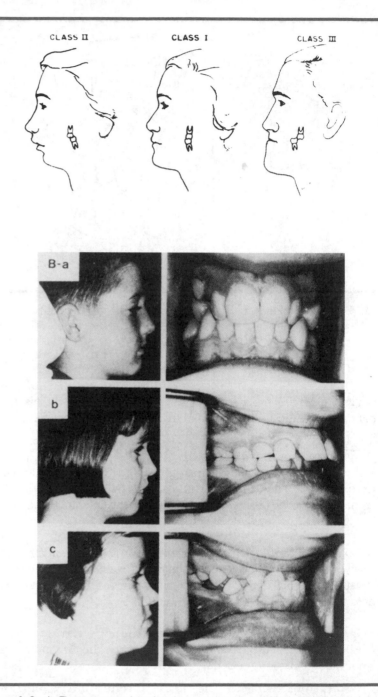

Figure 4–2. A. Three types of malocclusions showing Angle's classification, facial profile, and relationship of the first molars. Left to right are: distoclusion (Class II), neutroclusion (Class I) and mesioclusion (Class III). **B.** Photographs of dental occlusions and effects on profiles. **B-a** shows a balanced profile of a child with a neutroclusion; **B-b** illustrates a profile with a receding chin and a distoclusion with an overjet (note how the lips reflect the overjet); and **B-c** reveals a lip posture in profile which reflects the mesioclusion. From *Cleft Palate Speech* (2nd ed., p. 91) by B. J. McWilliams, H. L. Morris, & R. L. Shelton, 1990, Philadelphia: Mosby-Year Book, Inc. Reprinted with permission.

OVERJET	OVERBITE	OPENBITE

Figure 4-3. Illustrations of overjet, overbite, and openbite. *Overjet* is horizontal projection of the upper incisors in front of the lower incisors. *Overbite* is the overlapping of the upper anterior teeth over the lower anterior teeth vertically. *Openbite* is the vertical distance between the upper and lower incisors that are not overlapping. From "Orthodontic problems in children" by D. J. Hall & D. W. Warren (p. 966) in *Pediatric Otolaryngology, Volume II*, C. D. Bluestone, & S. E. Stool (Eds.), 1983, Philadelphia: W. B. Saunders. Reprinted with permission.

Overjet is the excessive horizontal distance between the surfaces of the incisors, as illustrated in Figure 4-3. The upper central incisors are normally 1-3 mm ahead of the lower central incisors. An overjet is sometimes seen in children who have a history of thumbsucking.

Underjet is a lack of normal horizontal distances.

In addition, there are terms that describe the relative positions of individual teeth in the dental arch. These are:

Labioversion (a tooth tilting toward the lip)

Buccoversion (a tooth tilting toward the cheek)

Linguaversion (a tooth tilting toward the tongue)

Edentulous space(s) (a missing tooth or teeth)

Supernumerary/extraneous teeth (extra teeth)

While you are conducting this portion of the speech mechanism examination, be sure to note the general, overall condition of the teeth. How clean do the teeth appear to be? Are there any spots or areas which could be caries, or cavities?

You also can encounter several different types of dental appliances or prostheses while conducting a speech mechanism examination. *Dentures* are commonly known as false teeth, and may be a full or a partial dental arch. There may be *orthodontic appliances* (braces). Don't be surprised to see orthodontic appliances on adults as well as children, as orthodontia is helpful to persons of all ages. *Obturators* and *palatal lift appliances* are similar in appearance to the more familiar dental retainers used in orthodontia, except that they are longer and have bulb-like structures at the end. These are special prosthetic appliances constructed to help the speech become easier to produce and to understand when there are problems with the function of the soft palate and velopharyngeal mechanism. These situations are addressed later in this chapter and in Chapter 14.

You need to evaluate dentition because of the possibility that dental abnormalities *may* have adverse effects on speech production. Sometimes you may conclude that there is a relationship between missing or misaligned incisors and erred productions of the fricative phonemes, such as the client who distorts sibilants (/s/, /z/, /ʃ/, /ʒ/, etc.) and who also has incisor dentition problems. Occasionally misaligned teeth also may intrude into the shape or the size of the mouth and result in speech errors. An example of this is a child who is unable to make the bilabials /p/ or /b/ because of an overjet of the upper incisors. Instead, the child may make a labiodental stop that closely resembles an /f/. The presence of dental appliances may cause some potential problems in how the tongue moves and where it is placed during speech attempts. However, the oral mechanism is able to compensate for many dental deviations.

Summary of Procedures

The dentition should be structurally assessed by:

1. Noting dental development and condition of teeth.

2. Observing the occlusion.

3. Observing any deviations in the positions of the anterior teeth.

4. Noting dental appliances or prostheses.

Tongue Structure

The tongue (Figure 4-4) is used in speech to channel and obstruct the air stream in the production of consonants. It also influences vowel productions and voice resonance by contributing to the shape of the oral cavity. Further, it is crucial in the process of swallowing.

Tongues vary in size and shape, as do overall mouth sizes. The size and shape of the tongue and mouth must be appropriately related to one another and they usually are. The determination of this relationship is a subjective judgment about which you will develop confidence with clinical experience.

You begin your assessment of the tongue's structure by observing it at rest. Note the size of the tongue. Does it appear to be atrophied (shrunken) or furrowed on one side? Are there any fasciculations (involuntary movements) seen with the tongue at rest? Are there any other involuntary contractions or twitches along the edges of the tongue? Next, ask the patient to protrude the tongue as far as possible. Does the tongue deviate to one side? If so, this may indicate a weakness in the musculature or innervation on one side. Should this be the case, the tongue deviates *toward* the side on which there is a problem. This is because the muscles on the affected side are unable to exert enough force to "balance" the force produced on the unaffected side — thus, the tongue moves toward the weaker side. Does

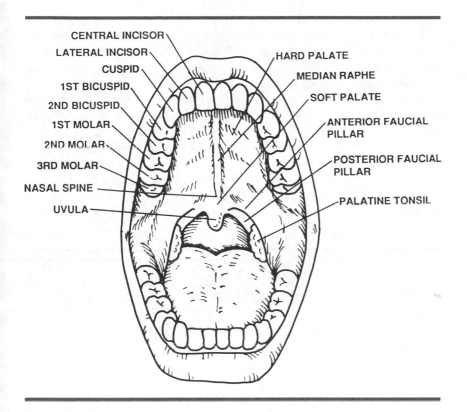

Figure 4-4. The physical structures of the mouth. Adapted from *Diagnosis in Speech-Language Pathology* (p. 43). I. J. Meitus, & B. Weinberg (Eds.), 1983, Austin, TX: Pro-Ed. Adapted by permission.

the tongue protrude very little or not at all? This may indicate a bilateral weakness in the musculature or innervation. Any of these problems may indicate that there is peripheral nerve damage, which can result in a neuromotor speech problem known as dysarthria, or in swallowing problems, known as dysphagia.

Dysphagia will be more completely discussed in Chapter 15.

You also will need to determine if there is tissue missing from the tongue. This information can be obtained during the case history or during the oral mechanism examination. Missing tongue tissue will have most likely resulted from injury or surgical removal, called a glossectomy. Total or partial glossectomy is performed when there is a disease process, notably cancer. Following glossectomy, the remaining part of the tongue is frequently very adaptable and capable of compensatory movements. The resulting speech may not be evaluated as "normal," but may be understandable, although the extent of the excision must be taken into consideration.

Next, look at the general condition of the tongue. Is there a coating? If so, what is the color? A coating on the tongue may reflect a disease process, the client's general health, or medication the person is taking. Also note whether there are any lesions on the surface, underside, or edges of the tongue. If so, medical consultation is needed, as the lesion(s) may be cancerous.

The *lingual frenum* or *frenulum* also needs to be assessed. The frenum is the web of tissue that connects the underside of the tongue to the floor of the mouth at the midline of the tongue. You can observe this structure as you investigate the underside of the tongue. You also need to observe the possible effects of the length of the frenum while the tongue is protruded. If the frenum is short, the anterior, or front, part of the tongue may be limited in the amount of protrusion it is able to make. The resulting appearance of the protruded tongue is that the anterior portion is "heart-shaped" because of the frenum's inability to allow for the extension of the midline of the tongue. The center of the tongue tip is thus unextended as the surrounding tissue of the tongue margin is extended, giving a heart-shaped appearance. When the lingual frenum is determined to be too short, and restricts tongue movement, a "tongue tie" may be said to be present.

Summary of Procedures

The structure of the tongue can be assessed by the following tasks:

1. Observe the tongue at rest for shape, completeness, and condition.

2. Ask the patient to protrude the tongue.

3. Observe the length of the lingual frenum.

Tongue Function

The normal tongue is highly mobile and is able to move rapidly and precisely. The next step in the evaluation of the speech mechanism is to assess these functions of the tongue. This is done to determine if there are limitations in tongue function and, if so, what these are and how the limitations might affect speech production. Some limitations in the function of the mechanism may be from underlying neuromotor problems. However, problems in performing tasks assessing tongue function do not always indicate a neuromotor etiology. Functional assessment of the tongue is done with both nonspeech and speech tasks.

Nonspeech Tasks

The first of several procedures you can use to evaluate nonspeech tongue function is to request that the patient open his mouth slightly, and make repeated elevations of the tongue tip to the alveolar ridge, while producing no sound. Observe how accurately and smoothly this task is performed. Because you will have no auditory cues, you will need to observe and count the number the times the elevation is completed within a selected time period. Thus, you will need to place your stopwatch near the mouth so you can monitor timing as well.

During this, as well as other diadochokinetic-type tasks, some clients may employ "mandibular assist." Assist is said to occur when the jaw, rath-

The average diadochokinetic rate for elevating the tongue to the alveolar ridge with no sound is 4.5 to 5.0 per second.

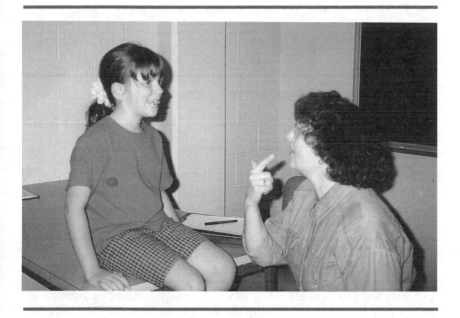

er than the tongue, makes the required movements. Use of mandibular assist needs to be noted, although the assist may be normal in clients below the age of 7 to 8 years. You should try to determine if the tongue movement can be made without the accompanying jaw movement. Have the patient attempt to stabilize the jaw by holding his chin to reduce or eliminate the movement of the mandible during the speech task. If this does not work, you should stabilize the jaw by holding it during additional trials of the task. By doing this, you can acquire information about whether the tongue is capable of making the movements or whether the assistance provided by the jaw movement is a necessary compensation for the patient to complete that particular movement.

The "tongue wiggle" is the second nonspeech procedure you can use. The "wiggle" consists of alternate lateral touching of the corners of the mouth during several trials. Again, because no sounds are being produced, you will need to watch the mouth to count excursions, so you also will need to place your stopwatch near the mouth. When counting, use only the full excursions from one side of the mouth and back again to signify a single unit. You also may find that the rate at which this task is performed is similar to the norms for the previously described elevation of the tongue tip to the alveolar ridge and for the diadochokinetic production of the syllable /tʌ/, which will be discussed later in this chapter. In addition to the rate at which the tongue can make these lateral moves, you will also want to evaluate how accurately and smoothly the trials are performed and to note if the performance deteriorates or remains consistent across trials.

The "tongue circle" is another nonspeech task that taxes the function of the tongue. The "circle" is completed by having the patient open the mouth slightly, and then attempt to move the tongue around the resulting circular-appearing mouth opening. Many patients find this a very difficult task because it involves a constant change in the direction of the tongue movement. There are no norms for the task. However, the procedure is an

The rate at which children and adolescents between 4½ and 14½ years of age can produce alternate lateral tongue movements is 10 repetitions in 3–5 seconds. Another norm is an average of 4.5–5.0 excursions per second.

excellent way to gain subjective judgments about the smoothness, accurateness, and coordination of the tongue. When repeated over several trials you also can check the consistency with which the client is able to do the task.

Summary of Procedures

Nonspeech tasks that may assist in the evaluation of the functional adequacy of the tongue are:

1. Repeated elevation of the tongue tip to the alveolar ridge without sound.

2. The tongue "wiggle."

3. The tongue "circle."

Speech Tasks

Typical diadochokinetic rates for /tʌ/ are 3.5–5.5 per second for children between the ages of 2½ and 5 years, and 5.5–6.5 per second for adults.

A speech task that can assess function of the tongue tip is the diadochokinetic production of /tʌ/. Typically, the syllable is repeated for several trials. Should you observe mandibular assist, attempt to stabilize the jaw to separate the tongue and jaw movements.

Several additional diadochokinetic tasks will help you assess tongue function. Diadochokinetic production of /kʌ/ assesses the function of the posterior part of the tongue in a speech task. Another diadochokinetic task that evaluates the patient's control of the tongue, as well as the lips, is production of the multisyllabic nonsense word /pʌtʌkʌ/. Some young clients may not be able to produce this nonsense string of sounds. They may be able to perform a similar task that has meaning to them, however. The words "patticake" and/or "buttercup" accomplish much the same purpose as /pʌtʌkʌ/ in your assessment procedures.

Average diadochokinetic rates for /kʌ/ are 3.5–5.5 per second for children and adolescents 2½ to 15 years of age, and 4–6 per second for adults.

In addition to the rate of production, the *accuracy* of the sequences of sounds in the multisyllabic words also is very important. For instance, observe if the correct order of the syllables is maintained over the repetitions, as well as being maintained over multiple trials. Problems with consistency in maintaining correct productions and syllable order is a characteristic of clients with apraxia of speech. A patient with apraxia might scramble the order of the syllables, such as: /pʌtʌkʌ/, /pʌkʌtʌ/, /tʌpʌkʌ/. Another client with apraxia might become inaccurate in the phonemes being produced, such as: /pʌtʌkʌ/, /bʌdʌkʌ/, /pʌdʌgʌ/.

Eight-year-old boys can typically produce /pʌtʌkʌ/ at a rate of 1.0–1.5 per second.

With some patients it also may be necessary to assess the impact of what appears to be a restricted lingual frenum, or possible tongue-tie. The tongue tip needs to move the furthest to produce the /l/, /n/, /t/, and /d/ sounds. During assessment you need to incorporate these sounds into speech tasks. Some clients with a frenum that appears restrictive may be able to produce these sounds accurately and with good rate. Other clients may have developed compensatory ways of producing the sounds to accommodate for the restrictive frenum. Still other clients may be unable to reach the alveolar areas or to compensate adequately to produce the sounds. In such a case, it is necessary to refer the patient for medical management, in which the "tongue tie" is "clipped" by a surgeon. However, it has been our experience that, although some clients show short frenums, these rarely impact negatively enough on speech skills to justify the surgery.

Summary of Procedures

The functional adequacy of the tongue can be assessed via use of:

1. Diadochokinetic productions of /tʌ/.

2. Diadochokinetic production of /kʌ/.

3. Diadochokinetic production of /pʌtʌkʌ/ or real words with a similar structure of their syllables.

4. In the case of a suspected restrictive frenum, production of the /l/, /n/, /t/, and /d/ in various speech tasks.

Tongue Strength

To assess tongue strength you will need to use a sterile individually wrapped tongue depressor. First, ask the client to protrude his tongue and then to resist your efforts to force the tongue to the right, left, and back into the mouth with the tongue depressor. A second task to assess tongue strength is done by asking the patient to place the tongue tip against the inside of the cheek, and then to resist your efforts to move the tongue toward the midline of the mouth with the flat of your fingers placed on the outside of the cheek. When a weakness is present, it is easier to force the tongue inward on the side which is opposite the weakness than it is to force the tongue on the side of actual weakness. Thus, if a weakness is on the right side, it will be easier to force the tongue inward from the left side of the mouth. This is because the force you apply on the left side meets little or no resistance from the weakened right side. If, during your assessment of tongue strength, you detect weakness, the speech and/or swallowing disorder that brought the patient to you may have a neuromotor basis or component.

Summary of Procedures

Tongue strength can be assessed:

1. Ask the client to protrude the tongue and provide resistance when you apply force with a tongue depressor on the left, right, and tip of the tongue.

2. Ask the patient to place his tongue against the inside of the cheek and provide resistance as you apply force.

Hard Palate Structure

The role of the hard and soft palates during speech and swallowing is to provide a barrier between the nasal and oral cavities. The hard palate, or roof of the mouth, is a bony structure that must be assessed for structural intactness or adequacy. If a hard palate is not intact, air may inappropriately escape from the mouth into the nasal cavity and out through the nose, resulting in nasalization of speech.

The structure and color of the center or midline of the palate need to be assessed. The normal midline structures may consist of a midline *raphe*, or indentation, or a bony line and bump, called a *torus*. The normal colors at the midline of the hard palate are pink and white. The posterior (back) edges of the hard palate usually are located near the last molar. Its shape should be scalloped and be continuous across the palatal vault.

Be sure to note the presence of an unrepaired, or a partially repaired, cleft in the hard palate. If the palate has been surgically repaired, be alert for the possible presence of small openings, or holes, along the repair line. These are called *fistulas*, which allow air to escape into the nasal cavity. You also will need to note the presence of lesions, or growths, on the hard palate, which require medical attention. Also note if there has been surgical removal of any of the hard palate because of disease or trauma. Finally, note the presence of any prostheses, such as dentures, obturators, or palatal lifts.

Fistulas are small holes resulting from breakdown of surgically repaired tissues.

A variation of cleft palate is the submucous cleft palate. The term *submucous* is descriptive, because the cleft is not apparent during visual inspection. The bone defect that constitutes the submucous cleft of the hard palate is beneath the intact mucous membrane (literally, submucous). The bony defect is a notch in the posterior margin of the hard palate, where the posterior nasal spine normally is found. The notch cannot usually be seen, and must be palpated, or felt, with a finger. The notch of the submucous cleft palate has no ill effects on speech or voice production.

The overall size and contour, or shape, of the hard palate or palatal vault also needs to be examined. Note the height and width of the vault. Make special note of hard palates that appear to have flat, low vaults or high, narrow vaults. These two contours can potentially result in problems with voice resonance and make articulation difficult for the lingua-alveolar sounds of /l/, /n/, /t/, and /d/. The impact of the vault shape on speech can be determined by assessing the ease and accuracy with which the patient can make these four speech sounds.

Velopharyngeal Mechanism Structure

The velopharyngeal port is known by several names, including the "VP port" and "palatopharyngeal mechanism." This mechanism is comprised of the velum, or soft palate, and the pharynx, which includes the "back wall" as well as the side walls of the throat. Please refer to Figure 4-4 to help you identify these structures and their relationship to one another. The velopharyngeal port mechanism opens and closes the area at the back of the throat that separates the oral and the nasal passages to allow safe swallowing and normal speech production. Specifically, the port is closed during swallowing so that food and liquid (including saliva) is forced downward into the esophagus and not permitted into the nasal cavity. Generally, the velopharyngeal port also is closed during the speech production of plosives and fricatives, but is open during production of nasals. However, it is important to remember that, even in normal speakers, there is considerable variation in the opening and closing of the port, depending on the speech task.

As is true elsewhere in the oral mechanism, there frequently is disparity between the structures and function of the velopharyngeal port mechanism. The structures may appear normal, but demonstrate disordered function. We need to remember that it is the function, not structure, that should be our focus during this part of the examination. Sometimes the apparent disparity between structure and function is because we are able to see only part of the mechanism. This is because the nasal surface of the soft palate and pharyngeal walls — the components of the velopharyngeal mechanism that cause closure — are hidden from our view by the oral surface of the soft palate. So, our view is incomplete, and we must be very careful in interpreting our observations. Still, examination of the velopharyngeal structures available to our limited visual inspection is worth our time.

It is important that the structures are in a position similar to that used when the client is talking, rather than distorted, as when the patient's head is tilted back. A tilted head distorts the musculature of the structures, as well as the typical way in which the structures move. You need to make your examination with the client's mouth at your eye level. With children, perhaps this can best be done by asking them to sit on a table or to stand. As well, the patient's mouth should be only three-quarters open, because full mouth opening also distorts the musculature that needs to be assessed.

A major observation is whether the soft palate, or velum, and uvula, (the most posterior portion of the soft palate) are intact, or whether there is a physical cleft or opening of another kind. Note if there is an unrepaired, or a repaired, cleft of the soft palate. If there is a history of a surgically repaired cleft palate, look for the presence of fistulas. The color of the soft palate at mid-line may give you a clue to a submucous cleft that is not detectable by visual inspection. Normally the soft palate is the same color as the hard palate. If there is a bluish color running throughout or partway through the palate at midline, suspect the possibility of a submucous cleft, which needs to be palpated. A submucous cleft of the soft palate consists of a muscle defect and results in diminished bulk, length, or movement of this component of the velopharyngeal mechanism. The client's speech may be uncontrollably nasalized. Also be suspicious of a submucous cleft if you see a bifid, or split-looking, uvula. You may need to use a sterile tongue blade to determine the degree of intactness or bifidness of the uvula. This is done by stroking the uvula forward in an effort to separate the individual-appearing parts of the structure. Also note scars, holes, or tears in the palatal tissue which have resulted from trauma.

While looking at the palate at rest, observe the symmetry. Should the velum appear to be asymmetrical, with one side resting at a lower level than the other side, ask the patient to produce sustained or repeated /a/ sounds and observe if the palate continues to appear asymmetrical. If so, a unilateral muscular weakness or a problem with innervation may be present. In this situation, the uvula will move toward the unaffected side. With other clients you may think that the palate is generally too low when at rest, which could indicate a bilateral weakness. In this situation ask the patient to produce a sustained /a/ or series of /a/s to see if there is any change in position of the velum. If bilateral weakness is present, you will see very little, if any, movement.

Other structures that need to be noted are the faucial pillars and tonsils, which, when present, are located between the anterior and posterior pillars (see Figure 4-4). Tonsils, one on each side, are usually very easy to identify in children, because the masses are often enlarged. The size of tonsils is not usually of concern *unless* they are red and inflamed and/or have white matter on them, indicating that they may be infected. Problems with the size of the tonsils also can occur if they are so large that the airway is obstructed, and if the movement of the posterior part of the tongue is affected. These problems may be severe enough to warrant a referral to a physician, whose management may include a tonsillectomy, or surgical removal of the tonsils. You may have to look very carefully for tonsils in many of your adult clients; this tissue naturally atrophies, or shrinks, as an individual matures and reaches adulthood.

You will need to make subjective judgments about the depth and width of the oropharynx, which is the space at the back of the mouth. Clinical experience will help you make these subjective judgments. The oropharynx must be shallow enough in depth to allow the soft palate to extend back and elevate slightly, for achievement of velopharyngeal closure with the back wall of the throat, or pharynx. As well, the velum must be long enough to reach the back wall of the pharynx. The width of the oropharynx is also important. The space must be narrow enough to allow the side walls at the back of the mouth to move inward, or mesially, a movement that helps to close off the nasal airway from the oral airway.

Not usually apparent during the speech mechanism examination, but important to the velopharyngeal structure and function, are the adenoids. Adenoids (and tonsils) are lymphoid tissues, and are presumably a part of the immunologic system protecting an individual against disease. Like tonsils, the adenoids are most prominent in childhood, and least prominent, if present at all, after adolescence. When the tissue is at maximum size, the enlarged adenoidal pad can provide considerable help in reducing the size of the velopharynx. In fact, if the adenoids are too large they may block the nasal passageway, creating denasal voice quality. If a patient's soft palate is short, the enlarged adenoidal pad may help the child compensate in closing off the velopharyngeal port; the velum makes contact with the enlarged adenoids rather than the back pharyngeal wall. However, if the child had an adenoidectomy, this compensatory mechanism for closing the port is no longer present, so velopharyngeal dysfunction may result because the palate is unable to reach the pharyngeal back wall. Likewise, adolescent patients may be referred to you because of concerns about the gradual increase in nasally emitted air during speech. This could be velopharyngeal dysfunction resulting from the gradual atrophy of the adenoids, which also reduces and eventually eliminates a compensatory means for closing the velopharyngeal port.

Hyponasality is another name for denasal voice quality.

The structural adequacy of the VP mechanism may be assessed by:

1. Observing the soft palate for intactness and symmetry at rest and during productions of prolonged and repeated /a/.

2. Evaluating width and depth of the oropharynx.

Velopharyngeal Function

As indicated earlier, assessing the ability of the VP port to function in its task to separate the nasal and oral airways is difficult to do. There are a number of structures that are involved in the necessary movements, and these movements must be made in a coordinated manner. You also need to be aware that some important movements are hidden from view during clinical physical examination of the mechanism. The function of the mechanism can be assessed by both speech and nonspeech tasks, as well as with instrumental approaches. The latter approaches are described in Chapter 14, which deals with cleft palate.

Speech Tasks

Important initial clues about the function of the VP port mechanism are gained by listening to your patient's speech as he is conversing with you. Is there hypernasality? (Does it sound to you as if too much air is coming through the client's nose during speech?) Is air actually escaping out the nose when the patient is producing nonnasal phonemes? Do you see the nares (nostrils) flaring when the client is talking with you? Do you hear "funny" sounding phonemes that could be transcribed as glottal stops or pharyngeal fricatives — speech sounds that are being made too far back, perhaps as a way of trying to help close off the nasal airway?

A simple assessment technique that can be helpful in determining if air really is escaping during nonnasal sounds is through use of a "nasal mirror." Ask the client to produce sounds in isolation, syllables or words that target the specific phonemes you think might be produced with "nasal emissions" during your general observations of connected speech. Hold a mirror under the patient's nares, or nostrils, and watch for clouding during nonnasal sound production. Clouding indicates that the VP port is not closing appropriately. This is, of course, not a precise measure of velopharyngeal function, but it is a very useful and inexpensive method to gain some information about the VP mechanism function during speech.

Have the client open his mouth (approximately three-quarters of the way) and observe the VP mechanism during two tasks — production of a prolonged /a/ and production of short, repeated /a/s. A sterile tongue depressor may be necessary for holding the tongue down so you can get a good view of the oropharynx during these tasks.

During production of the prolonged /a/ you should see two definite movements. The soft palate should move "up and back" so that the posterior pharyngeal wall is reached. You also should see the lateral pharyngeal walls and faucial pillars move mesially, or inward, toward the center of the throat. These two movements (posterior and mesial) should close the pharyngeal port, and the closure should be maintained as the /a/ continues to be produced. The movements occur simultaneously and quickly, so you need to be observant and know what you are looking for. As indicated earlier, it is possible to gain only part of the picture of the adequacy of velopharyngeal port movement during the oral examination; recall that many of the structural relationships and movement patterns within the velopharynx are not visible to you.

During the first /a/ produced in the series of short, repeated /a/s, you should see the posterior and mesial movements described for the prolonged /a/. However, these movements occur only on the first /a/; very minor movements occur during the remainder of the /a/ series.

Another speech task that can help assess the function of the VP mechanism is to determine if the diadochokinetic rates for /pʌtʌkʌ/ are better with the nares, or nostrils, closed or open. If the velopharyngeal mechanism is leaking air, the patient will find that having the nares closed may help the overall efficiency of the speech system and the diadochokinetic rate will improve.

Summary of Procedures

Speech tasks which can assist in the evaluation of the functional adequacy of the velopharyngeal port are:

1. Observation of conversational speech.

2. Use of the nasal mirror during simplified speech tasks.

3. Prolonged /a/.

4. Repeated /a/s.

5. Diadochokinetic rates for /pʌtʌkʌ/ with the nares (nostrils) open and closed.

Nonspeech Tasks

The functional adequacy of the velopharyngeal port also can be assessed by various tasks that do not involve speech. One such task is having the client blow out a birthday candle or a match in the usual oral way. Does air leak through the nose during the task? If it does, a comparison can be made with the nostrils open, requesting that the client make his best attempt to direct the air orally, and with the nostrils occluded (closed), as you manually prevent air from escaping nasally. If you can detect a difference in performance when the nostrils are open and when they are occluded, the chances are good that the patient has a velopharyngeal closure problem. *A caution:* Be alert for the possibility of nasal congestion from upper respiratory infections or allergies when performing these, or other, tasks in assessing how well the VP port is functioning.

A final nonspeech task you can conduct to assess functional adequacy of the VP mechanism is to attempt to elicit a gag reflex. This is an unpleasant experience for the client, so do not make this a part of your typical examination of the speech mechanism. Rather, elicit the reflex only if you hear hypernasality, have documented the presence of nasal emission during speech, and see little or no movement during the prolonged /a/ and repeated /a/ tasks. With these conditions, you need to estimate the maximal movement of the velopharyngeal mechanism in an attempt to establish if there is innervation to the port area. The gag reflex can be elicited in numerous ways by use of a tongue blade, such as touching the palate, touching or stroking the pharyngeal wall, or placing pressure on the back of the tongue. If the reflex is present, you will see a great deal of posterior palatal and mesial wall movement. If you see asymmetrical or little movement during the gag reflex, suspect neuromotor weakness. Place this task at the very end of your speech mechanism examination; few patients will let you have "another look" into their mouths after having had the reflex elicited!

Summary of Procedures

Functional adequacy of the VP port mechanism can be assessed by the following nonspeech tasks:

1. Impounding air to blow out a candle or match.

2. Eliciting a gag reflex.

The speech mechanism examination requires much practice — and the sooner you can start this practice, the better. You will need to overcome feelings of invading another person's very personal space. You will need to gain an important base that will help you learn to make subjective clinical judgments. You will need to begin acquiring the observations necessary to gain a concept of how large the range of "normal" structures and "normal" function really is. You will need to learn how to work efficiently when doing this examination; know what you need to look for when you ask the client to open her mouth and then gain this information with a minimal number of mouth-opening requests to your patient. Practice doing the procedures involved in the speech mechanism examination to become a proficient professional when you do it "for real" with your first client.

WHAT DO WE DO NEXT?

After we have made the observations and taken the measurements necessary to assess the structural and functional adequacy of the oral mechanism, we need to describe results. However, we must be *very* careful in relating these descriptions to the speech problems we have also observed and assessed. You must be very logical when thinking about cause-and-effect. The information you gain during the speech mechanism examination should be used to help you support or refute the hypotheses you've developed about the client's problems with communication. Some patients with structural problems of the speech mechanism also have articulation or resonance problems. However, the relationships among these aren't always predictable. For instance, remember that some individuals can compensate for very large abnormalities in the structure and/or function of the mechanism, while other clients seemingly are unable to compensate for what appear to be lesser problems with the mechanism. And, other patients may have problems with the mechanism that are so severe that the person's communication skills probably are not going to improve without assistance beyond what you will be able to provide. Finally, with some clients you will conclude that even though there are structural and functional deviations in the speech mechanism, these do not have any relationship to the communication problem.

You also must develop recommendations for your client as a result of your diagnostic evaluation. Recommendations may be based on your examination of the speech mechanism. Perhaps you will want to recommend a period of trial remediation, to see if the patient is able to improve speech skills despite the problems you may have observed in the structure or function of the mechanism. Or, you may want to determine if the client is able to learn some compensatory movements that will improve her speech skills. You may need to refer some patients to professionals in other fields, such as the family physician, dentist, orthodontist, or otolaryngologist. You also may refer some clients to other speech-language pathologists who have special expertise in dealing with specific kinds of communication or swallowing disorders. In some job settings these recommendations come from you alone, while in other job settings they are made by a team of professionals from different fields — each with input into the recommendation-making process on what needs to be done to best serve the client's present and future needs.

SUMMARY

An examination of the peripheral speech mechanism needs to be a part of the evaluation process for all clients. Through these results you will be better able to address the questions of whether or not there are problems with the structure and/or function of the mouth that might be the cause or contribute to the patient's communication or swallowing problems, as well as give you clues as to the specific nature of these disorders.

REFERENCES

Spriestersbach, D. C., Morris, H. L., & Darley, F. L. (1978). Speech mechanism examination. In F. L. Darley & D. C. Spriestersbach, *Diagnostic methods in speech pathology* (pp. 322–345). New York: Harper & Row.

RECOMMENDED READINGS

Examination Forms

Dworkin, J. P., & Culatta, R. A. (1980). *Dworkin-Culatta oral mechanism examination*. Nicholasville, KY: Edgewood Press.

Enderby, P. M. (1983). *Frenchay Dysarthria Assessment*. Austin, TX: Pro-Ed.

Mason, R. M., & Simon, C. (1977). An orofacial examination checklist. *Language, Speech and Hearing Services in Schools, 8*, 155-163.

Nation, J. E., & Aram, D. M. (1984). *Diagnosis of speech and language disorders* (2nd ed., pp. 354-360). San Diego: College-Hill Press.

Peterson, H. A., & Marquardt, T. P. (1981). *Appraisal and diagnosis of speech and language disorders* (pp. 191-192). Englewood Cliffs, NJ: Prentice-Hall.

Robbins, J., & Klee, T. (1987). Clinical assessment of oropharyngeal motor development in young children. *Journal of Speech and Hearing Disorders, 52*, 277.

St. Louis, K. O., & Ruscello, D. M. (1987). *Oral Speech Mechanism Screening Examination, revised*. Austin, TX: Pro-Ed.

Vitali, G. J. (1986). *Test of Oral Structures and Functions*. East Aurora, NY: Slosson Educational Publications.

Diadochokinetic Rates

Blomquist, B. L. (1950). Diadochokinetic movements of nine-, ten-, and eleven year old children. *Journal of Speech and Hearing Disorders, 15*, 159-164.

Canning, D. A., & Rose, M. F. (1974). Clinical measurements of the speed of tongue and lip movements in British children with normal speech. *British Journal of Disorders of Communication, 9*, 45-50.

Ewanowski, S. J. (1964). *Selected motor speech behavior of patients with parkinsonism*. Unpublished doctoral dissertation, University of Wisconsin, Madison.

Fairbanks, G., & Spriestersbach, D. C. (1950). A study of minor organic deviations in "functional" disorders of articulation. 1. Rate of movement of oral structures. *Journal of Speech and Hearing Disorders, 15*, 60-69.

Fletcher, S. G. (1972). Time-by-count measurement of diadochokinetic syllable rate. *Journal of Speech and Hearing Research, 15*, 763-770.

Irwin, J. V., & Becklund, O. (1953). Norms for maximum repetitive rates for certain sounds established with the Sylrater. *Journal of Speech and Hearing Disorders 18*, 149-160.

Kreul, J. E. (1972). Neuromuscular control examination (NMC) for parkinsonism: Vowel prolongation and diadochokinetic and reading rates. *Journal of Speech and Hearing Research, 15*, 72-83.

Lundeen, D. J. (1950). The relationship of diadochokinesis to various speech sounds. *Journal of Speech and Hearing Disorders, 15*, 54-59.

Robbins, J., & Klee, T. (1987). Clinical assessment of oropharyngeal motor development in young children. *Journal of Speech and Hearing Disorders, 52*, 271-277.

Sprague, A. L. (1961). *The relationship between selected measures of expressive language and motor skill in eight-year-old boys*. Unpublished doctoral dissertation, University of Iowa.

Yoss, K. A., & Darley, F. L. (1974). Developmental apraxia of speech in children with defective articulation. *Journal of Speech and Hearing Research, 17*, 399-416.

General

Haynes, W. O., Pindzola, R. H., & Emerick, L. L. (1992). *Diagnosis and evaluation in speech pathology* (4th ed., Chapter 9). Englewood Cliffs, NJ: Prentice-Hall.

Meitus, I. J., & Weinberg, B. (1983). *Diagnosis in speech-language pathology* (Chapter 2). Austin, TX: Pro-Ed.

Peterson, H. A., & Marquardt, T. P. (1981). *Appraisal and diagnosis of speech and language disorders* (Chapter 7). Englewood Cliffs, NJ: Prentice-Hall.

Shipley, K. G., & McAfee, J. G. (1992). *Assessment in speech-language pathology: A resource manual* (Chapter 4). San Diego: Singular Publishing Group.

APPENDIX 4-A
SPEECH MECHANISM EXAMINATION

1. Lips
   a. Structure:
      Touch when teeth are in occlusion: yes _____ no _____
      Upper lip length: normal _____ short _____ long _____
         (describe)
      Evidence of cleft lip or other structural deficit:
         yes _____ (describe) no _____
      Other structural deficiet: (describe)
   b. Function:
      Can protrude: yes _____ no _____
      Can retract unilaterally
         Left: yes _____ no _____
         Right: yes _____ no _____
      Equal retraction bilaterally: yes _____ no _____
      Number of times can produce /pʌ/ in 5 seconds:
         trial 1 _____ trial 2 _____ trial 3 _____
      Does stabilizing the jaw facilitate the activity?
         yes _____ no _____
   c. Adequacy for speech: 1 _____ 2 _____ 3 _____ 4 _____
2. Teeth
   a. Structure:
      Occlusion: normal _____ neutroclusion _____
         distoclusion _____ mesioclusion _____
      Anteroposterior relationship of incisors: normal _____
         mixed (some in labioversion, some in liguaversion) but all
         upper and lower teeth contact; all upper incisors lingual to
         lower incisors but in contact _____ not in contact _____
      Vertical relationship of incisors: normal _____
         openbite _____ closebite _____
      Continuity of cutting edge of incisors: normal _____
         rotated _____ jumbled _____ missing teeth _____
         supernumerary teeth _____
      If lack of continuity, identify teeth involved and describe nature
      of deviation:
   b. Dental appliance or prosthesis:
         yes _____ (describe) no _____
   c. Adequacy for speech: 1 _____ 2 _____ 3 _____ 4 _____
3. Tongue
   a. Structure:
      Size in relation to dental arches: too large _____
         appropriate _____ too small _____ symmetrical _____
         assymmetrical _____
   b. Function:
      Can curl tongue up and back: yes _____ no _____
      Number of times can touch anterior alveolar ridge with tongue
      tip without sound in 5 seconds:

trial 1 _____   trial 2 _____   trial 3 _____
above average _____   average _____   below average _____
Number of times can touch the corners of mouth with tongue
tip in 5 seconds:
    trial 1 _____   trial 2 _____   trial 3 _____
    above average _____   average _____   below average _____
Number of times can produce /tʌ/ in 5 seconds:
    trial 1 _____   trial 2 _____   trial 3 _____
    above average _____   average _____   below average _____
Number of times can produce /kʌ/ in 5 seconds:
    trial 1 _____   trial 2 _____   trial 3 _____
    above average _____   average _____   below average _____
Restrictiveness of lingual frenum: not restrictive _____
    somewhat restrictive _____   markedly restrictive _____
c. Adequacy for speech: 1 _____   2 _____   3 _____   4 _____

4. Hard palate
  a. Structure:
    Intactness: normal _____   cleft, repaired _____
      cleft, unrepaired _____
    Palatal fistula: yes _____ (describe)   no _____
    Alveolar cleft: yes _____ (describe)   no _____
    Palatal contour: normal configuration _____
      flat contour _____   deep and narrow contour _____
  c. Adequacy for speech: 1 _____   2 _____   3 _____   4 _____

5. Palatopharyngeal mechanism
  a. Structure:
    Soft palate:
    Intactness: normal _____   cleft, repaired _____
      cleft, unrepaired _____   symmetrical _____
      asymmetrical _____
    Length: satisfactory _____   short _____   very short _____
    Uvula:
      normal _____   bifid _____   deviated from midline
      to right _____   to left_____   absent _____
    Oropharynx:
      Depth: shallow _____   normal _____   deep _____
      Width: narrow _____   normal _____   wide _____
  b. Function:
    Soft palate:
    Movement during prolonged phonation of /ɑ/:
      none _____   some _____   marked _____
    Movement during short, repeated phonations of /ɑ/:
      none _____   some _____   marked _____
    Movement during gag reflex: none _____   some _____
      marked _____
    If some movement, is amount:
      Same for both halves _____   more for right half _____
      more for left half _____

Oropharynx:

> Mesial movement of lateral pharyngeal walls during phonation of /ɑ/:   none _____   some _____ marked _____
>
> Mesial movement of lateral pharyngeal walls during gag reflex: none _____   some _____   marked _____

Audible nasal emission while blowing out a match: yes_____ (describe)   no _____

Inconsistency in nasal emission during speech or blowing tasks: yes_____ (describe)   no _____

Patient stimulable to oral productions of pressure consonants: yes _____ (describe)   no _____

Nares constriction during speech or blowing tasks: yes _____ (describe)   no _____

Oral manometer ratio (instrument _____):

> Trial 1:   nostrils open _____   nostrils closed _____ ratio _____
>
> Trial 2:   nostrils open _____   nostrils closed _____ ratio _____
>
> Trial 3:   nostrils open _____   nostrils closed _____ ratio _____

c. Adequacy for speech: 1 _____   2 _____   3 _____   4 _____

6. Fauces

a. Structure:

> Tonsils: normal _____   enlarged _____   atrophied _____ absent _____
>
> Pillars: normal _____   scarred _____   inflamed _____ absent _____
>
> Area of faucial isthmus: above average _____   average _____ below average _____

b. Function:

> Posterior movement during phonation of /ɑ/:   none _____ some _____   marked _____
>
> Mesial movement during phonation of /ɑ/:   none _____ some _____   marked _____
>
> Restriction of velar activity by pillars: none _____ some _____   marked _____

c. Adequacy for speech: 1 _____   2 _____   3 _____   4 _____

From "Examination of the Speech Mechanism" by D. C. Spriestersbach, H. L. Morris, & F. L. Darley (pp. 339–343) in *Diagnostic Methods in Speech Pathology*, F. L. Darley & D. C. Spriestersbach (Eds.). New York: Harper & Row Publishers, 1978. Reprinted with permission.

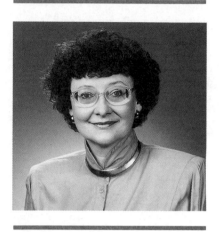

PENELOPE K. HALL, M.A.

M.A. 1967, The University of Iowa

Penelope K. Hall is an associate professor in the Department of Speech Pathology and Audiology at the University of Iowa. Her teaching, clinical, and research interests are in the areas of assessment and remediation of speech sound disorders and developmental language disorders, including developmental apraxia of speech.

Language Disorders

Amy L. Weiss, Ph.D.,
J. Bruce Tomblin, Ph.D., and
Donald A. Robin, Ph.D.

This chapter introduces you to the process of language diagnosis. We have included information for evaluating language abilities regardless of the age of the client or whether concern about language is one of many reasons or the only reason for referral. Language problems are pervasive in the individuals we serve and because of the need for language competencies in our activities of daily living the diagnosis of language disorder will be a common clinical challenge to you. Language diagnosis is particularly challenging because of the complexity of language and the varied nature of language disorders. Because of this complexity, it is essential that you have in mind a model, or road map, concerning the nature of language, a clear understanding of the diagnostic problem-solving process, and a clear sense of the clinical standards used to make decisions in this area. This chapter provides you with a usable framework to use in your diagnosis of language disorders.

Many clients referred to us for other reasons also may have a language disorder.

AN OVERVIEW OF LANGUAGE AND LANGUAGE DISORDERS

A Model of Language for Diagnostic Purposes

Our perspective is that *language* is a socially shared code comprised of a set of arbitrary symbols, used primarily for communication, and that language can be conveyed verbally, manually, or in written form (Owens, 1988). This definition emphasizes the first aspect of our model: the modalities of language usage. We believe that no assessment of our clients' language can be considered complete without evaluating both *language comprehension* (understanding) and *language production* (expression). Further, with some clients, particularly those with acquired language disorders, we include both the spoken and written forms of language in our evaluation. Our definition of language is not equivalent to, but instead is broader than, our definition of speech. *Speech* represents only one mode of language expression and, although it is probably the mode we spend the most time evaluating, it will not tell us the whole story about a client's language abilities. Broader even than the term *language* is the concept of *communication*. Our actual goal in evaluating the language abilities of our clients is to determine how successfully they can convey as well as interpret information in their activities of daily living because that is the all-important function that communication serves.

In keeping with current descriptions of the language system and to facilitate our discussions of assessment procedures, we have divided language into five different components: *phonology,* representing the sound system of a language and including the rules that organize the system and generate allowable sound combinations; *syntax,* which characterizes the allowable patterns of word combinations to form, for example, declarative or interrogative sentences; *morphology,* the set of inflections that allows us to alter words to indicate, for example, number, tense, and possession (bus*es*, walk*ed*, Mommy'*s*); *semantics*, which deals with vocabulary development as well as the roles that words can play when combined with one another (e.g., agent, action, object); and *pragmatics*, the use of language in context to express communicative intent, presupposition, and conversation rules (Roth & Spekman, 1984). This division of language into these component parts is done for the sake of convenience only. The student of language development and language disorders should appreciate the interdependence and influence we know that these parts of language actually exert on one another in language development (Prutting, 1979), language disorders (Panagos et al., 1979), and in day-to-day language use (Crystal, 1987).

Clinicians approaching language evaluation often differ in how they visualize the interactions and primacy of these different language components. Some believe that the components of language are equivalent and that, although these systems must interact for language to work properly, the status of these components can be evaluated separately. On the other hand, others propose that pragmatics determines the choices of specific words and sentence types to be used and, therefore, is the primary component of

The various interactions among the components of language make language evaluation even more challenging.

language. Advocates of the latter orientation are wary of the results gleaned from structured language assessment techniques that attempt to evaluate each component separately, often outside of the naturalistic contexts of pragmatics. Thus, we see how your approach to the nature of language is going to influence the way you go about your language diagnosis. Figure 5-1 illustrates the relationship among the component parts of language.

The Relationship Between Language, Sensation, Perception, and Cognition

There is nearly universal agreement about the close relationship between language and other systems required for successful language development and use. Obviously, if spoken language is to be acquired and understood, it is necessary for the person to be able to hear (*sense*) the auditory message

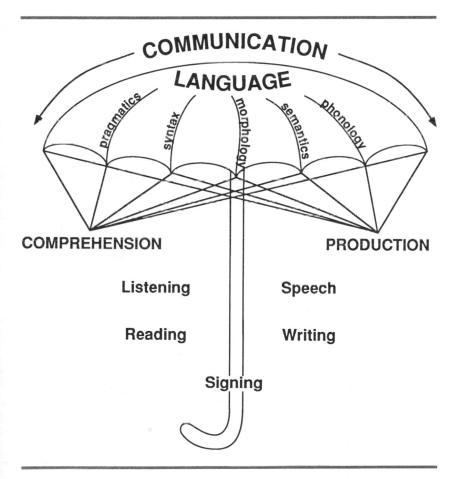

Figure 5-1. The relationships among communication and the component parts of language as they relate to the areas of assessment for language disorders.

and to *perceive* the complex frequency and temporal information contained in the signal. Further, higher level cognitive processes must be intact, including: the ability to represent experiences and ideas, or *concepts*; store this information (*memory*); and focus *attention* on information to accomplish *problem solving*. For many years researchers tried to determine if cognitive abilities were prerequisite for language learning, with impairment resulting from acquired language problems. Researchers also tried to determine whether linguistic operations depended on cognition. Today it is generally believed that cognition and language develop interactively and that this interaction continues in adulthood, meaning that the two areas are interconnected and mutually dependent.

Later we will be discussing the need to make a range of clinical decisions about the cause of a client's language disorder as well as its prognosis and treatment options. Information concerning the sensory, perceptual, and cognitive abilities of the client will be essential in making these decisions, and so we need to know about those abilities in our efforts to diagnose language problems. Some of this information you may be able to obtain yourself during the examination of the client; other information may come from colleagues in other professions. As a part of your professional education, you will be trained to perform basic audiometric testing to screen for a hearing loss; however, in most instances you should refer clients who may be at risk for hearing loss (e.g., those with language delay) to an audiologist for evaluation. Likewise, you may be able to obtain some information about general cognitive ability from your own tests, but most speech-language pathologists rely on psychologists for information about their clients' cognitive and intellectual functioning.

As you use information from cognitive testing, you need to keep in mind that many of the popular tests administered by clinical psychologists, such as the *Wechsler Intelligence Scale for Children — Revised* (WISC-R) (Wechsler, 1974), require the clients to have considerable prerequisite language ability. This requirement for language ability puts the client with a language disorder at a disadvantage, because language ability becomes confounded with intellectual ability in such tools. This is true for both clients with developmental language disorders as well as those with acquired language disorders (individuals who suffer a loss of language ability following their acquisition of the language system). For these clients who have language problems, tests that emphasize nonverbal performance rather than verbal skills are preferable. See Sattler (1988) for a comprehensive discussion of this issue. A note of caution must be extended here because even performance scale tests are not always a perfect solution. Careful examination of the particular performance measure should also be made because many "nonverbal" tests are performed with verbal strategies. For example, test developers often code nonverbal memory test items with names to assist in a task. This being the case, what may have been meant as a nonverbal performance scale to measure intelligence may actually invoke the use of verbal coding strategies and skew results for clients with developmental and acquired language problems.

We have now laid out a general model of language and its relationship to information processing systems. This model will guide you as you work through the complex terrain of language.

A DEFINITION OF LANGUAGE DISORDERS

We have just described language as a complex system of knowledge having to do with the function, meaning, and form of messages. Further, people must be facile in the use of this system of knowledge in the understanding and expression of ideas. When this complex system works well, people can engage in communication with few difficulties and with little effort. On the other hand, there are some children and adults for whom this system does not work well, and in such cases we regard the person as having a language disorder. These people may have difficulty understanding things said to them, they may have difficulties formulating messages, or both. Language disorders, therefore, occur when individuals do not possess the language skills required of them by their linguistic community and find themselves confronted with frequent communication failure.

This way of defining a language disorder emphasizes the relationship between the expectations and demands of the person's community and the person's language abilities to meet these expectations. By emphasizing the community expectations, we admit that there is no fixed standard of what is considered "normal" or "good" language performance. Rather, the standard is whatever the person's community expects. Notice that in this statement we mentioned the person's own linguistic community. If you are not very good at French and you go to Paris, you will face a good deal of communication difficulty. However, we would not say that you have a language disorder, unless you are a native French speaker and a part of the French society. This extends to instances of dialect. People are not considered to have a language disorder simply because they use a variant of a language that varies from the standard form, as long as the variant is viewed as acceptable within their own community.

In our definition of language disorder, we have been using the concept of expectations. Even within an individual society, the expectations may vary for different members. In Western societies, adjustments in expectations for language performance are made according to a person's age. Thus, we do not expect 2-year-olds to be able to talk at length on a topic, and furthermore, we are not surprised when they do not use adult phonologic and grammatic forms. On the other hand, if an adult were to have the language skills of a 2-year-old, it is likely that the adult would face difficulties. Because of this, the speech-language pathologist also makes adjustments in assessment of the language skills of children. This is often done by incorporating norm referencing in our interpretation of many of our language measures. This means the child's performance is compared with that by other children of the same or very similar age. Children who demonstrate language skills more than one standard deviation below the norm (below the 16th percentile) for their age are usually regarded by both speech-language pathologists and classroom teachers as having unacceptably low language abilities; and therefore, these children are likely to be diagnosed as language impaired. Similar adjustment for age may also be made for older clients, thus recognizing that language facility does decline with the normal process of aging. Many tests of adult language are normed on young adults aged 18–40, and thus, use of such assessments for comparison of the typical stroke victim age 60 or older is inappropriate.

We all speak a dialect or variant of some language; "nonstandard" dialects represent language differences, not disorders.

Subtypes of Language Disorder

So far we have been talking about language disorder in its broadest form; and many of the questions you will be asking during language diagnosis, as well as the methods you will use to address these questions, will be applicable to all forms of language disorders. However, we need to consider at this point that there are two major subtypes of language disorder, and at various points in this chapter we will be pointing out special diagnostic issues that pertain to these groups.

Developmental Language Disorders

As the term "developmental" implies, these are problems of language acquisition. These clients present with a pattern of delays in language development from the early stages of language learning that often persists throughout childhood and remain in adulthood in the form of a limited facility with language. Because a developmental language impairment can be viewed as a limitation in a growth or developmental process, we describe the language problem in terms of the level of development obtained by the client in the various domains of language function. Therefore, the assessment process for a developmental language disorder often involves varying language tasks along a continuum from early developing language skills to those that are acquired later in life. Notice that this approach to characterizing the language problem assumes that most clients with developmental language disorders are very similar to younger normally developing individuals — an assumption with a history of fairly strong support.

Acquired Language Disorders

In contrast, an acquired language disorder is characterized by a clear reduction in language abilities from an individual's previous level and is therefore viewed as a disturbance of an already successfully developed system. In most instances, the client has had normal language development but, as the result of trauma to the brain or some disease process affecting the brain, loses some degree of language ability.

Clients with acquired language disorders may have problems ranging in severity from subtle difficulties finding a word to a nearly complete inability to understand things said to them. In addition to variation in severity, acquired language disorders may differ in the areas of language affected. For example, some clients have considerable difficulties understanding things said to them, but have fairly good expressive language ability. In contrast, others may have considerable difficulty expressing themselves, but have good comprehension abilities. Individuals with right hemisphere damage or traumatic brain injuries may perform normally on tests of basic linguistic abilities but fail on higher level material involving such abilities as inferencing or sequencing. Some adults may have language impairments that are secondary to more general cognitive problems, such as attentional and memory problems. Many of these differences are related to the side and areas of the brain damaged, as well as the particular cause of the brain injury.

Unlike developmental language disorders, persons with acquired language disorders may not present with language skills that can be compared to normal language users at a younger age level. Instead, you will observe that their difficulties with language often appear in the form of language usage errors that are very uncommon for most normal language users. These errors are often associated with increases in the information processing demands of the particular language task. Thus, sentences that are long may place a heavy burden on the client's memory and can lead to frequent comprehension failure, whereas shorter sentences place less demand on memory and, as a result, are easier to understand. Because of this, when speech-language pathologists assess the language problems in acquired language disorder, they need to vary the information processing complexity of language tasks and then note the type and frequency of language errors made across the range of tasks. Moreover, as noted previously, many of the clients' problems may be related to more general cognitive problems. In this chapter, we will provide basic information on the diagnosis of acquired language disorders. Further details are in Chapters 7 and 13.

We emphasize that, although we are going to be looking at many of the same dimensions of language regardless of whether the client presents a developmental or acquired language impairment, our view of the basic nature of two forms of language impairment influences the way in which we characterize the language problem.

THE GOALS OF LANGUAGE DIAGNOSIS

The goals of language diagnosis are similar to the goals of diagnosis for any other disorder area: We are seeking to gain a clear understanding of the client's communication problem and to use this information to make decisions regarding the clinical management of the problem. In fact, our goals must fit into this broader diagnostic framework because our language evaluation usually will be part of a general consideration of the client's overall communication status. Often clients do not come to us already knowing that their problem involves the language systems concerned with communication. All they know is that they are having problems communicating. Also, many of the communication problems we see in the clinic are not isolated to language systems. For instance, many acquired language disorders also have problems of speech production in the form of dysarthria, apraxia, or cognitive impairments associated with them. Therefore, our diagnosis of language is usually placed within the broader context of the diagnosis of communication disorder.

Recall from Chapter 1 that several issues are often addressed as a part of diagnosis. Although all the issues listed are important, we will be addressing the following:

1. Determination of complaint.
2. Determination of the existence of a language problem.
3. Determination of concomitant factors.
4. Determination of the course of the problem.

We will look at each and consider what information we need for an answer and how we can go about obtaining this information.

Determination of the Nature of the Complaint

When a client with a language disorder comes to us with concerns about communication, our first step will usually be to guide whomever is the primary informant (the client, a parent or spouse, a teacher, a nurse, etc.) in describing the nature of the problems the client is having. It is during this initial conversation with the informant that you will begin to suspect that the problem may be one involving language. Complaints having to do with language will contain concerns over difficulties formulating ideas into well-formed utterances. If the client is a child, the parent may express concern that the child is using very limited word combinations or the child's sentences may have an immature quality. If the client is older and has had normal language, the complaint will contain comparative information about what the person cannot do now that he or she used to be able to do. Also, in the case of an acquired language disorder, there usually will be strong evidence of a medical event such as a head injury or stroke associated with the onset of the language impairment. Although informants initially are less likely to provide you with concerns about language comprehension problems, once you ask you often will be told that the client does have difficulty following directions and so on. It is also common to be told that the client has no problems with understanding. Accept this as a possibility, but realize that sometimes clients can appear to be understanding more than they are. This is something you will want to confirm later. You will be able to see rather quickly that you are going to have information that may suggest that at least part of the communication problem may be based on problems with language. If this is the case, you will then move to the next line of questioning, which has to do with establishing the presence of a language impairment. See Figure 5–2 for several suggestions of questions that might lead to a discussion of the complaint.

Clients often guess the meaning of things being said by using nonverbal cues. This may lead us to believe that they have better language skills than they actually have.

---

1. What are your concerns about (client's) communication?

2. When the person talks with you are questions asked, are you asked to get things, are you told about things that have happened?

3. Can you have a conversation with the client?

4. When talking with you, does the person speak in full sentences, short phrases, or mainly words?

5. When you talk with the client, do you believe the person can understand the things you say to him?

6. What situations make it easier or more difficult for the client to understand you?

Figure 5-2. Common questions you might ask while obtaining complaint information.

Determining the Existence of a Language Disorder

If the complaint suggests that there may be a language disorder, we then begin posing questions having to do with the client's language status in the various areas of language following the model of language presented earlier. This model guides us as we gather information about the client's language, and we will want to establish the client's status in each area of language provided by the model. This information can be obtained through the use of a variety of tasks, ranging from standardized language tests to very naturalistic conversations. Your job then is to select tasks that will provide you with reliable and valid information and provide you with this information efficiently. In so doing, you should consider some of the issues raised in Chapter 1 regarding the reliability and validity of measures.

GENERAL COMPONENTS OF THE ASSESSMENT BATTERY

By now it should be clear that a comprehensive characterization of the language abilities of a client will require you to employ several different tasks within which you can observe the client's language performance. As a result, you will need to construct a battery of tasks to be used for your evaluation. There are some standardized tests that cover both language comprehension and production areas. For example, the *Test of Language Development* (TOLD-2:P), a language test for young children, (Newcomer & Hammill, 1988) contains seven subtests, three of which address areas of language comprehension, with the four remaining tests serving to evaluate language production competencies. Comprehensive tests of aphasia such as the *Boston Diagnostic Aphasia Examination* (BDAE) (Goodglass & Kaplan, 1981) and the *Porch Index of Communicative Ability* (PICA) (Porch, 1968) examine both production and comprehension. Other standardized tests are more selective and focus either on language comprehension (e.g., the *Peabody Picture Vocabulary Test-R* [PPVT-R], Dunn & Dunn, 1981; *The Revised Token Test*, McNeil & Prescott, 1986) or language production (e.g., the *Carrow Elicited Language Inventory* [CELI]) (Carrow, 1974). So, it is important, when evaluating the usefulness of a test for inclusion in a particular client's test battery, that you identify which area or areas of language require assessment.

Within the general heading of language comprehension or language production, you need to know which subcomponent or subcomponents of language are evaluated by a given instrument. Getting back to the example of the PPVT-R, this test specifically addresses receptive, single-word, vocabulary. Carrow-Woolfolk's (1985) *Test of Auditory Comprehension for Language* (TACL-R), on the other hand, is a language comprehension measure that evaluates three aspects of receptive language: single-word vocabulary, sentences, and roles and relations of words within a sentence. Therefore, a clinician could argue that using both of these tests as part of the same test battery would be redundant and a waste of valuable time. Many speech-language pathologists, however, would consider the PPVT-R a more intensive clinical tool for evaluating receptive vocabulary, a well-respected test instrument because of its reliability and validity, and might decide to find the time for both tests. One additional rationale for using both tests could be that one measure of receptive vocabulary would have the potential of substantiating the findings gleaned from the other.

You will also be guided in your selection of testing materials by the presenting complaint. For example, if a child is perceived to have difficulty participating in classroom discussions, then a portion of the evaluation should focus on the child's classroom performance as described in Chapter 6. Similarly, if a wife's concern that her stroke victim husband appears to be most frustrated by his inability to respond to questions within a reasonable time frame, you will want to gather some data to evaluate this ability.

Informal Observation

In our desire to derive supportive numbers through test administration as evidence for diagnosis, we sometimes overlook the importance of observing our clients. As mentioned, scores resulting from standardized tests can be easily criticized for not reflecting typical behaviors of language use or for the limited sample of language skills they reflect. As a consequence, we usually need to supplement the information we can gain through formal testing by observing our clients in activities of daily living. Ideally, this would involve several different co-conversationalists in several different situations to provide the most comprehensive picture of how our clients' abilities correlate with their language needs. In addition, observation of clients with family members and other individuals even for 5 or 10 minutes enables us to form some opinion about the strategies used by other individuals to interact with the client.

Because language is a complex system, we need to observe it in natural settings to see how the system works as a whole.

For school-age children, observation in the classroom setting is strongly recommended to observe the child's ability to cope with the language demands of the classroom. Adults also should be observed in settings that more closely approximate their daily language use than typical testing situations to provide a comprehensive picture of whether and to what degree their language abilities are compromised. When working with adults with acquired language problems, it is also useful to observe the client in a variety of interactions between the client and other health-care providers (e.g., nurses, physicians).

THE TASKS USED TO COLLECT RECEPTIVE AND EXPRESSIVE LANGUAGE DATA

We cannot directly observe what clients understand when they hear an utterance. Therefore, we need tasks that allow the client to reveal what was understood.

From what we have said, you can see that you will likely be using several assessment methods to obtain information needed to determine a client's status in the various areas of language. Let's look at the most common methods used and see what information is provided by each. We will describe these methods in generic terms; however, as we do so, we will identify some of the common standardized tests that employ given methods (Leonard et al., 1978). Figure 5–3 illustrates all of the tasks for assessing receptive and expressive language abilities described here.

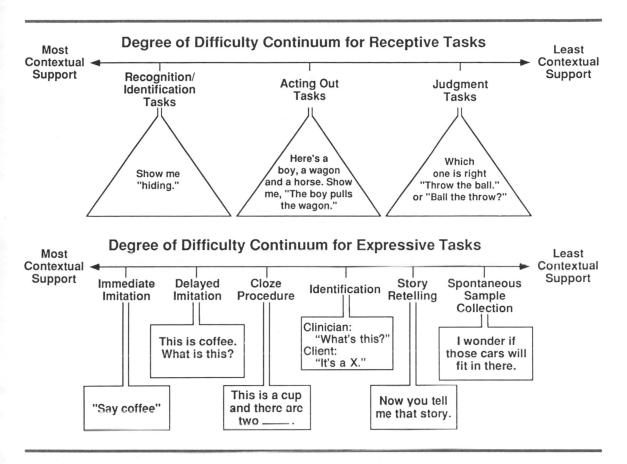

Figure 5-3. Tasks typically used to assess receptive and expressive language abilities depicted on a continuum representing most to least contextual support.

Receptive Language Testing

Three basic tasks can be used to evaluate receptive language. These are: *recognition/identification, acting out*, and *judgment tasks*. Because the tasks are designed to reflect receptive language testing, no client language production is required.

In *recognition/identification tasks*, the client is asked to listen to a language stimulus that may be a single word, a phrase, or a sentence. After hearing the language stimulus, the client is prompted to identify the object or event described in the word, phrase, or sentence from an array of nonverbal stimuli. These stimuli may be 3-dimensional objects such as toys, but more often they are sets of pictures. Figure 5-4 shows an array of items used to test the client's understanding of "the girl pushes the boy." Notice that the other pictures serve as foils for alternate meanings that could come from the sentence. When using pictured material, it is very important to consider how well the meaning is depicted in the picture; otherwise, you may find that you are measuring the client's ability to interpret the picture, rather than interpret the language stimulus.

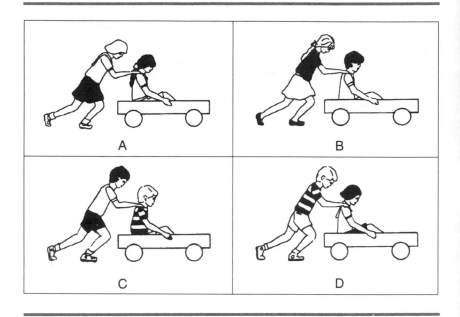

Figure 5-4. Picture material used to test comprehension of the sentence, "The boy pushes the girl."

Acting out tasks present clients with another venue for conveying information about language comprehension. Manipulable objects are made available to the client, who is then asked to perform some task like, "Show me the boy who pushes the wagon." Clients are then expected to maneuver the items to "act out" (or demonstrate) the sentence or word combination (e.g., "hug baby") presented. It should be noted that acting out tasks have been criticized because they may underestimate language comprehension because of the cognitive components that may be required to perform the task (Tyler, 1992). That is, abilities in addition to language comprehension are required for these tasks to be completed accurately. This potential problem has been tied to the testing of adults with aphasia (Tyler, 1992) and children with language disorders (Crain, 1982). In some quarters, then, caution has been recommended when judgments of language comprehension ability have been made based largely on the results of *acting out tasks*.

In the third type of task, *judgment tasks*, the client is asked to make a judgment if statements by the examiner are acceptable (according, presumably, to the client's internalized standards for language use). For example, the clinician says, "The sheeps are grazing" and asks the client for judgment of acceptability, such as, "Is that okay or not okay?" "silly or not silly?" "right or wrong?" and so on. The specific terms used should be selected based on the cognitive and language ability already demonstrated by the child or adult. In fact, the decision to use judgment tasks at all should be made carefully, because this is a task involving a metalinguistic use of language. Metalinguistics refers to a conscious, formal, and noncommunicative use of language. Metalinguistic tasks are cognitively demanding; therefore, as a general rule of thumb, judgment tasks may be too complex for children who have not achieved a mental age of at least 5 years or for an adult who demonstrates cognitive impairments. Using a judgment task with a child who is too cognitively immature to handle the task's demands or with an adult who has cognitive impairments could result in test scores that reflect poor understanding of the task, and not necessarily a lack of language comprehension for the targeted language items.

The responses we obtain on tasks involving identification, acting out, and metalinguistic judgment are usually scored on a right/wrong basis. Usually the client's overall performance on one of these tests takes the form of a total score (raw score) reflecting the number of correct or incorrect items. Sometimes, when time is limited, we use a shortcut in administration, called a basal-ceiling procedure. For example, the PPVT-R uses a maximum of 175 items to measure receptive vocabulary in individuals from 2 to 40 years of age. Because the items on this test are scaled from early learned to later learned, we can avoid employing all the items by using the basal-ceiling method.

The basic idea of this method is that many of the items on a test such as the PPVT-R will be either very easy for the client or very hard, that is, some tasks will be either well below the client's developmental level or well above it. There also will be a set of items that represent a transition from an individual's well-known words to words than are not known. If we can identify this region for a client and give only test items slightly below the transition region on up to items that are slightly above it, we can then determine the client's level of development without having to give all items. This is accomplished by establishing a basal level for the client. This is a set of test items in which we observe very high levels of accuracy. Therefore, we will credit the client with correct performance below this basal level because we assume that, if we had administered these items, the client would have gotten them correct. Once we establish the basal, we then progress through the test administering items above it that are increasingly difficult, expecting that the client will be making an increasing number of errors. Finally, we should reach a point at which the client's performance is simply a guessing game, because the items are unknown and, therefore, too difficult. This is the point of ceiling performance. Giving more items beyond the ceiling will not be useful because all we would be doing is measuring the client's guessing performance. Therefore, we can stop and assume that the client will get no more items correct, except by luck. The client's raw score, using this basal-ceiling approach, will be the number of items the client got correct up to the ceiling level plus the number of items below basal, because we are giving the client credit for these. You will find the basal-ceiling procedure used in many tests designed for developmental assessment of language and in particular those measuring receptive language skills. You will need to look at the test manual in each case to determine specifically how the basal and ceiling levels are to be determined, as this will vary from test to test.

Expressive Language Testing

There are a number of different tasks that can be used to assess a client's expressive language. Among these are: *confrontation naming, imitation,* both direct and delayed; the *Cloze technique, retelling,* and *spontaneous language sampling.* Each task can be viewed as a method of eliciting or increasing the likelihood that the client will produce language targets of interest.

In confrontation naming, the client is presented with a picture or an object and has to name that picture or item. *The Expressive One-Word Vocabulary Test* (EOWPVT) (Gardner, 1979) and the *Boston Naming Test* (Kaplan et al., 1983) are examples of tests that utilize this task. Most tests designed to assess the speech sound system also employ picture naming. Sets of pictured stimuli or 3-dimensional objects are presented and the clinician asks the client, "What's this?" or "Tell me what that is." Error responses from the client may come in the form of "not knowing" and therefore not giving the word, or they may be in the form of some type of response that is not correct. Clients with developmental language disorders will usually either give "I don't know" responses or an incorrect word. Clients with acquired language problems will also give these types of error responses, but they also may provide responses that are not real words. This latter type of error is *neologistic paraphasia.* Responses to confrontation naming can also be measured by the speed of the client's response, reflecting the client's facility with word retrieval.

Expressive language skills are usually impaired in individuals with language impairment.

Performance on these tasks may be used to establish the level of vocabulary development attained by the client. This is what is provided by the EOWPVT. Alternatively, you may use this type of task to determine if the client has difficulties retrieving and using words that the individual knows; that is, you are interested in determining if there is a *word-finding problem.* In instances in which we are using confrontation naming to evaluate for word-finding problems, we must have some way of demonstrating that the client knows the word for the pictures being presented. Therefore, when the client can't name a picture, we can assume that it is caused by a failure in retrieving the word rather than the word not being in the client's vocabulary. There are two common ways of determining whether the client knows a word. The first approach is to demonstrate that the client can recognize a word in a receptive vocabulary task. The other approach is to show that a client can use a word in other naming activities. Evidence for word-finding problems is usually based on frequent problems using words that are known, as well as slow response rates during confrontation naming.

Imitation tasks provide a quick way to elicit information from a client. The client is told to repeat what the clinician says; younger children are sometimes told that they are playing a "copycat" game with the clinician. When the expectation is for the client to repeat back the clinician's production without any delay or intervening language, this is a *direct imitation* task. When some delay factor is imposed, such as a brief time interval or additional language, the task becomes a *delayed imitation* task. Of the two imitation types, we assume that the *delayed imitation* task presents a greater challenge than the *direct imitation* task because it requires the client to hold information in stored memory longer before answering. The CELI is an example of a language test that employs a *direct imitation* task. The client is asked to repeat a set of 51 utterances one at a time after the items are spoken by a clinician, starting with very brief, simple sentence structures and ending with much longer, more complex sentence structures. Most comprehensive tests of aphasia include imitation (repetition of speech) subtests. Some speech-language pathologists assert that performance on imitation of words and high and low frequency sentences assists in classification of aphasic patients into various subtypes of aphasia or syndromes such as Broca's aphasia versus transcortical motor aphasia.

Some have criticized imitation tasks because they have concluded that the tasks may underestimate a client's language performance in more natural language usage tasks. This seems counterintuitive because imitation seems to be a simple task. However, imitation has some of the qualities of a metalinguistic task, as imitation is not a communicative use of language and, as we noted earlier, metalinguistic tasks tend to be demanding. Therefore, clients may fail to imitate sentences with certain grammatical structures correctly, but yet show clear evidence of being able to use the same grammatical form in spontaneous speech. Imitation tasks have also been occasionally criticized as more indicative of short-term memory than language ability. However, there are data to the contrary. There is considerable evidence among children and adults that performance on sentence imitation tasks correlates well with their level of grammatical use in spontaneous speech. Thus, clients who are more advanced grammatically or who have better language production skill following a brain injury tend to imitate sentences better than clients who have poorer grammatical skills. This means that we can use sentence imitation tasks to provide us with an index of a child's growth status or as an estimate of an adult's expressive language capability, but we need to be cautious about looking at specific grammatical errors made during imitation and assuming that they indicate that the client cannot use the form in spontaneous speech.

Sometimes imitation tasks are employed because they can elicit a language sample very quickly. When pressed for time, this can be a helpful strategy for clinicians to use as long as they remember that there is a potential "down" side to the collection of imitation data. Another strategy is to use imitation tasks in combination with another method of collecting expressive language information to cross-check the validity of the information between methods.

The *Cloze technique* is really a "fill-in" type of task and is commonly used for eliciting expressive language. The examiner presents a sentence or sentences in which one or more elements are missing. Usually the missing element(s) will be at the end of a sentence or a phrase. The grammatic closure subtest from the TOLD-2:P is a Cloze technique. For example, a client could be shown a photograph of a child climbing a tree and be told, "Yesterday the boy climbed the tree. Today he . . . ." and the client is expected to complete the sentence by saying, "climbs the tree." The portion of the sentence presented should provide the client with sufficient cues to produce the grammatical form or structure of interest that has been left out of the sentence. This technique is frequently used when testing adults with suspected language problems and is thought to be a good indicator of stimulability. When testing adults, the Cloze technique uses stimuli that vary along the convergent/divergent continuum. Stimuli that produce one or only a few possible responses (e.g., Grass is _____) are convergent, and stimuli that have numerous appropriate responses (e.g., I like _____) are considered divergent.

In *retelling tasks*, a story or some text is presented to the client either auditorily, visually (e.g., by pictures, video tape, written text, or film), or by a

Imitation tasks may be particularly helpful with clients who have poor intelligibility because you will know what the client is attempting to say.

combination of the two. The client is told to listen or watch carefully or read the presented material, and then to tell the "story" back to the examiner. Of course, the client has received some sort of model representation in a retelling task, but usually it is so lengthy that it would be largely impossible for the client to be using only imitation skills to complete the task. Sometimes, too, the client is permitted to have accompanying visual stimuli while retelling the story. This reduces the memory loading of the task and makes it more likely that the examiner is eliciting only information that reflects the client's expressive language abilities. The sounds-in-sentences subtest of the *Goldman-Fristoe Test of Articulation* (Goldman & Fristoe, 1986) is an example of a retelling task. Delayed recall has been used to distinguish dementing illness from other neurogenic language problems, such as aphasia (Bayles & Tomoeda, 1990). Used for that purpose, problems with specific memory may be determined by comparing immediate with delayed recall.

LANGUAGE SAMPLE COLLECTION

Language sampling is another expressive language task that can be employed to evaluate language production abilities. Because of its widespread use, this section is devoted to the collection and analysis of language sample data. Although language sampling is frequently used to obtain data for the evaluation of children's language abilities, it typically has not been part of adult language assessment. This may be because of time constraints that face clinicians in hospital settings or because of the lack of reliability data for such procedures with the adult population. Whatever the reason, neither elicitation nor analysis procedures for language samples has been well tested with adults.

Language Sampling Techniques

A spontaneous language sample is a set of client-produced utterances usually without examiner prompting, which are collected and analyzed by clinicians to help determine language production abilities. Our clinical goal is to collect a sample that is "representative" of the client's entire language repertoire. We recognize that we cannot gather every possible utterance a client can produce. Instead, we hope to collect a sample of at least 50 and preferably 100 or 200 utterances to represent the range of possible forms and structures we would find if it *were* possible to collect every single possible utterance.

Some clinicians attempt to collect samples that are chiefly monologues, with others preferring to collect samples from naturalistic conversations. Regardless of which form is selected, language samples should not contain imitated or rote-learned passages for much the same reason that imitation tasks, in general, are limited in usefulness (Miller, 1981). The examiner should also avoid eliciting too much of the sample through question-asking because responses to questions tend to contain diminished length and complexity. An open-ended request like, "Tell me about your favorite TV program" is better than a question like, "What is your favorite TV program?" Language samples largely comprised by answers to specific questions, memorized passages, and imitation may either under- or overestimate the client's true language capabilities and, therefore, should be avoided.

Typically, the examiner constructs situations in which the client can choose the topic and range of the conversation. For young children, provocative toys (e.g., a truck with a missing wheel, a doll with a missing limb) and unfamiliar objects (i.e., items that the child may not have previously seen or have a name for) are made available for play because such items often elicit interaction from the client (e.g., "What's that?" "How did that get broken?"). Toys that support "scenario," or role play, are also useful for this purpose (e.g., dollhouse, camper). Older children may prefer pictures and an interview format, with adults generally needing little prompting beyond some general, open-ended requests/questions like, "Tell me what you like to do in your spare time" to elicit a lengthy sample for analysis. Most clinicians are aware that individuals with language disorders tend to be reticent. Therefore, collecting language samples from these clients may require more time, patience, and planning than with clients whose language systems are intact.

Action figures, such as Ninja Turtles, are useful for eliciting language samples from young children.

We may also choose to use different types of discourse in collecting the sample. In addition to the quasi-monologues that speech-language pathologists often collect, *narratives, expository text,* and *conversation* are three examples of discourse types that can be utilized in language sample collection. For example, a clinician may want to collect a sample that reflects a client's understanding of story structures and will collect a narrative sample. To this end, a clinician can provide the client with the title of a story, a topic, or the first line of a story. In a series of story creation tasks, Stein and Glenn (1979) presented school-age children with the first line of three different stories, such as, "Once there was a boy named Alan who had many different toys." The children were told to make their stories as long or as short as they liked, but that the stories should contain all the things a good story should have. Another option is to give the client very little direction and tell the person to make up a story on any topic. Often, clinicians help put younger clients on the right track by telling them to start their stories with the phrase, "Once upon a time . . . ." This serves as a cue so that, even if the direction "tell me a story" does not make sense, "once upon a time" is often a sufficient reminder of what a story means and how to begin it.

Expository discourse provides an explanation to the listener and sometimes a clinician may ask a client to produce some expository discourse as part of sample collection. We may ask a child to explain to us how airplanes fly or how to make the best peanut butter and jelly sandwich. Explanation topics should be chosen carefully to match the client's age (chronological and/or developmental) and cultural background. For example, one of our recent graduates who was from Japan wanted to collect expository text samples from a group of school children there. She came up with a topic that gave her subjects very little trouble when she asked them to tell her how to prepare for an earthquake. With the frequent incidence of earthquakes in Japan, there is a high degree of public awareness of earthquakes, their disaster potential, and public preparedness. Thus, this is a procedure that each Japanese school child must know something about. On the other hand, for many adults in the United States, topics such as explaining how to grocery shop efficiently and how to parallel park may be useful, if expository discourse tasks are seen as needed.

There are considerable problems in trying to write down the sample during the interview. Not only is it difficult to write down the utterances and context notes quickly enough (except in a situation where a clinician works with clients who have minimal language output), but there is a tendency to write down sentences that are more complete than those the client actually produces or for the clinician to otherwise recall utterances incorrectly. Therefore, in most examining situations, interviews are audio or video taped for later analysis. Videotaping is a better format for recording a sample because it preserves the sample's contextual information along with the language content. That is, it is important to know what precedes a client's utterance, both linguistically and nonlinguistically, to determine the appropriateness of a client's utterances.

Elicitor Effects

It is reasonable to assume that some features of a conversation depend on the relationships between the people. When the focus is on the conversation of a client, we give some attention to the other person(s) in the conversation, whom we call the co-conversationalist(s). As already mentioned, clinicians need to guard against providing too much input and thereby biasing a client's sample unnecessarily. Samples collected with parents or other family members, such as spouses or siblings, may also be biased because a particular co-conversationalist may typically dominate conversations with the client or, conversely, may always be a passive co-conversationalist. If only one co-conversationalist is used for data collection, the picture of a client's expressive abilities that emerges may reflect only one type of conversation interaction for that client. One solution to this problem is to collect several smaller language samples in different settings with a variety of co-conversationalists. Some partners may be familiar to the client and some may be unfamiliar. Some may be older or younger than the client, with the co-conversationalist's language competence sometimes matching and sometimes being dissimilar to the client's. This way the clinician can determine if the client can demonstrate a number of different styles of language use, or if the client has one pervasive language use style that is relatively unaffected by the different demands placed by co-conversationalists who are more assertive in conversation than others or who may need more information and less sophisticated language. Fey's (1986) system of classifying language use in conversational contexts emphasizes the importance of determining how a client actually uses the language the individual is capable of using.

Language Sample Analyses

Analyses of a language sample can delineate information about semantics, morphology, phonology, pragmatics, or syntax. Historically, syntax and morphological measures have been the most widely used types of analysis, with *Mean Length of Utterance* (MLU) probably being the most commonly used measure of sentence length, and *Developmental Sentence Scoring* (DSS) (Lee, 1974), being a popular measure of sentence complexity (see Figure 5-5).

Each of these measures provides a quantitative index of the child's level of grammatical development. These quantitative measures, along with norms, can be used to evaluate the child's development status. There are several excellent resources for discussion of clinical language sample collection and analysis, among them Barrie-Blackley et al. (1978), Miller (1981), Miller and Chapman (1981), and Stickler (1987). You are encouraged to consult these references for a detailed explanation of a number of different analysis procedures, as well as information about the theoretical underpinnings of sample collection.

Clinicians select from among the available language sampling procedures for a number of different reasons. For example, a clinician may know a priori that a given client's ability to use language efficiently and successfully in conversation often is compromised. Rather than use a language sample analysis procedure that codes only syntactic structures, the clinician may choose to use a procedure that accounts for the functioning of the client's utterances in terms of topic maintenance or topic initiation (pragmatics), for example. Analysis of topic maintenance or topic imitation would not require a sample of complete sentences, but would require that the language sample be collected in a conversational context. Other sampling procedures might be selected because of the extent or type of normative data provided by the author(s) of the procedure. For example, if an analysis provided normative data for 8-year-olds, this sampling instrument might be a more attractive "fit" for a particular clinical situation.

A number of language sampling procedures are available in computerized form, such as *Systematic Analysis of Language Transcripts* (SALT) (Miller & Chapman, 1985), *Computerized Profiling* (Long & Fey, 1988), among others. By coding and inputting the samples in prescribed ways,

Measure	Description
MLU (Brown, 1973)	A measure of the average number of morphemes per utterance where an utterance consists of a simple sentence. MLU is a general index of grammatic development in the range between 1.01 and 4.49.
DSS (Lee, 1974)	A measure of grammatical development which scores a sentence based upon the presence of certain grammatical forms. Forms that are later developing receive higher values than early developing forms. Thus, the DSS score increases as more advanced grammatical forms are used.

Figure 5-5. Descriptions of Mean Length of Utterance (MLU), a commonly used measure of sentence length, and Developmental Sentence Scoring (DSS), a common measure of sentence complexity.

these computer programs tally different dimensions of language production. Depending on the program used, some calculate standard measures like MLU and DSS, and provide clinicians with a less laborious task than required by traditional hand analysis of language samples. Often, context notes can be placed directly into the sample so that no information helpful in the interpretation of the sample is separated from the analysis.

You should recognize that, even if computerized programs are employed for language sample analysis, it is you and not the computer that is responsible for understanding the underlying analyses being applied to the samples. Without an understanding of how the language sample analyses are applied and calculated, it is unlikely that you will be able to determine which type of analysis to apply, how to interpret changes in the analysis from calculation to calculation, and how to figure out if the results obtained from the computer may be indicative of a program or coding error.

INTERPRETATION OF INFORMATION

For quite a while now we have been talking about the ways in which we go about gathering information about the client's language performance. Remember, however, that all this information gathering is done for a purpose, which is to determine in what areas the client is having problems with language and the particular character of these problems. To draw some conclusions about these issues, we must begin to interpret the information we have gathered. Much of what we are discussing here builds on the information in Chapter 1 dealing with the interpretation of clinical measures. As you may recall, three common interpretive approaches are often used: *norm-referenced*, *criterion-referenced*, and *client-referenced*. Each of these approaches may be used by you in determining whether or not your particular client has a language disorder.

Norm-referenced Interpretation

The norm-referenced approach is often used when it appears that we are dealing with a developmental language disorder. Recall that a norm-referenced interpretation compares your client to some group of individuals referred to as the normative group. Further, norm-referenced interpretation leads to a quantitative statement about how the person stands within the normative group through the use of standard scores or percentiles. (See Chapter 1.) As developmental language disorders seem to involve impairments in the rate of development, we often base our decision about a child's language status on where the child is in the growth process and where we would expect the child to be. Thus, language impairment is determined by a discrepancy between the client's expected language status and the levels of achievement we have obtained from our observations of the client.

Two different approaches can be used as a basis for our expectations for clients, and these approaches are employed to compare the client to different normative groups. The first approach seems rather obvious: We use the client's *chronological age* as the basis of our expectations, and therefore, we compare our client to other individuals of a similar chronological age. One rationale for this approach is that our society bases its expectations on the age of the person. For instance, children are expected to enter elementary school at around 6 years, and they are expected to be able to perform much like an adult by age 15 or so. A child who presents language skills substantially below his age peers is likely to have difficulties meeting societal expectations.

In contrast to the use of chronological age, some have argued for the use of a child's level of *nonverbal development* or the adult's level of *nonverbal ability* as foundations for determining our expectations. In the case of the child, the level of language development, based on standardized measures, is compared with nonverbal intelligence, and the child is considered to have a developmental language disorder if the verbal development is substantially poorer than nonlanguage development. Adults with brain lesions may have differences between verbal and nonverbal skills, in either direction, with verbal skills being lower or higher than nonverbal skills. Information on verbal/nonverbal differences is used to understand the basis of a communication problem and to develop appropriate treatment goals. In some instances when working with adults, nonverbal skills are used to suggest potential for improvement, but in a guarded manner. The rationale for this approach has rested on the belief that language development is dependent on cognitive development and that language and cognition are inextricably linked in adults. Recently, with respect to children, this diagnostic standard has received criticism from several sources (Cole et al., 1990; Lahey, 1990). Regardless of which standard you use for basing your language development expectations, if you decide to use a norm-referenced approach in determining language impairment, then you will need to select measurement methods that provide the appropriate norms for your client.

Criterion-referenced Interpretation

Criterion-referenced standards for measurement interpretation compare the client's performance to a performance standard based on what is considered by some authority to be minimally adequate. Soon your clinical work will be evaluated and your supervisor will decide whether you are doing "acceptable" work. It is very likely that this judgment will be based on her beliefs about what kind of clinical work is necessary for appropriate service to the client. In so doing, this supervisor is using a criterion-referenced grading system. Criterion-referenced decisions for the determination of language impairment may be used for either developmental or acquired language disorders. Based on discussions with primary grade teachers, a speech-language pathologist may decide that first grade children must be able to express themselves in simple but grammatically acceptable sentences, to follow a set of basic commands, and to retell a simple short story. Failure by the child to do any of these things could result in a determination of a language disorder. Likewise, we know that adults should be able to carry out routine conversational activities. An adult who demonstrates several failures in the maintenance of the conversation, either because of an inability to formulate ideas or to comprehend things said, may be judged to have a language disorder on the basis of these criterion-referenced standards.

Client-referenced Interpretation

Client-referenced standards use the client's own performance as the basis for making a decision about a language disorder. This type of a standard frequently is used as the basis for evaluating acquired disorders. Although we rarely have formal language measures on clients prior to acquisition of a language disorder, we can obtain a reasonable sense of how a person was doing before a stroke or head injury. Some of this information can be obtained directly from an informant such as a spouse, but we can also make some inferences about the person's pre-injury language status based on the client's occupation and education. Using such information we can compare our observations of the client's current performance with levels of performance we believe to have existed before the brain injury. A substantial decline in language performance may be viewed as evidence of an acquired language disorder.

Arriving at a Conclusion: Is There a Language Disorder?

Using one or a combination of the interpretative methods just described, you should be able to arrive at a conclusion as to whether or not the client has a language disorder. In making this decision you will no doubt use your observations of the person's performance on both structured and informal language tasks. Further, you will draw on your knowledge of the client's background in interpreting the kinds of communication needs the person faces and the language abilities you have observed. Based on this information and the ways in which you can interpret it, you will ultimately need to arrive at answering the question: "Is this person likely to have difficulties in his or her life because of the language skills he now possesses or is likely to have in the future?" If the answer to the question is "yes," you have concluded there *is* a language disorder.

Determining Areas of Strengths and Weaknesses

The observations we make about the client's language status should allow us to go beyond a simple statement that the person has a language disorder. At the same time we evaluate the information obtained from our language evaluation to determine the presence of an overall problem, we look for patterns of strengths and weaknesses. This investigation provides an obvious opportunity for us to use a client-referenced approach to interpretation because we are comparing one area of language performance to another for the same person. As we noted earlier, some language assessment instruments comprise a set of subtests that cover several different areas of language performance. These test batteries are usually designed so that the client's scores can be arranged to form a profile of strengths and weaknesses. In other instances, the profile of performance will be derived from information obtained from different tests.

The use of profiles to display a client's strengths and weaknesses requires that the measures obtained be converted into a common format. For instance, if you have obtained an MLU score for a child and also have a receptive vocabulary measure based on the youngster's PPVT-R raw score, you will not be able to compare these two numerical results because you have been counting very different things. The typical solution to this problem has been to use norm-referencing. To do this, the client's raw scores for the two measures mentioned would be converted to standard scores, such as percentiles based on the client's chronological age. In this way, the scores can be compared, as each will now represent where the client stands in the normative population for MLU and receptive vocabulary. This should be a very familiar process to you, as you no doubt took college entrance exams as a high school student. These tests contain subtests. When you received your results, you were given a simple profile for your scores in each area. If you took the SAT (Scholastic Aptitude Test), results may have been reflected that you did better in the Quantitative subtest than the Verbal. The scores you were looking at in each case were standard scores, with a mean of 500 and standard deviation of 100. In a very similar manner, we can profile the relative strengths and weaknesses in the language status of our clients.

DETERMINATION OF CONCOMITANT FACTORS

Language problems do not exist in a vacuum. Instead, we must assume that a variety of factors can influence and, in some cases, cause a problem. These we refer to collectively as *concomitant factors*. These factors might be biological, psychological, and/or environmental. In considering these factors, we want to know not only what things might be working against the client's language status, but also what might be working for the client's language performance. To consider this, you need to develop a scheme that allows you to think about the factors that might influence the client's language status. Many of these concomitant factors will be shared between developmental and acquired language disorders; however, their impact on language performance or the relevance to performance may vary. Therefore, these two forms of language disorders are covered separately.

Examining for concomitant factors requires that you have a theory about what can influence language performance.

Concomitant Factors in Developmental Language Disorders

By now you have no doubt had some course work on language development, and it should come as no surprise to you that there is a lot we do not know about the factors that influence language development. This forces us to work with partial knowledge, but the clinical world often requires that we do the best we can with what we do know.

The hearing status of the child with a language impairment must always be determined.

One concomitant factor that must be considered when thinking about developmental language disorders is *hearing*. We know that a child needs to hear language to learn it. Thus, any time we find a child having problems with language development we want to know if there is a hearing loss. This is one of those concomitant factors that can directly cause a language problem. Further, by treating hearing loss either medically or with a hearing aid and thus improving the child's hearing, the child's language learning should improve. Notice that it is just as important clinically for us to know that a child has normal hearing as it is for us to know that the child has a hearing loss. It is the child's hearing status, not just the presence of a hearing loss that is important to us. Many of our language measures assume that the child has heard what we said. Unless we know the child's hearing status, we will not be able to be sure our test results are valid.

Another concomitant factor we want to know about is the child's *home environment*. We know that children need to be exposed to language to acquire it. At this time, we do not know which circumstances are absolutely necessary for adequate language learning. We can say, however, that in the white, middle-class culture, better rates of language development are found in homes in which the parents talk with their children about things the child is doing and saying. There are probably only a very few children who present with language disorders because they have been denied even minimal levels of language exposure; however, there are probably many children whose unfavorable home environment is compounding their language learning problem. Unfortunately, we have few ways, short of visiting the home, to learn about the rearing environment. It is possible, though, to talk with parents about the ways they talk with their child; and in some clinical settings you can observe the parent interact with the client. There are no clear guidelines as to when you would want to conclude that the environment is contributing to the problem or is likely to exacerbate the course of therapy. At this point, however, you should recognize the need to think about the child's language exposure and its potential impact for good or ill on the child's language development.

Earlier we noted the interrelationship between language and *cognition*. It is at this point in the diagnostic process that you may bring this notion into play. The relationship between language and cognition is sufficiently complex that we are unlikely to be able to make absolute, strong claims about a child's cognitive skills as restricting language development. Many clinicians have made the reasonable assumption that children with developmental language disorders who have normal or above normal nonverbal intellect will fare better in language acquisition than those who have subnormal nonverbal skills. If this is true, even though you might not attribute the language impairment to the cognitive status of the child, you may employ this information in making predictions about the child's expected progress. Recently, there has been some evidence that the beneficial influence of higher cognitive ability on language development is not necessarily true (Cole et al., 1990). More research is required before we know how or under what circumstances the child's nonverbal cognitive abilities limit or promote language development. Thus, just as with language exposure, you will need to keep this factor in mind and, as new information becomes available, you can determine how you will use it in your clinical decision making.

There is one concomitant factor with which many parents of children with developmental language disorders will be concerned. This is the neurological status of the child. Many of the children you will see who have language problems will have normal hearing, seem to have been provided with sufficient exposure to the language of their community, and have adequate nonverbal cognitive skills. Through a process of elimination one could argue that these children have something about their brain that must be causing them to have language problems. Others have argued that this conclusion, based solely on negative evidence, is not sufficient to claim that we know that the child has a neurological problem. There is beginning to be research evidence suggesting that at least some children with developmental language problems may have some subtle differences in their brain structure. This evidence comes from imaging studies of the central nervous system (CNS) which require very expensive equipment and unusual expertise. Therefore, this type of examination is currently not conducted as a part of routine clinical examinations of clients with developmental language disorders. Furthermore, we don't know whether these differences in brain structure are actually causing the child's language learning difficulties. As a result, in the typical clinical setting, we usually do not know whether the child has any unusual brain characteristics. We said earlier that parents will ask about this issue. When this topic comes up, what do you say? Currently, the best answer is that we do not know if there are subtle brain differences contributing to these language problems, and there is, at this time, no good way of answering the question.

For some children, there may be evidence of brain damage that can be obtained without the use of sophisticated imaging examination methods. For example, if the client demonstrates certain neurological signs, such as very poor motor skills or evidence of seizures, you should refer the client to a neurologist. You should also refer a client if you have evidence that he is regressing in language status. Recall that developmental language problems reflect limitations in the rate of language growth, but we do not expect affected individuals to lose skills that they have developed. If this happens, there may be an active disease process, and the client should be seen by a neurologist.

The concomitant factors just covered are the principal influences on developmental language disorders. There are others that you may also want to keep in mind, such as the client's attitudes and concerns about the problem, the presence of behavioral or emotional problems, or the presence of other health factors. These things and many more may have an impact on the client's general status and may influence the decisions you make.

Concomitant Factors in Acquired Language Disorders

As indicated earlier, the concomitant factors in acquired language disorders (which you will most often see in adults) are similar to those already mentioned for children with developmental disorders, but there are a few important differences. Among the similarities are hearing, home environment, and cognition. As with children, hearing status is important. This is particularly true for older adults, who frequently suffer sensorineural hearing loss in growing older. As with children, it is important to know if the client has a hearing loss or normal hearing for best interpretation of the results of our language testing.

Also, similar to children, is the need to know something about the home environment. Thus, when assessing adults we should gain enough information about the home environment to determine the presence of factors that may facilitate or impede communication. As well, with adults we need to gain information about the work environment to determine the employment needs and factors that may exacerbate the client's problems.

As is also the case with children, the interrelationship between language and cognition must be considered in the evaluation of adult language skills. In some instances, one may need to consider whether the basis of the language problem is in the cognitive domain. For instance, a number of the communication problems seen in individuals with traumatic brain injuries may stem from cognitive problems such as memory loss or poor attentional abilities. Moreover, many persons with right hemisphere involvement demonstrate language problems when asked to address sophisticated, abstract language tasks, such as an inability to make logical inferences that may go beyond verbal stimuli. Thus, knowledge of nonverbal skills is an important aspect of understanding acquired language disorders.

In the case of acquired language disorders, sensory modalities other than hearing may be disturbed as a function of aging or brain injury. For instance, assessment of visual status is as important as assessment of hearing. Because we frequently test reading and writing ability in adults with acquired language problems, knowledge of visual status is critical. Changes in vision can affect the interpretation of any stimulus (e.g., object or picture) placed before the client and thus change performance. Visual changes to be alert for in adults with acquired problems include sensory changes as a result of the aging process as well as visual function change as a result of neurologic insult. Common types of problems related to neurological lesions include visual field deficits (i.e., patients may be blind in a portion of their vision) and color, depth, or form perception problems. Tactile and proprioceptive sensory changes may also follow brain damage and need to be considered in interpretation of performance on language tests.

Another important concomitant factor when evaluating adults is the motor ability of the client. Many persons with brain injuries suffer paralysis of all or part of their body. Thus, movement of body parts may be impaired, making results of clinician prompts for the client to point difficult to interpret. The clinician will need to find ways to assess language that do not rely on a fine motor response. In other words, the reliability of the client's motor response must be carefully considered in evaluation of adults with acquired language problems. In addition, most adults with aphasia have concomitant motor speech problems. For instance, individuals with lesions of the left frontal lobes and aphasia frequently have apraxia of speech as well. This makes delineation of the language and speech components of the overall communication problem difficult.

A particular problem with adults with acquired language problems is the emotional status of the client. Many neurologic problems result in changes in emotion and personality. Thus, the person may not be motivated to cooperate during an evaluation or may be inappropriately angry or euphoric (catastrophic response). In addition, because the individual has suffered a potentially life-threatening event and is coping with a host of other physical problems, he or she may be less motivated to engage in communication testing. For instance, the person with concomitant paralysis is often more concerned with lack of arm control than with a difficulty in talking.

Finally, as is the case with children, the presence of other behavioral, health, or financial factors may have an impact on the client's current and future communication ability as well as his ability and willingness to seek appropriate special services. All concomitant factors should be considered by the clinician.

PREDICTION OF THE COURSE OF THE LANGUAGE PROBLEM

In discussion of identification of concomitant problems, we began to talk not only about the client's current language status, but also the client's future status. In fact, one of the principal uses of the information gathered about concomitant factors is for use in predicting the future course of the problem. You will discover that clients and family members are very interested in your answers to questions about the future. In most instances, the client's current status is well known and, therefore, your determination that the client has a language problem is not surprising. What is desired, however, is to know how the client will be doing in the future. Many clients with developmental or acquired language disorders will improve in their abilities over time, whether treated or not. However, even if they improve, they may never achieve normal status. The question, then, is often how much improvement can be expected and whether the outlook can be improved by therapy? The approach to this question will depend, in part, on whether the disorder is developmental or acquired.

One of the important clinical services you can provide is to help the client and family build reasonable expectations of the future.

Predicting the Course of Developmental Language Disorders

As usual, the best guide to the future is the past. Thus, a child who presents evidence of very poor language development at age 4 is likely to continue to show very poor language development in the future; whereas the child with marginally normal levels of language development is likely to continue at that level. These predictions can be made assuming that none of the concomitant factors influencing language change. However, if we believe some of the concomitant factors have had a negative impact on the child's language development, and we believe the negative influence can be removed, such as by the use of hearing aids, then our prognosis can be more positive.

There is one group of children who especially present prognostic challenge. These are toddlers and preschool children who show signs of slow language growth, but because even normally developing children show uneven rates of language growth, we have difficulty determining whether a more persistent language problem will continue or whether they are going to "catch up" with their normal peers. The problem for us in such a case is determining whether a young child with poor language skills will continue to have such a problem. Fortunately, this problem has received the attention of researchers and we now have some ways of improving our guesses. One of the most consistent positive signs for potential language development is the child's language comprehension abilities. Children whose language delays are limited to expressive language only are likely to do better with long-term language growth than those who have problems in both receptive and expressive language usage. This is a good example of how the information you obtain in the assessment of language and, in particular, the client-referenced interpretation of strengths and weaknesses can be used to aid in an important clinical decision.

So far, we have covered prediction of the course of the language problem without intervention. We also must predict whether the client will improve with therapy. Our professional ethics dictate that we will provide therapy only when we believe that the client will benefit from it.

In the case of a young child, cooperativeness during the evaluation can be a predictor of how easily the client adapts to the treatment setting. With young children, the transition into treatment may require more time and patience, with structured and less play-like activities introduced gradually. So, if a child demonstrates some eagerness to participate in activities planned by the clinician during the evaluation and a willingness to try tasks obviously difficult or impossible for the youngster to complete correctly, the clinician has obtained some valuable information: the client is a risk-taker, at least where new skills are concerned, and the forward progress of therapy may not be impeded by fear of failure. Therefore, it is a good idea for a clinician to plan some activities during an evaluation that are clearly beyond a given client's easy capability. This provides an opportunity for the clinician to observe the client's perseverance and willingness to be wrong on the road to learning how to be right.

The Prognosis of Acquired Language Disorder

Patients who have an acquired language disorder from neurological damage will usually demonstrate considerable variability in language status and other behavioral characteristics during the course of recovery. This is particularly true for those who have suffered from a stroke or traumatic event. For most of these patients there is a period immediately after the insult during which there are many neurophysiologic responses to the trauma. In particular, there will be swelling of the brain tissue, referred to as edema. During this early phase of recovery, you will often observe much poorer language function than you will later on. As the edema and other physiological responses to the trauma resolve, we can expect some return of language function. The challenge for clinicians is to determine how much recovery can be expected.

When working with adults with acquired language problems, judgments about prognosis should be made with extreme caution, particularly in the early stages following neurologic insult. Although some clinicians suggest that age, gender, education level, and premorbid intelligence (to name a few) are predictors of outcome, recent data do not support these claims. Likewise, more research is needed on type, size, and site of lesion information in dealing with prediction of outcome, particularly for adults. Only one standardized test, the PICA (Porch, 1968), purports to have prognostic value. However, numerous concomitant problems including physical problems, rate of physiological recovery, emotional problems, cognitive impairments, and client motivation impede our ability to accurately and reliably predict eventual language outcome. Prognosis, then, is a continually changing activity, and we constantly need to assess and update our information by contact with colleagues and research sources.

In the later stages following brain trauma (at least 1 year after insult), when the client's abilities in all areas have begun to stabilize, prognosis can become more accurate. The lack of outcome forecasting ability is often frustrating for clients and family members. These individuals require our most supportive efforts during the client's recovery course.

An evaluation also needs to include information-gathering on the degree to which the client can self-monitor language performance. That is, if it becomes obvious to the clinician during evaluation that the client can identify the desired language target and can accurately evaluate the acceptability or unacceptability of attempts to produce the target, then the clinician knows that the rehabilitation process, in the case of an acquired language problem (or the habilitation process, in the case of a developmental problem), has begun. Often, such monitoring skill is demonstrated by the client's ability to self-correct. Learning to monitor or make accurate judgments about one's own language is an essential component in the therapeutic process. In a sense, the clinician's goal is to make therapy and the clinician's participation obsolete by teaching the client how to become his or her own clinician. If the clinician's input for judging client productions is not needed or only needed intermittently, then the clinician has evidence of a positive prognosis.

Conveying Diagnostic Information to the Client and Others

Clients should receive at least some information from the clinician at the end of each evaluation session. It is true that additional testing sometimes must be scheduled and that, after an initial meeting with a client, it is not always possible to speak very much about the client's problem. However, clients should be told where things stand and any impressions the clinician may have formulated at the time. If there is a plan to obtain more information, the client must be informed about the plan status. Depending on the age and cognitive and/or language status of the client, it is sometimes appropriate for the clinician to convey outcomes of the evaluation to a person other than the client or other than to the client, alone.

Options for Treatment

Depending on the amount and type of information a clinician is able to glean from the language evaluation, plans can be made following the evaluation to set up a treatment schedule. Of course, a number of different variables influence recommendations for that schedule. Clinician availability, as well as the availability and willingness of the client to participate, are two initial factors that need to be addressed. When caseloads are crowded, clinicians may need to place a client on a waiting list until space is available for providing clinical services. If the client presents with a severe or profound disorder, existing cases may need to be reprioritized. Sometimes, clients who have been on the caseload for a while and who have not made significant progress can be given a hiatus in their treatment schedule to make space available for new and needier clients more amenable to treatment. Such decisions are likely to be among the most difficult decisions you will have to make. The only way to decide fairly is from results of in-depth evaluation of reassessments of your caseload (Fey, 1988).

TRANSITION FROM ASSESSMENT TO TREATMENT

What Assessment Data Can Tell You About the Plan of Therapy

It is wise to view test battery planning as more than solely an avenue to get information about the presence of a language problem. In addition to providing numerical support for inclusion or exclusion from treatment, language evaluations should also be designed to answer questions about client capabilities and preferences for different therapy materials, to provide tasks for eliciting productions or facilitate learning, and to result in gathering behaviorial baselines.

To that end, different types of materials should be used during evaluations to determine potential treatment tools' and tasks' meaningfulness for a client. One example of this is using the evaluation to determine whether 3-dimensional or 2-dimensional stimuli or both could be employed as therapy materials for a particular client. For some young children, presumably those who have had limited experience with books, the use of 3-dimensional stimuli (objects) will be the most appropriate for therapy use. For these children, the use of 2-dimensional stimuli (pictures) may not be all that meaningful, especially if the pictures are line drawings. Likewise, with adults diagnosed with acquired problems, line drawings may be too abstract, and 3-dimensional stimuli may need to be used to facilitate testing. Photographs may serve as a viable middle ground between line drawings and objects, providing an acceptable method for presentation of 2-dimensional materials. That is to say that when limited experience with books and/or reading is suspected, photographs may best elicit responses in treatment. When working with adults, the prototypicality of a given stimulus item may need to be considered, because some clients may have difficulty with items that are not the best examples of a category (e.g., use a *robin* instead of a *wren* for a *bird*).

Similarly, the evaluation should be utilized as a testing ground for the different task types for potential use in therapy. As noted in the discussion of the different task types that can be used for assessing receptive and expressive language, some tasks are more demanding than others. A number of tasks require the clinician to provide more or less cuing and other support for the client to complete them. Remember that the tasks illustrated in Figure 5–3 were arranged according to which contexted support could be utilized. If the clinician can establish which tasks are feasible for use with a client from information gleaned at the time of the evaluation, this information could be employed in therapy planning. In Chapter 2, Westby more fully discusses this issue of dynamic assessment.

The collection of baseline measures during an evaluation and early diagnostic therapy can inform you about a client's existing knowledge that can be the foundation of probable therapy goals. That is, goals that will be addressed in therapy rarely reflect targets that are entirely absent from a client's pretherapy repertoire. It is more likely that the targets will have been partially learned and inconsistently used by the client. With the help of baseline measures that probe the scope of the target's current usage by the client, you can better set appropriate levels of expectation for the client's performance during the therapy course. For example, a client who demonstrates inconsistent use of plural markers (60%) during evaluation is more likely to achieve a 90% criterion level earlier (all other factors being equal) than a client who shows no evidence of any plural marker production during assessment. For the latter client, setting a criterion (goal) of 50% usage as therapy begins would be appropriate.

How Reassessment Differs From Initial Assessment

It is important to reevaluate treatment programs periodically to determine if changes are occurring, and, if they are, is improvement rapid enough or in as far-ranging a manner (with generalization) to recommend ongoing treatment. Such an evaluation is another rationale of assessment. Reassessment will probably focus on both the specific goals being addressed in therapy and in overall changes to the client's language system that treatment may have led to. As speech-language pathologists we are very much aware that the natural human cognitive tendency to generalize to new settings and new instances of the language target is the basis of the treatment we provide. That is to say that we know we cannot provide all possible needed examples in therapy. Instead, we present a representative sample of all the possible examples of therapy targets and hope that we are teaching a general rule that allows the client to expand what has been learned to all other possible examples. Reassessment allows us to figure out how close we are to dismissing the client from therapy, and it also should help us to troubleshoot the therapy procedures we are using to determine if adequate progress is being made (Fey, 1988). If adequate progress is not being made, this troubleshooting should provide clues for the aspects of therapy that need to be changed to enhance therapy efficiency. For example, reassessment may indicate a lack of generalization stemming from the selection of too few or too many examples for rule learning. Also, adults with a language disorder may not be ready for treatment after a first evaluation, but their condition can change enough to warrant intervention later. Thus, periodic reevaluation is highly recommended for adult brain-injured clients.

REFERENCES

Barrie-Blackley, S., Musselwhite, C., & Rogister, S. (1978). *Clinical oral language sampling: A handbook for students and clinicians.* A monograph of the National Student Speech and Hearing Association, Danville, IL: Interstate Publishers and Printers.

Bayles, K., & Tomoeda, K. (1990). Delayed recall deficits in aphasic stroke patients: Evidence of Alzheimer's dementia? *Journal of Speech and Hearing Disorders, 55,* 310–314.

Brown, R. (1973). *A first language.* Cambridge, MA: Harvard University Press.

Carrow, E. (1974). *Carrow Elicited Language Inventory* (CELI). Austin, TX: Learning Concepts.

Carrow-Woolfolk, E. (1985). *Test for Auditory Comprehension of Language* (TACL-R). Allen, TX: DLM Teaching Resources.

Cole, K., Dale, P., & Mills, P. (1990). Defining language delay in young children by cognitive referencing: Are we saying more than we know? *Applied Psycholinguistics, 11,* 291–302.

Crain, S. (1982). Temporal terms: Mastery by age five. *Papers and Reports on Child Language Development, 21,* 33–38.

Crystal, D. (1987). Towards a 'bucket' theory of language disability: Taking account of interaction between linguistic levels. *Clinical Linguistics and Phonetics, 1,* 7–22.

Dunn, L., & Dunn, L. (1981). *Peabody Picture Vocabulary Test-R* (PPVT-R). Circle Pines, MN: American Guidance Service.

Fey, M. (1986). *Language intervention with young children.* Needham Heights, MA: Allyn & Bacon.

Fey, M. (1988). Dismissal criteria for the language impaired child. In D. Yoder & R. Kent (Eds.), *Decision making in speech-language pathology.* Toronto: B.C. Decker.

Gardner, M. (1979). *The Expressive One Word Picture Vocabulary Test* (EOWPVT). Novato, CA: Academic Therapy Publications.

Goldman, R., & Fristoe, M. (1986). *Goldman-Fristoe Test of Articulation.* Circle Pines, MN: American Guidance Service.

Goodglass, H., & Kaplan, E. (1981). *Assessment of aphasia and related disorders* (2nd ed.). Philadelphia: Lea & Febiger.

Kaplan, E., Goodglass, H., & Weintraub, S. (1983). *The Boston Naming Test.* Philadelphia: Lea & Febiger.

Lahey, M. (1989). Who shall be called language disordered? Some reflections on one perspective. *Journal of Speech and Hearing Disorders, 55,* 612–620.

Lee, L. (1974). *Developmental sentence analysis.* Evanston, IL: Northwestern University Press.

Leonard, L., Prutting, C., Perozzi, J., & Berkeley, R. (1978). Nonstandardized approaches to the assessment of language behaviors. *Asha, 20,* 371–379.

Long, S., & Fey, M. (1988). *Computerized profiling.* Ithaca, NY: Steven Long.

McNeil, M., & Prescott, T. (1986). *The Revised Token Test.* Baltimore: University Park Press.

Miller, J. (1981). *Assessing language production in children.* Baltimore, MD: University Park Press.

Miller, J., & Chapman, R. (1981). The relation between age and Mean Length of Utterance in morphemes. *Journal of Speech and Hearing Research, 24,* 154–161.

Miller, J., & Chapman, R. (1985). *Systematic Analysis of Language Transcripts* (SALT). Madison, WI: Waisman Center.

Newcomer, P., & Hammill, D. (1988). *Test of Language Development-2 Primary* (TOLD-2:P). Austin, TX: Pro-Ed.

Owens, R. (1988). *Language development: An introduction.* Columbus, OH: Merrill.

Panagos, J., Quine, M., & Klich, R. (1979). Syntactic and phonological influences on children's articulation. *Journal of Speech and Hearing Research, 22,* 841-848.

Porch, B. (1968). *Porch Index of Communicative Ability* (PICA). Palo Alto, CA: Consulting Psychologists.

Prutting, C. (1979). Process: The action of moving forward progressively from one point to another on the way to completion. *Journal of Speech and Hearing Disorders, 44,* 3-30.

Roth, F., & Spekman, N. (1984). Assessing the pragmatic abilities of children: Part 1. Organizational framework and assessment parameters. *Journal of Speech and Hearing Disorders, 49,* 2-11.

Sattler, J. (1988). *Assessment of children* (3rd ed.). San Diego: Jerome M. Sattler.

Stein, N., & Glenn, C. (1979). An analysis of story comprehension in elementary school children. In R. O. Freedle (Ed.), *New directions in discourse processing* (Vol. 2, (pp. 53-120). Norwood, NJ: Ablex.

Stickler, K. (1987). *Guide to analysis of language transcripts.* Eau Claire, WI: Thinking Publications.

Tyler, L. (1992). *Spoken language comprehension: An experimental approach to disordered and normal processing.* Cambridge, MA: MIT Press.

Wechsler, D. (1974). *Wechsler Intelligence Scale for Children — Revised* (WISC-R). New York: Psychological Corporation.

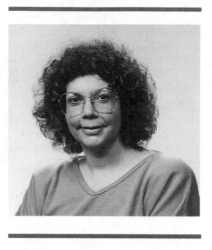

AMY L. WEISS, Ph.D.

M.A. 1976, The University of Illinois at Urbana
Ph.D. 1983, Purdue University

Dr. Weiss is an Associate Professor in the Department of Speech Pathology and Audiology at the University of Iowa. She was previously at the University of Colorado. Her special interests are in language development and disorders of preschool children, as well as the language and communication performance of children who stutter.

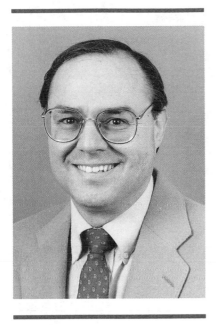

J. BRUCE TOMBLIN, Ph.D.

M.A. 1967, University of Redlands
Ph.D. 1970, The University of Wisconsin at Madison

Dr. Tomblin is a Professor in the Department of Speech Pathology and
Audiology at the University of Iowa. He was previously at Syracuse
University. His special interests are in language development and
disorders of children, including possible genetic influences on specific
language impairment.

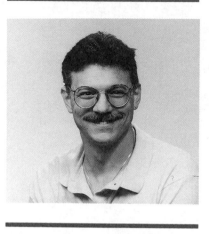

DONALD A. ROBIN, Ph.D.

M.S. 1981, University of Redlands
Ph.D. 1984, Case Western Reserve University

Dr. Robin is an Associate Professor in the Department of Speech Pathology and Audiology at the University of Iowa. His special area of interest is in neurogenic communication disorders.

CHAPTER

Assessing Language in the Classroom and the Curriculum

Frank M. Cirrin, Ph.D.

LANGUAGE AND LANGUAGE-LEARNING DISORDERS IN THE SCHOOLS

Did you know that more than 50% of speech-language pathologists work in a school setting? Perhaps you remember a speech clinician in your school who helped students with articulation, voice, or fluency problems. Today, students who have *language learning disorders* make up the majority of school speech-language pathologists' caseloads. Children with language learning disorders are a heterogeneous group who have difficulty acquiring, comprehending, or expressing themselves with spoken or written language. The difficulties that these students have with language also place them at severe risk for academic and learning problems. That is not surprising, given that language is the basis for virtually all learning, both in and out of school. Language is so embedded in school curricula that it is often difficult to separate learning the concepts of a subject from learning to use language to talk about these concepts. All aspects of the classroom environment are important to the learning process, but the most crucial ingredient is language.

A RATIONALE FOR ASSESSING LANGUAGE INTERACTIONS IN THE CLASSROOM

Do not assume that poor language abilities are the cause of a student's learning problem. Find out if the language used by the teacher and the language required by the lesson are contributing to the problem.

Gruenewald and Pollak (1990) suggest that there are three interacting language components in every learning or instructional task. There is a continuous interaction between the student's language, the teacher's language, and the language and concepts in the curriculum or instructional materials. Many teachers assume that the causes of a student's learning problem lie in the language abilities and conceptual skills that the student brings to the task. A more accurate assumption is that the student's learning is also influenced by the other two language components always present in the classroom environment.

An example may help to clarify these language interactions. Jerry, a third grader, is typical of a student whose language learning problems place him at risk for academic failure. In casual conversation, Jerry is spontaneously verbal, uses a mix of complete and incomplete sentences, and communicates messages effectively most of the time. However, in class he presents language and learning differences that affect his ability to participate in many learning activities. Jerry often engages in self-distracting behaviors, such as rocking in his chair or playing with pencils and paper clips. On these occasions Jerry needs repetition of directions that seem to be within his cognitive and language capabilities. He has difficulty following verbal and written directions for independent work sheets, and often turns in incomplete assignments. When he does not know what to do, he usually copies random words and sentences from the work sheet or the text. When participating in structured speaking tasks such as describing a sequence of directions, Jerry's verbalizations are short, incomplete, and difficult for a listener to follow. Although he often requires teacher repetition of directions and their sequence, Jerry has little difficulty remembering the gist of a story read to him, especially when the teacher uses a slow, conversational speaking style that includes periodic pauses for story-related comments from the class. For this task he can recall key vocabulary, characters, episodes, and other essential information. This suggests that when provided with a structure for remembering information (as in a story recall task) he has fewer problems retaining information, which, in turn, facilitates his understanding. Jerry's teacher was confused by the inconsistencies in his learning and was uncertain how to devise teaching strategies that would be more effective in helping him learn. The teacher needed to understand how Jerry's language abilities interacted with the classroom task (the curriculum) and differences in teacher language and interactional style and how to help him in the context of the regular classroom.

The main goal of language intervention for students with language learning disorders is to improve their functioning in real-life contexts, such as the classroom. This may seem obvious, but sometimes it is easy to lose sight of this basic tenet. Speech-language pathologists must make sure that language interventions are relevant to the classroom and that they will actually help students use language to communicate and learn in that context. To help students with language learning disorders to use language for learning, you (as a speech-language pathologist) must learn to observe and analyze the learning activities that students routinely encounter in school.

The need to assess the language interactions in classrooms is also related to a major change in service delivery that has affected virtually all school speech-language pathologists. Recently, we have begun to provide services to students with language learning disorders *in their classrooms*. These classroom-based language services include team teaching with the regular classroom teacher, working with large and small groups of students in the regular classroom, and collaborating with teaching staff in creating classroom environments that foster language development, higher level thinking, and literacy. By working with students in the classroom, we are helping them use new skills and knowledge in the actual learning context. Speech-language pathologists and teachers need assessment information that can be used to connect language intervention to the day-to-day learning activities that the student encounters. This can only be accomplished by systematically analyzing the language interactions between the student, teacher, and instructional materials in various classroom learning tasks.

This chapter focuses on specific assessment questions that you need to answer about classroom language interactions. As we have seen, information should be gathered on at least three important language variables:

1. The student's ability to use language effectively in classroom speaking and listening tasks,

2. The teacher's language during teaching and other instructional tasks, and

3. The concepts, vocabulary, and sentence structures that are found in the lessons and student's textbooks.

The process of assessing classroom language interactions is focused on understanding how each of these three variables may be contributing to the student's communication and academic difficulties. The teacher and the speech-language pathologist can then generate hypotheses about possible intervention strategies and modifications that can take place in the regular classroom to help the student.

COLLABORATING WITH TEACHERS

The first step in gathering relevant assessment data is to collaborate with those who know the child well. Although this appropriately includes parents and peers, this chapter is geared to working with teachers. Speech-language pathologists need to collaborate with teachers to identify key classroom learning situations if communication and academic problems are evident and to describe the language abilities of our students.

It is important that assessment of classroom language interaction be a collaborative venture between the teacher and the speech-language pa-

Effective language assessment *and* intervention requires you to be *in the classroom.*

thologist for at least two reasons. First, the teacher is the professional who has the primary responsibility for students' education. In this sense, the classroom is the teacher's "territory." An observation of a student, an examination of instructional materials, or an analysis of the teacher's language in that territory by the speech-language pathologist may be threatening. This is especially true if the teacher has not been an equal partner in identifying the problem, asking the assessment questions, and designing the assessment and observation plan.

Second, the teacher is usually very familiar with the student's language strengths and weaknesses as they affect that student's learning in the classroom. This is only natural because it is teachers who spend the most time with students. In school settings, teachers are also the main referral source for students with language learning disorders. They tend to be the first professionals to recognize that a student may be having difficulties with language and learning. Teachers will also have important information on students' academic performance, learning styles, social abilities, and other aspects of performance that must be integrated to obtain a picture of the "whole" child. Through collaboration, the teacher can add critical information to the analysis and ultimately participate in seeking solutions to our students' language and learning problems.

Although a detailed discussion of collaborative classroom-based services is beyond the scope of this chapter, it is important to recognize that collaboration is a *voluntary* interaction between colleagues having a parity of knowledge and skills. This means that two (or more) professionals contribute their strengths and abilities to the assessment-intervention process. The intent of collaboration should be to solve identified problems using the knowledge and skills of all professionals involved and effect lasting changes in the student's behavior and instill the ability to handle similar problems that may arise in the future.

Because collaboration is based on the premise that individuals have entered into a voluntary, nonsupervisory relationship, it does not work to *require* teachers to engage in collaborative activities with speech-language pathologists, or vice versa. This caveat applies to the collection and analysis of assessment data on classroom language interactions. In this regard, speech-language pathologists may find interactions with teachers less problematic if they view their role as one of empowering teachers rather than one of simply giving advice. We need to recognize the teacher's strengths and needs in providing an atmosphere that is communicatively rich and language-sensitive for students. There may be a tendency for a speech-language pathologist to view his or her role as language expert too narrowly. Identifying what teachers do not do "right" or often enough may justify to ourselves our role as "helper," but it does little to raise the awareness, competence, or acceptance of the teacher.

> Speech-language pathologists and teachers must *share their professional knowledge* with each other for students to be successful with classroom language demands.

ASSESSING STUDENT LANGUAGE USE IN THE CLASSROOM

Student language use is the first of the three interacting language variables we address. Teachers expect students to be able to comprehend, produce, and use language competently in classroom speaking and listening tasks.

Even though educators realize that learning is affected by both the teacher's language and the curricular materials themselves, students with language learning disorders may not have all of the language skills that the learning task requires. To help a student who has been referred, you will need to examine the particular learning task that the youngster is having problems with and determine if the student has the necessary speaking and listening skills. Several specific assessment questions must be asked about a student's use of language in the classroom.

Does the Student Have Sufficient Oral Language Skills to Do the Instructional Task?

Each instructional task requires the student to have knowledge of specific language forms (sentence structures) and language content (word and sentence meanings). To use language as a tool for learning and problem solving requires that students be able to produce a wide variety of simple, compound, and complex sentences and to use age-appropriate vocabulary. Most students enter school with the ability to combine words into phrases, clauses, and sentences. Teachers are sometimes misled into assuming that, because a student uses language for social purposes (such as getting needs met or interacting with family and friends), the child will be able to use language for the more formal types of verbal communication required in school. For example, a student with a language learning disorder may not be able to use verb tense markers when asked to give an oral report about an activity that took place in the past, as the following monologue of a third grade student illustrates.

> Well, the kids get on the bus and we go to the mall and have some money to buy some stuff. Oh, and this man wants us to stop running in the store.

Retelling stories, another common classroom language task, requires students to use complex and compound sentences to talk about temporal and cause-effect relationships (*Well, the wolf tried to trick the sisters because he wanted to eat them*) and use pronouns as devices to help link the sentences of the story together (*The wolf climbed the tree to eat a nut. When he fell, the sisters escaped*). Many students with language learning disorders do not have the expressive language abilities to perform adequately in retelling and other oral expression activities in the classroom.

Listening and language comprehension abilities are also required for academic success. Language learning disordered children often have difficulty drawing inferences about meanings that are not explicit. This limits their comprehension of what they hear and read. The ability to go beyond the information given to make inferences or conclusions is expected at all elementary grade levels. An example is the following question from a fourth grade workbook exercise:

Henry shook his dimes out onto the bedspread	Henry is _____.
His expenses had been heavy.	(a) in the store.
He wanted to buy Ribsy a new collar.	(b) in the house.
	(c) in his backyard.

In this exercise, students must not only understand the meanings of the printed words and sentences, but must go beyond these meanings to reach the appropriate conclusions.

Children with language learning problems also experience difficulties using grammatical rules to understand sentences produced by their teachers. They may try to rely on such strategies as identifying one or two key words and responding on that basis, rather than getting enough syntactic and semantic cues to understand the intent of the speaker or author. For example, the teacher's direction "Before you go outside, make sure to finish your work packet" may be interpreted as the teacher giving permission to go outside and then returning to finish the class task. This is because the student uses the order in which events have been mentioned as the order in which they are to occur.

What Information Do You Need to Gather?

You need to gather information on the student's ability to communicate effectively meanings and ideas with sentence forms when *speaking*. Does the student use a variety of simple, compound and complex sentences when speaking in the classroom? Information should be obtained on the student's use of appropriate verb tenses, plurals, prepositions, and other parts of sentences. You also need to find out if the student uses vocabulary that is appropriate for his or her age and grade level, and uses words that have more than one meaning. Classroom language also requires the student to appropriately use humor (such as puns) and figurative language.

In addition to data on oral expression, information must be gathered on the student's ability to understand a variety of sentence forms and vocabulary when *listening* in the classroom. You need to obtain information on the student's general ability to attend to the teacher's explanations and instructions. It is important to know if the student can understand classroom directions and a variety of sentence structures. The student's ability to understand the concepts and main ideas presented in stories and lectures also needs to be assessed. Specific information that can be gathered on a student's classroom speaking and listening abilities is listed in Figures 6-1 and 6-2.

How Do You Gather the Information?

Teachers have information on student language in the classroom that *you need*. Approach them as a partner, *not as an expert*, and you will find that they are willing to collaborate.

It is likely that some information on a student's expressive and receptive knowledge of language forms and content will be available from previously administered language tests and language samples. It is still necessary to find out, however, how the language learning disordered student performs in actual classroom speaking and listening tasks.

Two assessment methods may be used to determine if a student has sufficient oral language skills to do a particular instructional task. First, checklists (see Figures 6-1 and 6-2) that contain the relevant behavior categories can be used to interview the student's teacher. As previously noted, the classroom teacher has the best opportunity to observe the student's comprehension and use of language in daily learning situations. By interviewing the teacher or having the teacher fill out the checklist before

Classroom Speaking Checklist	Yes	No	Sometimes
1. Uses correct grammar and sentence structure			
a. Formulates sentences correctly			
b. Uses verb tenses correctly			
c. Forms plurals correctly (regular and irregular)			
d. Uses pronouns correctly			
e. Uses prepositions correctly			
f. Uses negation correctly			
g. Forms compound sentences correctly (with *and, but, or*)			
h. Forms complex sentences correctly (with *when, if, because*)			
i. Asks grammatically well-formed questions			
2. Meaning			
a. Uses age appropriate vocabulary			
b. Uses concepts of location, time, quantity, etc			
c. Uses and understands multiple meaning words			
d. Uses humor, sarcasm, and figures of speech appropriately			
e. Produces complex sentences that contain			
subordinate relationships			
relative clauses			

Figure 6-1. Student Language Checklist for Speaking. Teacher Interview and Observation Guide.

your observation, you will obtain information on how the instructor perceives the student's use of language in the classroom. Second, you need to observe the student using language during a specific instructional task. The same checklist that the teacher completed can guide your direct observation of the student. The main purpose of observing the student in one or more classroom speaking and listening tasks is to gain insights into how the student's language abilities interact with the language requirements of a specific learning situation.

Can the Student Use Language for a Variety of Academic Purposes?

Recently, we have become more aware of the language demands that are placed on children in school. It is not sufficient to be able to use language to communicate with others. In school, language must be used to regulate

Classroom Listening Checklist	Yes	No	Sometimes
A. Attention			
1. Attention span for oral presentations is adequate			
2. Attends to all or most of what is said in class			
3. Ignores auditory distractions			
4. Responds after first direction or presentation of information			
5. Asks for things to be repeated in class			
B. Comprehension			
1. Understands stories presented in class			
2. Understands material presented verbally (lecture) as well as those presented visually (written or drawn)			
3. Responds to questions within expected time period			
4. Follows a sequence of directions presented in class			
5. Understands concepts: temporal (before/after), position (above/below), quantity (more/several)			
6. Understands subtleties in word or sentence meanings (idioms, figurative language)			
7. Understands a variety of sentence structures			
8. Interprets meaning from tone of voice and other context cues			
9. Understands (verbally or nonverbally) the main idea of a verbal presentation			
10. Understands teacher questions presented in class			
11. Understands words (vocabulary) used in class			

Figure 6-2. Student Language Checklist for Listening: Teacher Interview and Observation Guide.

thinking, to plan, reflect, evaluate, and to acquire knowledge about things that are not directly experienced. The language demands of social conversation are comparatively simple, because people comment, request, state, and in other ways refer to events and activities *as they occur*.

The task demands in school are much different extending to the literate end of what has been called the "oral-to-literate continuum" (Westby, 1985). The use of language in school is often *decontextualized*, relating to things not in the here-and-now. This requires that students use language that is more specific, less repetitive and redundant, more reflective on experiences, and more related to topics that the student may not have directly experienced. Students with language learning disorders are likely to have difficulty using language to formulate ideas, compare and contrast, plan how to do a task, verbalize their experiences and feelings, and obtain information by asking questions. As teachers and speech-language pathologists, one of our most important jobs is to encourage students to use oral language for these purposes and to develop language as a tool for learning.

What Information Do You Need to Gather?

You need to determine how the student obtains information needed for school learning tasks and how effectively the student provides information to others. In addition, data should be gathered on how the student uses language to interact with teachers and classmates throughout the school day. For example, does the student use language to ask permission? Can the student use language to say what he or she wants to do or to explain how he or she feels?

Information also needs to be collected on how the student uses language for academic purposes and learning. For example, it is important to know if the student can use language effectively to describe an object or event. Other lessons may require students to use language to make predictions and inferences, make and defend judgments and opinions, and to compare and contrast. Figure 6-3 presents a language use inventory that can be used to record the student's use of language in a variety of structured and unstructured situations in the classroom.

How Do You Gather the Information?

Because the classroom teacher has many opportunities to observe the student's use of language in learning situations, information can be obtained from the teacher using a checklist that contains the relevant behaviors (see Figure 6-3). The teacher can focus on the student's overall ability to use language as he or she has observed throughout the school year.

Information should also be gathered by direct observations. A language use inventory will help you record the student's use of language in specific instructional tasks. Because the use of language depends so much on the task, it usually makes sense to use this inventory to obtain information during several days or in a variety of learning situations.

Get into the classroom at least once per week for all students on your caseload. Watch how classrooms work and what it takes for a student to be successful. Don't feel guilty about doing lots of observation.

What Does the Student Know About the Classroom Rules and the Various Routines or Scripts Followed in the Classroom?

Children's performance on many learning tasks is affected by what they know about how to act and interact in specific situations in the classroom. This knowledge is referred to as a script. Script knowledge includes information on the actors (who can participate), the props (what materials and tools are needed), the routine or required actions (what each actor is supposed to do and when to do it), and all of the possible variations.

I. How the Student Gives Information

1. Student gives information to others

   _____usually on his or her own

   _____sometimes on his or her own

   _____only when asked

2. Student gives information

   _____in classroom discussion

   _____one-to-one conversation

   _____play or free time with other students

3. When student gives information or explains something, people

   _____usually understand

   _____sometimes understand

   _____have difficulty understanding

II. How the Student Gets Information

1. Student gets most of his or her information (learns best) through:

   _____listening

   _____seeing

   _____reading

   _____doing it on student's own

   _____a combination of all of these

2. If student doesn't know something,

   _____he or she usually asks

   _____sometimes asks

   _____rarely asks

Figure 6-3. Student Language Use Inventory: Teacher Interview and Observation Guide. Adapted from Gruenwald, L., & Pollak, S. (1990). *Language interaction in curriculum and instruction* (2nd ed.). Austin, TX: Pro-Ed.

Scripts can be used to describe virtually all classroom learning tasks. For example, the script for quiet in the classroom may include the teacher flicking the light and counting to 10. Students may be expected to know that they need to have the tops of their desks clear and be sitting quietly facing the front of the room by the time the teacher reaches the number

III. How the Student Uses Language in the Classroom	Yes	No	Sometimes
A. Using Language for Basic School Communication			
1. Student uses language to ask permission.			
2. Student uses language to refuse to do something.			
3. Student uses language to criticize something/someone			
4. Student uses language to praise something/someone.			
5. Student uses language to say what he or she believes.			
6. Student uses language to explain how he or she feels.			
7. Student uses language to say what he or she wants to do.			
B. Using Language for Learning			
1. Student uses language to instruct, and provide sequential directions for how to do something.			
2. Student uses language to inquire, and gain information by asking questions.			
3. Student uses language to describe, or to tell about something; to give necessary information to identify.			
4. Student uses language to compare and contrast, or to show how things are similar and different.			
5. Student uses language to explain, or to tell why and provide specific examples.			
6. Student uses language to predict, or tell what might logically happen as a consequence.			
7. Student uses language to infer, or arrive at a conclusion from facts that are provided.			
8. Student uses language to evaluate, and judge the relative importance of an idea.			

Figure 6-3 *(continued)*

10. Other common classroom scripts include how teachers give directions for homework assignments and the rules for participating in class discussions, such as knowing when hands should be raised and when it is permissible to speak out.

Some classroom rules are stated by the classroom teacher. Other rules are implicit and, therefore, never communicated directly to the student.

Most children learn the stated and unstated classroom rules easily. Other children may have difficulty learning the rules given to the class as a whole, may be unable to generalize stated rules to new situations, or may not pick up on subtle verbal and nonverbal cues for learning the teacher's unstated rules.

Knowledge of the script enables the student to determine what is appropriate to do and say during the event or task. Some language learning disabled students may have difficulty following classroom directions or participating verbally in classroom activities because they have not learned the appropriate scripts. The information that we gather during our assessment can be used to help students develop stronger school scripts.

What Information Do You Need to Gather?

To answer this question you need to obtain information on the scripts necessary for a variety of classroom instructional tasks, and on the student's knowledge of various classroom scripts. It is important to determine if the student does not know the rules, perceives the rules and scripts differently from the teacher and classmates, or is not able to recognize subtle clues for identifying the teacher's rules for various classroom tasks and for the teacher's mood.

Figure 6-4 presents some questions that can help determine the behavior scripts for a particular classroom. Answers to these questions will give you an idea of the explicit and implicit classroom rules that students are expected to follow.

How Do You Gather That Information?

Information can be obtained on the teacher's perceptions of rules in the classroom by posing the questions in Figure 6-4 as part of an interview. You can also gain insight into classroom scripts by making direct observations of various classroom routines. Select a specific lesson and attempt to answer the questions in Figure 6-4. Through observation, you are attempting to discover the classroom rules and scripts, both explicit (stated by the teacher) and implicit (not stated). It is important to talk with the teacher after the observation to verify the accuracy of what you saw, heard, and concluded about the script requirements of the particular classroom.

After determining the script requirements of a specific learning task, you should examine the teacher's cues for defining the script and alerting the children when a given script is to begin. It is helpful to compare the cues for those scripts in which the child is successful and those in which he or she is not. This may allow you to identify specific teacher cues that facilitate the student's performance in the learning task.

Finally, you need information on the child's awareness of the script and the teacher's cues. For example, does the student know when to be quiet? Does the student know when questions are allowed? Does the student know when it is okay to talk out without raising his or her hand? This information can usually be obtained by directly asking the student.

Student problems with "following directions" may relate to their lack of script knowledge of what to do and how to participate in the classroom.

A. Questions for determining the **behavior script** for a particular classroom

　1. When is talking allowed?

　2. When is it okay for the student to ask a question in class?

　3. What are students supposed to do when they need help? Is it permissible to get help from peers?

　4. When is it okay for the student to talk out without raising a hand?

　5. What is the first thing the student should do when class begins?

　6. When are students supposed to give a short, specific answer, and when is an elaborated answer expected?

　7. How important is it to use correct grammar and complete sentences when talking? Writing?

B. Questions for determining the **teacher's cues** for a classroom script

　1. How does teacher communicate satisfaction/dissatisfaction with student?

　2. What does the teacher say or do to indicate that something is really important?

　3. How does the student know when the teacher is joking or teasing?

　4. What does the teacher do when it is time for a lesson to begin?

C. Questions for determining the **child's awareness** of classroom scripts and teacher cues

　1. Does the student know when to be quiet?

　2. Does the student know when to ask a question?

　3. Does the student know when to raise his or her hand, and when it's okay to talk out?

　4. Does the student know when it's okay to answer in single words, and when to use complete sentences?

　5. Does the student know when the teacher is joking? Dissatisfied? About to say something important?

Figure 6-4. Classroom Script Inventory. Adapted from Creaghead, N. (1992). Classroom interactional analysis/script analysis. In J. Damico (Ed.), *Best practices in school speech-language pathology: Descriptive/nonstandardized language assessment.* San Antonio: The Psychological Corporation/Harcourt Brace Jovanovich.

Section Summary

It is important to assess the student's language use in the classroom because usage is one of the critical language components for interacting in all learning activities. There are three specific assessment questions that need to be answered. Does the student have sufficient oral language skills to do the instructional task? Can the student use language for a variety of academic purposes? What does the student know about the various routines and scripts followed in the classroom? Formal tests of language can provide us with some information on student language abilities. Teacher interviews and direct observation, however, must be used to gather information on how the student uses language in real classroom contexts.

ASSESSING TEACHER AND INSTRUCTIONAL LANGUAGE

Teacher language is the second of the three interacting language variables we address. The talk that students encounter in school can be quite different from the conversations they experience with family and friends outside of the classroom. School discourse places additional demands on the student's ability to understand language, which continues to become more context-free as age and grade level increase. Communication in the classroom relies heavily on the meaning expressed by the teacher's spoken words. In school there are fewer opportunities for the student and teacher to engage in communicative repair if a breakdown has occurred in the child's comprehension. At home, parents may make revisions and repetitions as often as necessary tailored to fit the child and the situation. In the classroom, however, teachers must try to accommodate the varying needs of all the listeners in their classrooms, and they often must do this with little prior knowledge of the individual student's experiences.

Other differences between school and home discourse are also apparent. The style of teacher talk can affect a student's ability to process incoming verbal information. Teachers often adopt an expository style that includes numerous directions and explanations, plus a variety of questions all centered around topics in the curriculum. Finally, the complexity of the sentence structures that teachers use, in addition to suprasegmental variables such as rate of speech, intonation, and stress, can either facilitate making the intended meaning of the message clear to the listener or interfere with processing rather than aiding it.

The language used by the classroom teacher influences the responses of students in an instructional task. It is important to analyze the effect of teacher talk within an instructional task. This analysis provides clues about how a teacher's language interacts with the language abilities of a student who is having communication and academic problems. This information can help teachers become more aware of how their language affects the performance of students in their classrooms, and allows them to tune in closely to the multiple verbal and nonverbal signs that individual children in their classrooms are comprehending or not. At least three specific questions should be asked about teacher language.

What Is the Length and Rate of the Teacher's Verbal Instructions? How Much Talking Does the Teacher Do?

An excessive amount of teacher talk can create students with language learning problems who are passive or confused listeners. These students may have difficulty focusing on the important information if it is embedded in a lengthy discourse. Students may process academic information better if opportunities for student talk and questions are built into the lesson. Repeating or paraphrasing a direction may help some students who did not understand something the first time. Although it may be beneficial to repeat instructions, lengthy or complicated repetitions may not positively affect student comprehension. It is important to determine if the length of the direction is affecting the response of the student with a language learning disorder. The rate of the teacher's speech also may affect the student's understanding of the message.

What Information Do You Need to Gather?

Information should be gathered on the rate and on the amount of teacher talk that occurs during a particular instructional task. First, identify those aspects of teacher talk that seem to match and support the student's comprehension in the task (strengths). Focusing on strengths of teacher talk is important for several reasons. Teacher talk behaviors that appear to facilitate student performance in one learning situation may be applied to other contexts. In addition, discussing facilitative language behaviors with the teacher builds rapport and trust. This may make teachers receptive to examining their own language as it interacts with the language abilities of his or her students.

When a student does not understand verbal directions, find out if changes in teacher talk improve comprehension.

Teacher talk behaviors that do not appear to match the level of the student's comprehension should also be described (potential mismatches). When potential mismatches are observed, they should be accompanied by a hypothesis of a modification that might foster a better match between teacher talk and student listening. For example, you might note that a teacher effectively used intonation to highlight important concepts or vocabulary words in a lesson (strength). This is an important strategy to use with students who have language learning disorders. At some point in the lesson, the teacher might have asked three questions in a row without pausing for students to respond (potential mismatch). In this case, it would be appropriate to explore if a strategy of pausing for several seconds between each question might facilitate the comprehension of the student with a language learning disorder (hypothesis). The speech-language pathologist and the teacher might brainstorm about other possible hypotheses or strategies for increasing student comprehension and systematically try these techniques in future lessons.

How Do You Gather That Information?

Information on teacher language can be gathered by observing an instructional task in the classroom and using the format in Figure 6-5 to take notes and write down examples in each category. To save time, try to limit your observations to classroom tasks that seem to be especially difficult for the student with language learning problems. Consultation with the teacher before the observation can provide useful information about which task(s) to observe.

The Use of Tape Recording Equipment

Because it is difficult to write down everything that a teacher says during an observation, you may sometimes tape record the lesson for later analysis. If you and the teacher are in a collaborative relationship and he or she voluntarily agrees to participate, try to tape record a 5- or 10-minute segment of a lesson with an individual student who is experiencing difficulty in learning the task. The lesson should be an exchange between student

Teacher Language During Lesson	Strengths	Potential Mismatches	Hypothesis

1. Rate of teacher talk:
 	
  Amount of teacher talk time:
 	
2. Teacher's instructional language
 	
a. Questions
 	
  Number of questions asked:
 	
  Pauses for students to answer:
 	
  Types of questions
 	
    Close-ended:
 	
    Open-ended:
 	
b. Directions
 	
  Number of directions given:
 	
  Single concept directions:
 	
  Multiple concept directions:
 	
c. Explanations
 	
  Length of explanations:
 	
  Clarity of explanations:
 	
3. Teacher's sentences
 	
a. Sentence Complexity
 	
  Simple Sentences:
 	
  Complex Sentences:
 	
b. Sentence Length
 	
  Short Sentences:
 	
  Long Sentences:			

Figure 6-5. Recording Format for Teacher's Language. Adapted from Gruenewald, L., & Pollack, S. (1990). *Language interaction in curriculum and instruction* (2nd ed.). Austin, TX: Pro-Ed.

and teacher. Initially, you can listen for examples in one or two teacher talk categories each time the tape is played. With practice, it is possible to chart several items during one listening session.

As a general rule, recording equipment should be considered when the communication is unfolding so quickly that it simply cannot be reliably heard and written down in real time. Recording equipment is also used when the language and communicative behaviors of interest are so complex that all aspects of language cannot be focused on simultaneously. The analyses of tape transcripts can provide insights that may not be available solely by listening to an exchange between a teacher and a student.

Cautions When Analyzing Teacher Language: Empower Rather Than Judge

It is important to keep in mind that one of our main goals is to help teachers become skilled in analyzing their lessons to obtain insights into and control over the language of teaching. Increased knowledge can also provide teachers the opportunity to acknowledge their strengths or, if they think it necessary, to modify their instructional style as a tool for facilitating student learning. The overall purpose of analyzing teacher talk should not be viewed as judgmental.

There are several reasons why teachers might be reluctant to participate in such activities. Recording and analyzing language can be quite time-consuming. It also may make some persons uncomfortable or embarrassed to listen to their voices. In some cases, it may be frustrating, disappointing, and/or threatening for a teacher to hear that what he intended to convey did not occur. For these reasons, teacher participation must be voluntary.

How Syntactically Complex Are the Teacher's Messages in the Classroom?

The length and complexity of teachers' sentences may not match the language form comprehension abilities of some students with language learning disorders. When this occurs, these students may encounter difficulties when engaged in a specific instructional task. Sentence complexity refers to whether the teacher uses mostly simple, compound, or complex sentences. A simple sentence is defined as containing a subject, verb, and object; a compound sentence is composed of two or more simple sentences; a complex sentence includes dependent and independent clauses connected by conjunctions.

What Information Do You Need to Gather?

It is necessary to obtain information on the number of simple and complex sentences that have been used by the teacher in a specific instructional task. You also want to know the approximate number of sentences that were short (e.g., 7 words or less) and those that were long (e.g., 8 words or more).

How Do You Gather That Information?

This information can be obtained by direct observation and/or a tape recording of a specific teacher-student interaction. The recording format presented in Figure 6–5 guides the observation.

What Instructional Style Does the Teacher Use and How Varied Are the Teacher's Questions, Directions, and Explanations?

The expository style that most teachers use in the classroom contains many explanations, directions, and questions. Students with language disorders may not be able to process and remember directions and explanations that are lengthy or contain multiple concepts. It is also difficult for some students to understand a rapid series of directions all given at one time.

Teachers spend a great deal of time asking questions during instructional activities. Students with language disorders may be overwhelmed by many questions unless sufficient pause time is left between questions. A pause time of at least 3 seconds gives students time to think and formulate an answer.

Questions may be close-ended or open-ended. Close-ended questions usually require "narrow thinking." This means they often have a single answer that is correct. Teachers usually know the answers to the close-ended questions they ask students. In most educational systems, these close-ended "knowledge" and "comprehension" questions allow students to demonstrate their knowledge verbally to teachers. This is a skill related to academic success and something that students with language learning disorders need to know how to do. Close-ended questions typically involve recalling facts, naming places, or providing yes or no responses. Open-ended questions are those that focus on broader, higher level thinking skills such as making inferences and generalizations, predictions, or evaluations. Open-ended questions usually have many possible responses.

Both types of questions are appropriate depending on the lesson, the teacher's goals for the lesson, and the language abilities of the students. Selecting to pose primarily close-ended questions, however, can hamper students with language learning problems in using language to develop the higher levels of thinking required in the upper grades. When teachers vary their question types, they allow students to practice using language to develop higher levels of thinking. Figure 6–6 presents examples of some close- and open-ended questions that might be used in the curricular areas of language arts, science, and social studies.

The taxonomy of questions for "higher level thinking" (see Figure 6–6) makes an excellent tool to include in both classroom language assessment and intervention. Find out how your students answer these questions.

What Information Do You Need to Gather?

Information should be gathered on the instructional talk that teachers use in the classroom. You should analyze the types of questions that were asked for a given instructional task. Information should also be obtained on how the teacher gives directions or instructions and if they appear to match student comprehension abilities. The approximate length and number of concepts expressed in teacher explanations should also be noted.

Type	Definition	Language Arts	Science	Social Studies
Close-Ended/Narrow				
Knowledge	Memorizes and repeats information presented; answers simple questions.	What was the little girl's name in Charlotte's Web? Where did Templeton the rat live?	What kind of rock is made of mud and clay pressed together?	Where did the Alaskan oil spill occur? What company owned the boat that caused the spill?
Comprehension	Demonstrates understanding by paraphrasing or stating information in another form.	What was the story about? Tell me the story you just heard.	Explain how metamorphic rock is produced.	Describe how the Alaskan oil spill occurred.
Open-Ended/Broad				
Application	Uses information or principles in new but similar situations.	Charlotte and Wilbur are friends. How can friends help each other?	(After discussion of the characteristics of granite) What could we use granite for?	What are some other ways that the wildlife could have been rescued?
Analysis	Identifies components, gives reasons, identifies problems.	How did Wilbur change over the course of the story?	How are limestone, shale, and sandstone alike?	What types of problems were caused by the spill?
Synthesis	Generalizes from previously learned knowledge to generate new solutions to problems.	What would have happened if Templeton hadn't found words for Charlotte to weave in her web?	How would the world be different if there were no volcanoes?	What kinds of problems would occur if there were a chemical spill in our town?
Evaluation	Compares alternatives, states, opinions, justifies responses.	Which character do you like best in this story and why?	If you had to create a monument, what type of rock would you use and why?	Discuss who should be responsible for the clean-up and why they should be responsible.

Figure 6-6. Examples of open-ended (narrow) and close-ended (broad) questions in several curriculum areas. Based on: Bloom, B. (1956). *Taxonomy of educational objectives: Cognitive domains.* New York: David McKay Co.; Westby, C. (1985). Learning to talk–Talking to learn: Oral-literate language differences. In C. Simon (Ed.), *Communication skills and classroom success: Therapy methodologies for language-learning disabled students.* San Diego: College-Hill Press; and Gruenewald, L., & Pollak, S. (1990). *Language interaction in curriculum and instruction* (2nd ed.). Austin, TX: Pro-Ed.

How Do You Gather That Information?

This assessment data can be obtained by direct observation and/or a tape recording of a specific teacher-student interaction. The recording format presented in Figure 6-5 is a guide for observation.

Teacher Language Example

The following example from Gruenewald and Pollak (1990, p. 11) illustrates how teacher language can interact with students' ability to solve a math story problem using subtraction.

Teacher: I have a story problem I want you to do. I will do it, too. First, I want you to listen. Then, I will give you a copy of it and we will do it together and then we will do the figuring. The first thing we are going to do — I want to ask you to think whether or not you have to do addition or subtracting first. Think really hard. Just do the whole problem. Don't just write down plus or minus. Just do the whole problem whether you think it is adding or subtracting.

Yesterday Sue traveled 36 miles. Today Ed traveled 53 miles. How many more miles did Ed travel than Sue?

Teacher: Okay, let's see. Would you please put your sign down so I know exactly what you did? Okay, and let's see — David, you said you plussed 36 and 53, and Debbie, you said you plussed also. Okay what were the key words in that story?

Debbie: How many.

David: How many more.

Teacher: How many more. Does that tell you that you had to be adding?

Students: Yes.

Teacher: We want to know how many miles. Are we going to put them together or find a difference? Ed traveled more miles. Right? When we are finding more miles are we adding or subtracting?

Students: (no response)

Even though these students may have been able to perform the operation of subtraction when presented as a standard math problem (e.g., $53 - 36 = ?$), the language of the math story prevented them from solving the problem. The length and grammatical structure of the teacher's explanations did not appear to match the students' comprehension abilities. Also, the teacher asked a series of three questions without waiting for a response. A preliminary hypothesis might ask if opportunities for the students to use verbal language to solve the problem or ask questions would have aided student performance?

Section Summary

It is important for teachers to analyze the language they use during instruction, because it interacts with student language and the curriculum in all learning tasks. Speech-language pathologists can help gather data on instructional language for teachers who choose to participate in these activities. There are three specific assessment questions that can be answered about teacher talk. What is the length and rate of the teacher's verbal instructions? How syntactically complex are the teacher's messages in the classroom?

How effective are the teacher's questions, directions, and explanations? This information can help teachers become aware of how their language affects the comprehension of students with language learning disorders.

ASSESSING LANGUAGE REQUIREMENTS IN THE CURRICULUM

The language of the curriculum is the third component interacting with student language and teacher language in all learning tasks. What is the curriculum? As used in this chapter, the term "curriculum" refers to the lessons, textbooks, worksheets, and the scope and sequence of the actual content of what is being taught (and learned) in the classroom. For example, a third-grade class will have a curriculum for math, language arts (including reading, writing, and spelling), and science, among others. Nelson (1989) points out that there are other curricula in schools besides this "official" curriculum. She suggests that students must have knowledge of "school culture" curriculum (e.g., implicit and explicit classroom scripts) and "defacto" curriculum (e.g., lesson content determined by a *Teacher's Guide* to a particular textbook series), among others. The official curriculum is the focus of this section.

To help students with language learning disorders, speech-language pathologists and teachers must analyze the language of the lessons and textbooks that students are expected to use and understand. The language requirements of specific lessons and texts can be analyzed in at least two ways. The concepts and vocabulary embedded in the lessons can be examined, as well as the sentence structures that students encounter in the oral lessons and written materials. Both of these variables will affect the ability of students to learn and understand the lesson.

Language Content, Vocabulary, and Concepts in Curriculum Materials

Embedded in every instructional task and textbook is a set of *explicit vocabulary words* relating to the content or concepts being taught. For example, locating a city on a map in a social studies lesson requires that the student use and understand explicit vocabulary words for spatial relations, such as *north, south, near, closer,* and *far.*

In addition, each instructional task requires the student to have knowledge of some *implicit concepts and operations.* These underlying concepts and operations are just as important to learning as the explicit vocabulary words, but may not be as obvious to the student or the teacher. For example, the implicit skills required for using a map include the knowledge of spatial concepts and the ability to represent space in a 2-dimensional pencil-and-paper task. To be successful in instructional tasks, students must have knowledge of the required underlying concepts and operations, as well as ability to use and understand the explicit vocabulary words contained in the task. In determining how the conceptual content of a lesson interacts with a student's language abilities, the following assessment question needs to be asked.

Effective assessment of the language of curriculum materials requires that you read the books and worksheets that the student is expected to read.

What Concepts and Vocabulary Do the Curriculum Materials Contain, Both Explicitly and Implicitly?

In this chapter it is not feasible to cover all the possible concepts and vocabulary taught in the various curricula in the schools. However, there are several basic concepts that you can describe and analyze in a variety of curricular materials in the classroom.

Classification

Classification operations are strategies for organizing and grouping objects, symbols, and events. Classification requires the ability to manipulate, order, and group and regroup symbols and objects. Classification skills, including the knowledge that objects can be members of certain categories (class inclusion and exclusion), are present in all academic tasks.

Each classification task has its own specific vocabulary. For example, classifying objects by perceptual attributes requires the use of words to describe color, shape, size, texture, and form of the objects. Classifying objects by function requires vocabulary words for addressing the uses of objects and how they function. If objects are grouped into categories, the relevant vocabulary words include the names of classes of objects (e.g., fruits, animals, words that start with the letter "A").

Students must be able to demonstrate that they can group according to one or more attributes (i.e., size, shape, color, etc.). Students should also be able to talk about their decision process for classifying. After a student has grouped a series of objects or words in any fashion, asking the student to tell "why these go together" is a critical part of the learning process. Children can progress to more abstract classification tasks by using language to express the concept.

Classification skills are embedded in many academic areas including math (formation of sets, story problems), social studies (outlining, historical concepts, geography), language arts and reading (grouping letters to make words, combining syllables to make words), reading comprehension (main ideas, part/whole relationships), and science (classes of plants and animals).

Conservation

Conservation is defined as the ability to realize that certain attributes of an object are constant, even though that object may change in appearance. For example, pouring liquid from a short, fat glass into a tall, thin glass may change the appearance but not the volume. You can rearrange or combine objects in a group without changing the number of objects. In both examples, nothing has been added or taken away. The ability to conserve is basic to the understanding of number, measurement, and space.

The vocabulary items associated with conservation concepts differ, depending on the nature of the instructional task. For example, the vocabulary for number includes the terms *more, less, the same as, all, half, whole, few, before*, and *after*. The vocabulary for size includes the terms *tall, short, thin, fat, wide, narrow, high*, and *low*. The explicit vocabulary for length includes the terms *taller than, shorter than*, and *the same length*.

Time

Time, or temporal concepts, can be expressed in two ways: temporal order (sequence) and duration (the time interval between two events). Vocabulary words used to express temporal order include *first, second, before, during, after, next, last, earlier,* and *later.* Vocabulary words used to express duration or time include *morning, afternoon, old, young, long time, today, tomorrow, yesterday, hour,* and *day.*

Time concepts are found in the academic areas of social studies (dates, times), language arts (order of events in a story), math (measurement), and science (seasons, changes over time).

Seriation

The concept of seriation involves the ability to learn the relationships between objects and put them in order. Vocabulary associated with seriation includes number (*first, second, third,* etc.), size (*big, bigger, biggest*), length (*long, longer, longest*), height (*tall, taller, tallest*), space/time (*in front of, behind, before, after*), and amount (*least, most*).

Seriation is a part of all subject areas. Instances of seriation in academic tasks include science (ordering items by attributes), math (counting), and language arts (ordering of events in a story, ordering letters of the alphabet for dictionary and library skills).

Space

Spatial concepts are required to locate the position of objects in relation to one another. This requires the ability to view an object from different points of view. Vocabulary used to talk about the location of an object in space includes *over, under, above, below, in front of, in back of, behind, next to, right and left, in, out, on, off, inside, outside, top,* and *bottom.*

Causality

Causality involves the knowledge of cause/effect relationships. The vocabulary used to express causality includes the words *because, if/then, when, therefore,* and *why.*

What Information Do You Need to Gather?

Information should be obtained on the implicit and explicit concepts and operations in the instructional task for which the student is having problems. You need to analyze specific curriculum materials for the underlying operations of classification, conservation, time, seriation, space, and causality. You should also record the explicit conceptual vocabulary that the materials require the student to use and understand.

How Do You Gather That Information?

It is important to confer with the teacher and decide which specific curriculum materials should be examined. Once that decision is made, list the important vocabulary or concept words in the materials. Vocabulary words also serve as cues to determine the implicit concepts and operations present in a particular task. Examples of the vocabulary and conceptual content of lessons can be recorded on an analysis guide like the one in Figure 6-7.

Language Forms and Sentences in Curriculum Materials

The language in a reading assignment or in the instructions on a worksheet may include sentence structures that do not match the comprehension abilities of students with language learning disorders. Complex sentence forms that the student can understand in spoken social communication may be incomprehensible when encountered in written form. Thus, it is important to analyze the sentence structures and grammatical forms em-

---

I. Explicit - Vocabulary

    List vocabulary in the instructional task:

Comments:

II. Implicit - Concepts and operations

    Check appropriate line for concepts and operations required in the instructional task

        _____Conservation (number, size, length, amount)

        _____Time (temporal order, duration)

        _____Spatial

        _____Causality (cause/effect)

        _____Classification (sorting, inclusion/exclusion, regrouping)

        _____Order/seriation (number, length, height, space/time, amount)

Comments:

Figure 6-7. Format for Recording Language Content/Concepts in Curriculum Materials. Adapted from Gruenewald, L., & Pollak, S. (1990). *Language interaction in curriculum and instruction* (2nd ed.). Austin, TX: Pro-Ed.

bedded in curriculum materials. The following assessment question should be asked.

What Sentence Structures Do the Curriculum Materials Contain?

What Information Do You Need to Gather?

To answer this question, you need to obtain information on the major sentence structures and the constituent parts of sentences in the curriculum materials. Constituent parts of a sentence include verb tenses, comparatives, prepositions, conjunctions, negatives, questions, and modifiers.

There are two ways to analyze this information. First, you should determine what sentences forms the task requires the student to *produce*. For example, is the student expected to write the answers to reading comprehension questions in complete, syntactically correct sentences? If so, does the student need to use simple, compound, or complex sentences? Second, you should determine what sentence structures the materials require the student to *understand*. For example, does the student need to understand prepositional phrases and comparatives? Are the instructions written in simple sentences or are they complex?

Figure 6–8 presents a list of major sentence types and constituent parts of sentences that guide the analysis of curriculum materials.

How Do You Gather That Information?

The only way to determine the conceptual content and the sentence structures in curriculum materials is to analyze carefully the materials themselves. Examples of the major sentence structures and sentence parts required by the curricular materials, texts, or lessons can be listed on an analysis guide like the one presented in Figure 6–8.

The classroom teacher can help select those curricular materials that seem most difficult for the student. These may come from a wide variety of learning tasks, such as written instructions on a worksheet, an assignment in a textbook, or even sample class tests and quizzes.

Curricular Concepts Example

The following example from Gruenewald and Pollak (1990, p. 26) illustrates concepts and sentence forms embedded in a fourth-grade math lesson.

> A turkey is to be cooked 20 minutes for each pound. If a turkey weighing 10 pounds is to be done at 5 p.m., what time should it be put in the oven to cook?

The explicit vocabulary representing the temporal concepts in this example are *5 p.m.* and *20 minutes*. The underlying temporal concepts and operations (implicit) include duration of time (length of cooking time is 20 minutes × 10), number of minutes to the hour (200 minutes/60 = 3⅓ hours),

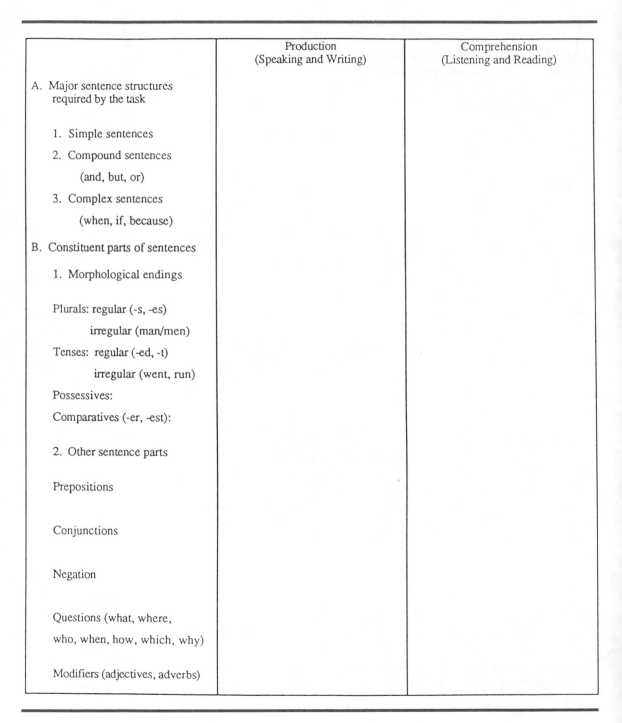

	Production (Speaking and Writing)	Comprehension (Listening and Reading)
A. Major sentence structures required by the task		
1. Simple sentences		
2. Compound sentences (and, but, or)		
3. Complex sentences (when, if, because)		
B. Constituent parts of sentences		
1. Morphological endings		
Plurals: regular (-s, -es) irregular (man/men)		
Tenses: regular (-ed, -t) irregular (went, run)		
Possessives:		
Comparatives (-er, -est):		
2. Other sentence parts		
Prepositions		
Conjunctions		
Negation		
Questions (what, where, who, when, how, which, why)		
Modifiers (adjectives, adverbs)		

Figure 6-8. Guide for Analyzing Sentence Structures in Curriculum Materials. Adapted from Gruenewald, L., & Pollack, S. (1990). *Language interaction in curriculum and instruction* (2nd ed.). Austin, TX: Pro-Ed.

and reversibility (working backward from 5 p.m. to 1:40 p.m.). Syntax requirements include complex sentences with *if-what then* constructions.

There are several possible reasons why a fourth-grade student with a language learning disorder might have difficulty with this problem. One reason is that the student may not understand that the concepts of *a.m.* and *p.m.* are equivalent to morning, afternoon, and evening (for example, the concept of a day). It is also possible that the student may not have the concept of *duration* as being equivalent to the interval between two points. Another possibility is that the student might not understand complex sentences with if-then constructions.

This type of analysis allows teachers and speech-language pathologists to hypothesize if aspects of the language in curriculum materials match the level a student can process. From these hypotheses, we can systematically implement one or more interventions that might result in a better match between the materials and the student's cognitive and language level. For example, instructions for an assignment could be rewritten or rephrased using a different syntactic construction. The teacher might try having a peer read instructions to the student. The student could be asked to paraphrase the instructions and ask clarification questions, if parts were not understood. The speech-language pathologist might try preteaching the required concepts or vocabulary to the student.

Section Summary

The language embedded in texts, lessons, and other instructional materials in the curriculum must be carefully examined. These language forms and content will interact with student language and teacher language and affect the ability of students to learn. There are at least two specific assessment questions that can be asked. What concepts and vocabulary do the curriculum materials contain, both explicitly and implicitly? What sentence structures do the curriculum materials contain? Answers to these questions can lead the speech-language pathologist and the teacher to generate hypotheses about possible interventions to help students with language learning disorders.

PREPARING TO GATHER INFORMATION IN THE CLASSROOM

Speech-language pathologists need to collaborate with teachers and observe in the classroom to answer specific assessment questions about classroom language interactions. Strategies that can make the assessment of language interactions more effective include:

1. Before the observation, set up a 15-minute block to interview the teacher using one or more of the checklists presented in this chapter, in the recommended supplemental readings, or one that you and the teacher have designed. If it is difficult to find a time to meet, it may be easier to leave the checklist with the teacher and have it returned to you in a day or two. Once the teacher returns the checklist, it is important to meet briefly to plan the observation.

The teacher and you should agree on which classroom activities will be observed, when the observation(s) will take place, and the length of observation. For example, it may be possible to obtain the necessary information by observing one session or it may be necessary to observe different sessions over several weeks. The instructional tasks that you select to observe should be those in which the student is having difficulties.

2. You may want to visit the classroom as a helper one or two times before your observation. This will allow you to become familiar with the general layout of the classroom, as well as for the children to become familiar with you. An observer's presence in the classroom is soon forgotten by the children. There should be close coordination with the teacher to keep classroom disruption to a minimum.

3. Record information such as the child's name and contextual features that may be important for interpreting the assessment data at a later time. The following contextual information should be noted: time of day; information about the instructional activity; a sketch or map of the classroom including the student's, teacher's, and peer's place/position; the types of instructional materials used; and other information that will allow you to analyze the physical, temporal, and social organization of the activity, including its communication requirements.

4. Check with the teacher the morning of the observation to confirm that the student is present and that the learning activity will take place at the scheduled time as planned.

How long should the observation be? The amount of time per observation should be kept within reason. Start off with 10- or 15-minute observation periods. In limiting the observation to a student's specific problem in an instructional task, extensive observational time is not required.

5. It is necessary to compare notes with the teacher sometime shortly after your classroom observation. This allows you to integrate the viewpoint of the teacher and confirm the accuracy of your own observations. Discrepancies in the viewpoint of the teacher about the accuracy of your written records should be discussed.

If the teacher has previously volunteered to collaborate and analyze a tape recording of a lesson, schedule time for this activity. The teacher's role is to stop the tape when the child (or the teacher) is engaged in behaviors that are related either to the reason for a potential referral or to the initial problem. The tape should also be stopped when a contrast is noted between the target child's behaviors and those of other children in the activity or when something occurs that the teacher would like to comment on.

SUMMARY

Formal or standardized language tests cannot provide you with all of the information you need to help students with language learning disorders succeed in school. Spending time in classrooms and becoming familiar with the language requirements of instructional activities allows you to gather relevant assessment data. Current classroom-based service delivery models emphasize the need for collaboration with regular classroom teachers, both to plan and carry out valid assessments and to design intervention strategies and classroom modifications. Assessing language interactions takes time, effort, and training. Given the time constraints on all teachers and speech-language pathologists who work in schools, it is sometimes tempting to limit language assessment to an initial assessment battery focusing primarily on student strengths and weaknesses. Classroom-based language assessment is well worth the time and effort. The information you gather in the classroom is the most relevant to the real-life language and learning problems the student faces. Language interventions based on relevant classroom assessment data have the best chance of making a real difference for students with language learning disorders.

REFERENCES

Bloom, B. (1956). *Taxonomy of educational objectives: Cognitive domains.* New York: David McKay.

Creaghead, N. (1992). Classroom interactional analysis/script analysis. In J. Damico (Ed.), *Best practices in school speech-language pathology: Descriptive/nonstandardized language assessment.* San Antonio: The Psychological Corporation/Harcourt Brace Jovanovich,.

Gruenewald, L., & Pollak, S. (1990). *Language interaction in curriculum and instruction* (2nd ed.). Austin, TX: Pro-Ed.

Nelson, N. (1989). Curriculum-based language assessment and intervention. *Language, Speech, and Hearing Services in Schools, 20*(2), 170–184.

Westby, C. (1985). Learning to talk — Talking to learn: Oral-literate language differences. In C. Simon (Ed.), *Communication skills and classroom success: Therapy methodologies for language-learning disabled students.* San Diego: College-Hill Press.

RECOMMENDED READINGS

Silliman, E., & Cherry Wilkinson, L. (1991). *Communicating for learning: Classroom observation and collaboration.* Gaithersburg, MD: Aspen Publications.

Simon, C. (Ed.), (1985). *Communication skills and classroom success: Assessment of language-learning disabled students.* San Diego: College-Hill Press.

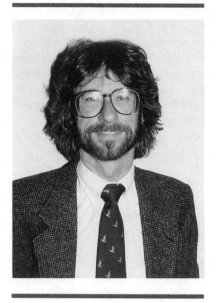

FRANK M. CIRRIN, Ph.D.

Ph.D. 1980, The University of Iowa

Dr. Cirrin is a Resource Teacher in the Speech-Language Program in the Department of Special Education, Minneapolis Public Schools. Previous fellowships and positions were at Parsons Research Center, Bureau of Child Research, University of Kansas, and Idaho State University, Pocatello. His current duties include development of classroom-based service delivery modes for language intervention and organization of school-based collaborative teams to provide special education services for students with language learning disabilities.

C H A P T E R

7

Aphasia

Linda Smith Jordan, Ph.D.

"Yes, yes," says Mrs. Fraizer, nodding vigorously as you introduce yourself as the speech pathologist, "I have it. It's all here, but I can't talk it." To a similar introduction, Mr. Andrews responds, "Damn, don't need it," and closes his eyes to dismiss you.

Welcome to the world of assessment of aphasia. If you find pleasure in working with puzzles, I am sure you will enjoy working with individuals with aphasia. An individual appears before you. Her family complains about her sudden loss of verbal skills. She has lost the ability to interact with people using verbal abilities. You are about to assume the task of describing her skills that were impaired or lost. You want to describe problems in enough detail for rehabilitation efforts to follow quite naturally. This is a goal of assessment of aphasia.

WHAT IS APHASIA?

Aphasia is an acquired disorder of communication affecting the ability to comprehend and produce language. It occurs secondary to damage to the brain. Disruption of brain function results in the concomitant disruption of language functions subserved by the affected areas of the brain. This formal definition means that your client, following some kind of brain damage, has lost the ability to ask and answer questions, to give and follow directions, to share feelings and emotions. As a result, she can no longer

Mrs. F. has a room full of visitors. Her son observes that visitors talk until his mother objects to the facts they "tell wrong."

"visit," entertain friends by sharing plans and memories, or give directions to other people.

Damage to the brain is responsible for the sudden and unexpected development of aphasia in a person. It is important to remember that the problem of aphasia occurs in an individual who had previously exhibited what, for that individual, were "normal" language skills. In other words, the damage to the brain is responsible for altered language performance abilities.

YOUR ROLE WITH AN INDIVIDUAL WHO HAS APHASIA

As a speech pathologist, you may become a member of the professional team working with an individual with aphasia. The team working with the individual and the involved family should address the problem of aphasia on several levels. Specifically, the individual can be viewed in terms of the impairment, the disability, and the handicap.

The *impairment* is a disruption of, a loss of, or a change in physiological structure or function. The impairment is identified by the name of the disease state. For example, "hemorrhage," "blood clot," "vision loss," or "hypertension" label a part or all of the impairment for various individuals. The goal of treatment for an impairment is prevention of future impairments (Frey, 1984) or avoidance of exacerbation of the present impairment. The treatment is directed, for the most part, by members of the medical community. The speech pathologist must understand the impairment and help ensure that the patient understands the information given about the impairment.

At a second level, people working with individuals with aphasia need to address the *disability* that accompanies this symptom of damage to the brain. This requires assessment of what Frey refers to as an individual's ability to "perform activities, tasks, skills and behaviors . . . 'within the range considered normal for a human being'" (p. 33). As a speech pathologist, you might describe manifestations of the disability as "inability to think of names, inability to follow directions, inability to read printed words," or "inability to write checks," and so on. Your assessment may indicate that the individual with aphasia could benefit from rehabilitation, "the improvement (or enhancement) of functional capacities" (Frey, 1984, p. 32). After your initial assessment of the communication status has been obtained, a speech pathologist (perhaps you) will provide treatment to enhance the individual's ability to compensate for impaired or lost skills and to maximize use of residual skills. It is frequently helpful to provide counseling to assist the patient's or family's adjustment to the changes in abilities and life style that the brain damage has necessitated. Such counseling may be your responsibility.

At a third level, you must consider the *handicap* that the individual with brain damage experiences as a result of the impairment and disability. The handicap incorporates the attitudes and responses which "limit or prevent the fulfillment of a role that is normal for that individual" (Frey, 1984, p. 33). Your role as a member of the treatment team may involve educating others in the patient's environment, as well as the person with aphasia, about the impairment, the disability, and the handicap. You will want to influence the family, service providers, policy makers, the voting and tax pay-

---

Mrs. A. reports that Mr. A. has become "cranky," since his stroke. "He doesn't understand what I tell him."

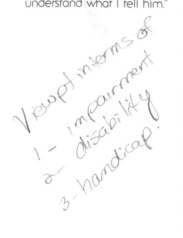
Viewpt in terms of
1 - impairment
2 - disability
3 - handicap.

Mrs. F. has mild weakness of her right hand and arm.

Mrs. F. produces choppy speech that lacks specific words. She is aware of a word-finding problem. Mr. A. produces neologisms (new words) and is unaware of his errors.

Because of Mr. A's anticipation of failure with communication he avoids social contacts.

ing public. Hopefully this education will have an impact on children as they begin to develop attitudes about individuals with communication disabilities. If society is to be taught how to respond appropriately to individuals with communication difficulty, distinctions must be made between the three levels just discussed: the impairment, the disability, and the handicap.

Before her stroke occurred, Mrs. F. was considered a leader in the social groups in which she participated.

HOW WILL YOU KNOW WHERE TO BEGIN?

Your professional knowledge and understanding of the impairment will allow you to anticipate the resulting disability, an asset when selecting aphasia assessment tools for individual clients. With such insight, you will have the skill to choose from a variety of tools available to help you with your task of assessing a particular disability. Your selection will be based on the model of aphasia that you decide to endorse as you become familiar with the aphasia literature. Remember to share your insights about the disability with your client and the involved family.

You might suggest to the family that Mrs. F. may be able to talk more easily with only one person at a time rather than try to deal with three "competitors."

Because a great deal hinges on your assessment of aphasia, you should view the process as a problem-solving activity. To do so you will need to ask a series of questions. The answers will paint a picture of your client for you, including the nature of her language disorder, the coping strategies that she uses, and her adjustment to the change in her language status. The picture you will get will depend on the questions you have asked and answered during your assessment.

You may use these results to resolve a series of management issues. A primary concern frequently is, "Does this individual have aphasia?" If the answer to this question is "Yes," follow up with questions such as, "How does the aphasia explain her behavior? What does the future hold for her? Are rehabilitation efforts recommended? What should the focus of rehabilitation efforts be?"

To answer the question "Does she have aphasia?" it is helpful to contrast her current skill levels with her premorbid language skill level (before brain damage was experienced). The difference between premorbid abilities and status on examination helps you decide if a diagnosis of aphasia is justifiable. A description of premorbid abilities is seldom, if ever, available. Therefore, you will need to estimate her past performance abilities. To do so, it is helpful to consider the individual's education and vocational history. Reductions in the levels of understanding and production of language in the oral, written, and gestural modalities are consistent with the diagnosis of aphasia. With any individual with aphasia, all modalities such as listening, speaking, reading, and writing will not be equally affected. Some modalities will be more impaired than others. An important point here is that it is rare to find one modality completely spared. If your assessment is sensitive enough, you will demonstrate that each modality has been affected by brain injury in some way.

Mr. A. refuses to attend the weekly meeting of his men's club. "Nobody talks to me anymore."

WHAT WILL YOU WANT TO KNOW ABOUT THE INDIVIDUAL AS YOU BEGIN?

The change in an individual's level of performance from premorbid levels depends on many factors, all of which you need to understand. First, these factors include characteristics specific to the brain damage, itself. Second, you need to consider characteristics unique to the individual who experiences the brain lesion. Finally, the responses to all of an individual's communication efforts by those in the person's environment are key features in determining recovery.

Characteristics of Brain Damage

Characteristics of the brain damage have implications for the pattern and severity of the resulting aphasia. Three characteristics will be discussed more specifically: type of brain damage, location of brain damage, and size of lesion.

Type of Brain Damage

The nature of the lesion has implications for the type of brain damage. The causes most frequently associated with aphasia are cerebrovascular accidents (CVAs), traumas, neoplasms in the brain (brain tumors), or infections.

There are two primary types of CVAs (strokes), which disrupt blood flow to brain tissue. With a *hemorrhagic stroke*, the patient experiences a rupture of a cerebral vessel and blood escapes into the surrounding tissue. Because improved function must await reabsorption of the blood in the tissue, the patient with the hemorrhagic stroke is slower to regain function than the patient who experiences an *ischemic stroke*. An ischemic stroke is characterized by an interruption, or blockage, of the blood supply to an area of the brain. For the patient with an ischemic stroke, recovery begins as the cerebral swelling (edema) subsides and blood flow to undamaged tissue is restored. Both hemorrhagic and ischemic strokes are acute events. The common term "stroke" well describes the sudden impact that these CVAs have on the patient's life.

Assessment of language behavior in an individual with a head injury may reveal impairment of mental functioning from traumatic brain injury (TBI). A more thorough discussion of TBI may be found in Chapter 13. TBI is secondary to "stroke" as a common cause of sudden onset aphasia. A non-penetrating head injury (closed head injury) leaves brain coverings (meninges) intact. These tissues protect the parenchyma (functional tissue) of the brain from invasion by foreign substances. The individual with a penetrating head injury (open head injury) has a fractured or perforated skull with torn or lacerated meninges. As a result, in addition to the swelling, bruising, and tearing that may occur with any head injury, foreign substances such as hair, skin, bone fragments, dirt, bacteria, and organic material may be introduced into the brain and result in infection. Because of damage to the brain and the resulting change in function, the individual may experience aphasia.

Slower, more insidious neurologic events gradually disrupt the central nervous system. Slow changes may allow the patient some time to adjust to, and initially to compensate for, deterioration in skills. Examples of such events are primary and secondary (metastatic) brain tumors. As the changes in skill levels become more profound, the initial compensation is

Mr. A. had a hemorrhagic stroke.

Mrs. F. experienced an ischemic stroke.

not adequate to allow the individual to continue to mask the deterioration in performance abilities as a tumor grows.

Each of these causes of brain damage present potentially different medical problems. Recovery varies, depending on the type of brain damage, the cause of the brain damage, and concomitant medical problems.

Location of Brain Damage

The specific location of brain tissue disrupted by brain damage influences behavior altered by damage. For most individuals, the damage responsible for aphasia occurs in the left hemisphere of the brain, the language-dominant hemisphere. However, the relationship between symptom and location is not as certain as had once been predicted. Brown and Perecman (1985) present a current review of theories of localization and language processing.

Size of Brain Lesion

The size of the lesion may have implications for changes in neurological behavior. A small lesion may result in "a critical hit," with no substitute for the damaged tissue likely. In some situations, other neural pathways may permit reasonable compensatory function. A large lesion may contain "critical hit" damage, but so many additional fibers may have also been damaged that other pathways cannot be expected to provide satisfactory alternative function. Larger lesions, therefore, reduce the number of brain cells available for alternative neural pathways that might be capable of providing acceptable compensatory function.

Characteristics of the Individual

An individual has certain unique characteristics that determine her response to her altered ability to execute an intended act following brain injury. Failure to think of a word, understand an instruction, or read the name on an envelope are examples of frustrations that can trigger a variety of different responses from different individuals with aphasia. You will certainly be interested in her language performance. Her responses to altered language abilities also will be of interest to you during your assessment of total performance. You probably will find that you develop an interest in her ability to cope with all of the changes caused by brain damage, not just those that are language-related. You will observe reactions that range from lack of awareness to impaired ability to attend to a task and catastrophic emotional responses.

Premorbid Language Abilities

As noted earlier, you will want to gain an appreciation of your client's premorbid language status. A good source of that information is through interviews with your client and people aware of her background. Ask about her recognition/perception of the changes in ability to communicate. Such insight, on her part, may be instrumental in determining the success of her participation in rehabilitation.

Your client's ability to recognize the need to produce and accept alternative responses may reflect past language experiences. Richer and more varied communication experiences may open more rehabilitative approaches and solutions to a variety of problems an individual is seeking to overcome. For example, more experiences with competitive situations may provide a wider selection of phrases which can be used to substitute for the word, "win." Terms such as "victory," "bull's-eye," "score," or "triumph," are meaningful alternatives for a sports fan.

During your assessment of her post-traumatic language abilities, you will have opportunities to observe examples of the strategies she uses to cope with changed abilities. As your skills increase, you will find that language behavior provides you with an opportunity to witness the strategies that she uses to deal with frustration and failure. Although tears, anger, resignation, and denial may be exhibited, she may tap other skills to compensate for an elusive word. For example, if she has maintained an active interest in continuing to expand her vocabulary, she may exhibit a wide range of techniques in selecting alternative words. She may have developed these techniques by reading in a variety of areas and conversing about a wide range of topics. She may have many synonyms available to her ("pretty" = "lovely" = "beautiful"). She may find it meaningful to search for semantic cues by exploring category relationships (furniture for sitting = chair = bench = couch). She may find that word associations provide strong cues ("I read a good _____"). You may note that she purposefully uses such techniques for self-cuing. The client with more diverse premorbid experiences may use memories of these as resources to provide additional stimulation for self-cuing.

General Physical Health

You will want to explore the health history of the individual and be sensitive to his self-perception of the relative importance of the different impaired systems with which he must attempt to cope. An individual's general physical health may dictate his overall energy level. Knowledge of physical health may reveal other conditions requiring patient attention and concern. For example, the laborer may be worried about whether he can maintain employment because of right-sided weakness and paralysis. At the same time, he may not exhibit much apparent concern about language status and may display poor motivation to attend speech therapy. Such an individual may identify weakness and coordination problems as primary limitations to continued employment. Physical therapy can address these concerns. As a result, his motivation to participate in physical therapy is relatively high compared to concentrating on speech therapy. You may also encounter the reverse scenario. The loss of verbal skill is particularly distressing for the individual accustomed to controlling his environment with his verbal skills. In view of your own academic achievement, you may find yourself identifying easily with the individual who is highly dependent on verbal skills. The skills that we believe our independence depends on are the skills that we prize most highly.

Age at the Onset of Brain Damage

An individual's age when a brain lesion is incurred can have an indirect effect on his ability to cope with the concomitant change in abilities. A characteristic of the younger brain is the potential for greater adaptability. The younger brain may be better able to compensate for impaired neural function because of vicarious functioning of undamaged areas of the brain.

Furthermore, the younger individual may be better able to deal with the experience of a change in the ability to perform a function. The more youthful client may not view the change with certainty as a "loss." Rather, it may be viewed more optimistically as a "temporary" inability while working toward recovery of functions. The age at which such attitudes prevail varies from individual to individual and from event to event.

Influence of the Environment

The attitudes expressed by others in her environment influence your client and how she addresses the changes necessitated by the aphasia and the brain damage. Her past experiences help determine the support from her family and friends. Explore these relationships. Consider her influence on the people in her environment. Be sensitive to the response of those in the environment to her needs and demands. You must recognize the environment as a dynamic, ever-fluctuating influence on her.

WHERE CAN WE GO FOR INFORMATION?

The personal history of educational, vocational, avocational, and personal experiences is revealing about the client's achievements before the injury to the brain. Experiences relevant to physical and emotional health also may provide insights into an individual's coping strategies. All of this information contributes to your assessment of the client with aphasia and your development of a plan of treatment for the disability.

Various examinations have been developed to help us assess aphasia. Various authors choose different behavioral characteristics to diagnose aphasia. A variety of formats are available to assist you with the appraisal process. Some instruments are designed to help us perform a differential diagnosis of aphasia through structured examination. A tool for differential diagnosis separates the condition from other language problems that occur in adults. Examinations developed by Goodglass and Kaplan (1983), Kertesz (1982), Porch (1981), and Schuell (1965) represent four of the more commonly used published tests for differential diagnosis. In contrast, there are instruments developed to expand or refine our descriptions of one or more specific aspects of behavior associated with aphasia. Examples of such instruments are represented by Goodglass and Kaplan (1983), McNeil and Prescott (1978), and LaPointe and Horner (1979).

Different examinations have varying definitions for assessing "mild" versus "severe" aphasia. They differ in the training necessary to correctly score and evaluate the procedures. Many experienced clinicians use a variety of instruments, selected on requirements of their work facility or their perception of the needs of a given client. Some professionals report that they do not administer all tests in their entirety, but select portions based on the clinicians' perceptions of clients' strengths. As you develop a personal model of language functioning, you will find specific instruments of value to you in the assessment process.

It is not my purpose in this chapter to direct you to any one examination or model of aphasia. Rather, I hope to encourage you to read widely in the literature about aphasia and to search critically among the instruments available for use in assessment. Extensive chapters and books by authors with somewhat different views on aphasia are available. A sample of relevant resources is presented in Additional Readings at the end of this chapter.

Obtaining a Discourse Sample

Common features exist among the available tests. Discourse samples provide valuable data. These can be obtained through a conversational interview, probe questions, or requests for picture descriptions. The productivity of these instruments varies, depending on the stimulus questions or visual stimuli used and your sensitivity in posing appropriate probe questions. A discourse sample is of value early in your contact with your client because it gives you the opportunity to observe how she uses language to communicate, how she reacts to deficits and errors, and how she attends to the task. As you listen to her, you will become aware of word retrieval errors and her reactions to them when she is aware of errors. The fluency with which she is able to produce verbal efforts and her response to her changed patterns of fluency enrich your knowledge about your client. Your observations will help you plan the future course of the assessment.

Auditory Comprehension

Before responses to auditory stimuli can be evaluated, auditory sensitivity must be ensured and, if questioned, must be documented by an audiologist.

Once you have a reliable means of presenting the stimulus material to your client, a variety of tools are available for assessment of auditory comprehension. Stimuli range from individual words and short sentences to single and multistep commands and paragraphs. Errors in response to auditory stimuli may be noted when the stimuli are increased in complexity or length, or when sequences must be responded to in order.

Because there is some redundancy in most longer verbal units, the brain-injured client may be able to compensate for what she does not actually hear. Her ability to predict what you are saying relieves her of some of the responsibility of hearing and understanding you. A task requiring that she hear and comprehend every element of the stimulus to respond accurately provides you with a powerful assessment instrument. Various versions of the Token Test (such as McNeil & Prescott, 1978) have this reputation.

Because a task or subtest has been designated as one with a specific purpose, clinicians sometimes cannot recognize other client problem(s) with stimulus materials that may be ignored. For instance, an individual with aphasia may be asked to attend to a visual array of pictured nouns and select an item named by the examiner. The correct response is assumed to indicate good auditory comprehension skills at a single-word level. Frequently, an error response is then interpreted as reduced auditory comprehension when, in fact, your client's vision may be impaired and the stimuli are not easily visible. Therefore, careful assessors must always check that basic perceptual abilities of hearing and vision are intact.

Visual/Reading Comprehension

Before responses to visual materials can be evaluated, visual acuity must be ensured.

Oral Expression

Before you evaluate oral responses you must complete a speech evaluation to satisfy yourself that you appropriately identify problems of speech sound production, articulation, apraxia of speech, or dysarthria. You do not want to confuse such errors with oral language errors.

Oral language may reveal variations from predicted performances. You should be aware of a client's difficulty in word retrieval. Note what type of cues assist in retrieval of a word and if your client spontaneously self-cues. Such observations are helpful in planning future remediation.

"I know what I want to say but I can't think of the word."

You may observe that she has difficulty producing words in correct syntactic order. Sentences may be agrammatical or she may be able to produce words easily, yet the combinations of words result in meaningless utterances. She may produce near-normal attempts at language, but lack the ability to produce the specific words that give meaning to sentences, "I drive over the side is wrong." Pronouns frequently are in error and contribute to listener confusion, "On Mother's Day, I forgot to send him pretties, but she knew it was O.K." On the other hand, despite multiple attempts, she may produce few words, "Ah, . . . don't remember . . . when broke." Recognize the apparent effort necessary for her to make an attempt at verbal communication. Be aware of the type of errors made.

"I went to . . . well there . . . but they were out so I didn't get some."

Written Expression

Before written responses are evaluated, any weakness of the preferred hand must be determined. The ability of your client to use visual skills to monitor attempts at writing needs to be recognized. Failure to perform an activity should be attributed to the appropriate cause. Special problems may need to be accommodated; for instance, an arm may need to be supported, a larger pencil may make a necessary grip possible, or better light may need to be provided. The written modality provides a window that is sensitive to language problems. Writing skills are learned late and, for many individuals, are infrequently practiced. Therefore, writing appears to be vulnerable to disruption by brain damage. Analysis of written efforts is another important rationale for attempting to acquire some appreciation of premorbid skill performance. Your client's attempts to translate verbal attempts into a written modality provide you with valuable observations.

Assessment of Functional Communication

Although there is growing appreciation of the need to assess the functional communication needs and abilities of an aphasic individual, there is, now, no standard test generally accepted as a satisfactory tool for such an assessment. In part, this is because clinicians value different windows for looking at the disorder. As I have noted, some look at language processes. Others value the ability of the individual with aphasia to achieve communication with any compensatory strategy at the individual's disposal.

Frattali (1992) has written that "functional communication is the ability to receive a message or convey a message, regardless of the mode, to communicate effectively and independently in a given environment" (p. 64). The recognition by the health care community of the need for functional assessment and the pressure for such assessments by public policy mandate foretells the demand for functional assessment as a supplement to the traditional aphasia test batteries. You will need to stay abreast of assessment tool developments to meet this demand in your professional life.

Let's consider two clients. Your assessments of both Mrs. Fraizer and Mr. Andrews confirm initial hypotheses of aphasia. Mrs. Fraizer had an ischemic stroke and began to show almost immediate recovery of language functions. She demonstrated good self-awareness of errors, allowing her to self-monitor speech/language production. She was frequently able to provide necessary cuing to facilitate self-correction of errors. Her local family was very supportive. An out-of-state daughter profited from encouragement to allow her mother to perform as independently as the client was capable.

Mr. Andrews had suffered a hemorrhagic stroke. For the several weeks he was severely impaired, he withdrew from verbal interactions and rejected attempts to assess his disability. As he became able to participate in assessment activities, he displayed little awareness of language comprehension deficits.

As both of these vignettes illustrate, one assessment does not adequately portray the aphasic individual with whom you are working. The changing influence of family and improvement affected by neurological recovery and the rehabilitation program, as well as the emotional state of the individual with aphasia, necessitates reevaluation or expanded evaluations at a number of points during the course of your interaction with an individual with aphasia. Such evaluations may confirm impressions of improvement or lack of improvement. Ongoing assessment may provide information to redirect rehabilitation efforts or terminate treatment. Reevaluation allows you to maintain current and relevant records about the performance of your client.

THE END OF THE STORY OR AN ALTERNATIVE ENDING?

It is time to summarize what you have learned in your assessment. Are the observed and tested behaviors consistent with the diagnosis of aphasia? Be sure to record the dates of assessment. Describe auditory comprehension, reading comprehension, oral expression, written expression, and compare performance on each of these behaviors, providing available normative data. Give recommendations about needs for further assessment and suggestions for future rehabilitation goals.

SUMMARY

This chapter has described aphasia, an acquired disorder that affects the ability to comprehend and produce language, secondary to damage to the brain. The client is evaluated at three levels: the impairment, the disability, and the handicap. I emphasize that your role is to facilitate the interaction of clients with you, the entire treatment team, society defined as the family, service providers, policy makers, and the voting and tax-paying public.

In the case of any aphasic client, information about the brain damage, the manner in which she or he is responding to diminished abilities, and status of language behavior are all important. Before you begin to assess language performance, you are encouraged to gain an appreciation of the client's underlying, premorbid abilities in auditory sensitivity, visual acuity, manual dexterity, and speech production. Specifically, as you progress to evaluation of language performance, you need to make maximal use of a discourse sample and to evaluate auditory comprehension, visual/reading comprehension, oral expression, and written expression. Careful assessment of functional communication abilities is important; you are encouraged to continue to monitor our field's increasing sophistication in this area. Finally, I emphasize the potential value of test-retest information to document improvement (or lack of it) to direct rehabilitation efforts or to terminate treatment.

Best wishes for your pursuit of truth in assessment of aphasia.

REFERENCES

Brown, J. W., & Perecman, E. (1985). Neurological basis of language processing. In J. Darby (Ed.), *Speech and language evaluation in neurology* (pp. 45–81). New York: Grune & Stratton.

Frattali, C. M. (1992). Functional assessment of communication merging public policy with clinical views. *Aphasiology, 6,* 63–83.

Frey, W. D. (1984). Functional assessment in the 80's: A conceptual enigma, a technical challenge. In A. E. Halpern & M. J. Fuhrer (Eds.), *Functional assessment in rehabilitation* (pp. 11–43). Baltimore: P. H. Brookes.

Goodglass, H., & Kaplan, E. (1983). *Boston Diagnostic Aphasia Examination* (BDAE). Malvern, PA: Lea & Febinger.

Goodglass, H., & Kaplan, E. (1983). *Boston Naming Test.* Malvern, PA: Lea & Febinger.

Kertesz, A. (1982). *Western Aphasia Battery.* Orlando, FL: Grune & Stratton.

LaPointe, L. L., & Horner, J. (1979). *Reading Comprehension Battery for Aphasia.* Tigard, OR: CC Publications.

McNeil, M. R., & Prescott, T. E. (1978). *Revised Token Test.* Baltimore: University Park Press.

Porch, B. E. (1981). *Porch Index of Communicative Ability* (3rd ed.). Palo Alto, CA: Consulting Psychologists Press.

Schuell, H. (1965). *The Minnesota Test for Differential Diagnosis of Aphasia.* Minneapolis: University of Minnesota Press.

RECOMMENDED READINGS

Brookshire, R. H. (1992). *An introduction to neurogenic communication disorders* (4th ed.). St. Louis: Mosby-Year Book.

Darley, F. (1979). *Aphasia.* Philadelphia: W. B. Saunders.

Helm-Estabrooks, N., & Albert, M. (1991). *Manual of aphasia therapy.* Austin, TX: Pro-Ed.

Kitselman, Kurt P. (1985), Assessment of aphasia: Speech pathology. In J. K. Darby (Ed.), *Speech and language evaluation in neurology: Adult disorders* (pp. 216–217). Orlando, FL: Grune & Stratton.

Wertz, R. (1985). Neuropathologies of speech and language: An introduction to patient management. In D. F. Johns (Ed.), *Clinical management of neurogenic communicative disorders* (pp. 1–96). Boston: Little, Brown.

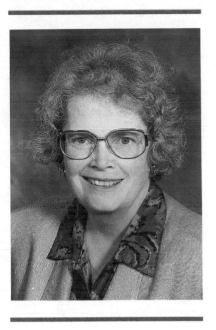

LINDA SMITH JORDAN, Ph.D.

M.A. 1964, The University of Iowa
Ph.D. 1972, The University of Iowa

Dr. Jordan is a Senior Speech Pathologist in the Department of
Neurology and Adjunct Professor in the Department of Speech
Pathology and Audiology, The University of Iowa. She has special
interests in the evaluation and treatment of patients with communication
problems related to neurogenic problems and shares these interests
through supervision of students in the clinical master's degree
program. In 1989, in recognition of her clinical skills, she was the
Iowa nominee for the Louis B. DiCarlo Award.

CHAPTER

Speech Sound Disorders

Ann Bosma Smit, Ph.D.

Difficulties in producing speech sounds can cover a very wide range, from the speech errors that are the result of a cleft palate to the severely unintelligible speech of certain deaf speakers. This chapter focuses on the types of disorders illustrated in the following examples:

- a young woman who distorts the /r/ slightly (a phonetic error). In her case, the exact nature of her distortion may be obvious only to a trained listener, and the distortion may not interfere with either her communication or her success on the job.

- a teenage boy who produces /s/ and /z/ laterally (a phonetic error). This distortion typically is a very prominent one, and it may interfere with communication by calling a listener's attention to the medium (speech) and away from the message.

- a girl in second grade who was born with cerebral palsy that resulted in weakness and incoordination of the speech production mechanism (developmental dysarthria). She communicates orally, but her speech is effortful and is intelligible only with careful listening.

Speech sound disorders — a very diverse set

- a man who has suffered a cerebral vascular accident (CVA, stroke) resulting in significant weakness in the oral and laryngeal systems. The stroke

179

has left him able to produce speech only with great difficulty (adult-onset dysarthria). The speech he can produce is obviously labored and is very difficult to understand.

- a boy entering preschool who is extremely reluctant to talk and whose speech is virtually unintelligible to listeners who are not familiar with him because of many systematic errors, such as omitting sounds (phonological disorder). His speech is surprisingly effortful, and he appears to use very short utterances, although his comprehension of complex commands appears to be intact (possible developmental verbal apraxia).

These examples illustrate that we can have speech sound production disorders for a number of reasons: failure to learn the sound system of the language (phonological problems), difficulties making the necessary movements because of neuromotor impairments (dysarthria), difficulties with sequencing the movements needed to produce speech sounds (apraxia), or difficulties producing the sounds of speech due to other structural problems (such as cleft palate). Some of these difficulties are discussed in greater detail in other chapters of this book.

Each of the above-mentioned clients provides an example of one of the traditional diagnostic groupings, which are based on what we understand the etiological (causal) factors to be. These diagnostic groups can occur in relatively pure forms, such as a dysarthria without complications of hearing loss, aphasia, or loss of intelligence. However, as a speech-language pathologist, you will more often find that the client exhibits one or more complicating factors. For example, a child who simplifies many words by leaving out sounds may also have mild oral-motor difficulties and/or difficulties in speech perception, and/or general difficulty in language use.

The range of severity that may be found in clients with disorders of spoken communication is very wide, ranging from mild to profound. And the degree to which the disability is handicapping also varies considerably.

As the speech-language pathologist who must assess the communication abilities of these clients, your challenge is to determine the scope of each client's speech sound difficulties, which potential etiological factors are involved, to determine the likely effects of this communication disability, and the prognosis (outlook) for change with and without intervention and then to make recommendations concerning treatment and referrals to other professionals as needed.

A FRAMEWORK FOR DIAGNOSIS

The starting point for our diagnosis of a client is a set of concepts that describe levels of functioning. These concepts were introduced in Chapter 1, and they include *impairment, disability,* and *handicap.* Briefly, *impairment* is the loss or abnormality of any function or structure that we think is basic to normal speech sound production. Many potential impairments appear to have a causal relationship to impaired speech sound production. For example, weak oral musculature would represent a type of impairment, as would difficulties in speech perception.

Impairment/disability/
handicap

At another level, we find *disability*, which is a reduction in the ability to communicate effectively using speech sounds. Disability can refer to completely unintelligible speech. Disability can also refer to intelligible but obviously defective speech.

Finally, the term *handicap* represents the effect that the disability has on a person's life. For example, a stroke resulting in severe dysarthria is handicapping for a woman whose speech is so unintelligible that very few persons understand her. She is at a disadvantage because she has trouble making her wants, needs, and ideas known. Less severe difficulties also can be handicapping, as in the case of a third-grader whose classmates tease him about his babyish speech.

As a practical matter, speech-language pathologists usually begin their evaluation with estimates of disability, and they investigate the components of that disability. They also evaluate potential sources of impairment, judge the degree to which the situation is handicapping, and determine a prognosis after evaluating prognostic indicators. At the end of the diagnostic process, they make recommendations based on all of their findings.

We can think of the diagnostic process as including five questions we need to answer:

1. **To what extent is this client limited in ability to communicate using the sounds of speech?** At this point, we are trying to estimate the *degree of disability* in oral communication, and for this task we use listener judgments, quantitative measures of connected speech, and standardized tests, as well as less formal measures.

2. **What characteristics of this client's speech and language contribute to this limitation in ability to communicate orally?** The goal of answering this question is to determine the *components of disability* in oral communication. For example, perceived unintelligibility in a young child may be related to extensive use of phonological processes, to the presence of phonetic errors, and to concomitant difficulties in voice, resonance, prosody, or fluency. The content, form, and use of the child's language may also be related to the overall disability.

3. **For this particular client, what potentially related variables are evident?** This question looks at *impairment of function*. Such impairment may be present if the client has chronic otitis media, if the status of the speaking mechanism is compromised, if cognitive and language abilities are reduced, if there is a history of medical difficulties, or if there is a history of abuse or neglect.

4. **To what extent is the difficulty in oral communication likely to have psychosocial, educational, or vocational consequences?** When we explore this question, we are estimating the *degree of handicap* experienced by our client. To do this, we might use the reports of parents, teachers, and significant others in the client's environment, as well as our own judgment of the degree of handicap.

5. **What positive and negative prognostic indicators characterize this client?** To answer this question about *prognosis*, we may use information from the client's medical, developmental, and psychosocial his-

Handicap: "Aw, don't listen to him. He still says *wabbit!*"

tory. We may examine the client's response to stimulability tasks, and we may also evaluate variability of errors.

Our Goal — The Comprehensive Diagnostic Statement

The goal of our evaluation is to develop a comprehensive statement in terms of the answers to the questions we have asked. We assume that all relevant factors will be mentioned in our statement. Furthermore, the statement will be followed by recommendations, and we assume that the recommendations will address all factors for which we are able to initiate change.

Of course, we will cover some areas of this evaluation in greater depth than others, depending on the traditional diagnostic category our client falls into. When we are evaluating an adult who has had an injury resulting in the neuromotor difficulties we call dysarthria, we will certainly assess his respiration and phonation in considerable detail. In the case of a young child whose speech sound difficulties have no known etiology, we most likely would assess respiration and phonation in only a cursory way, but we would spend a large portion of our assessment time documenting her patterns of speech sound use.

AN EXPANDED VIEW OF DIAGNOSIS

Estimating the Degree of Disability

As we begin to think about the ways in which we might assess disability, it is important to remember that many aspects of communication may be affected *by* the speech sound difficulties or *in addition to* the speech sound difficulties. These aspects all combine to produce a communication disability. We also need to keep in mind that disability includes not only difficulty in conveying a linguistic message, but it can also refer to speech that is obviously defective or distorted, although still understandable. In such cases the speech draws undesirable attention to itself — attention that may even interfere with communication of a message.

To estimate the degree of disability in oral communication, we may use one or another *index* (indicator) of the client's ability to communicate using speech (Figure 8–1). These indexes may be estimates of intelligibility (how understandable the client is), or they may be estimates of perceived severity or defectiveness. We may use categorical scales ("speech is intelligible only to familiar persons") or we might decide to use a percentage scale ("the client's speech was judged to be intelligible about 75% of the time"). Finally, we can use equal-interval rating scales that are anchored at both ends ("on a scale of 1 to 6, with 1 being most intelligible and 6 being least intelligible, the intelligibility of this client's speech was ranked 3").

Global Listener Judgments of Disability

Listener judgments are of two types. In the first, a person in a child's everyday environment, perhaps a parent, makes an estimate of how much is un-

Our goal: A comprehensive diagnostic statement

Using descriptive categories*

Sound errors are occasionally noticed in continuous speech.

Speech is intelligible although noticeably in error.

Speech is intelligible with careful listening.

Speech intelligibility is difficult.

Speech usually is unintelligible.

Speech is unintelligible.

Using percents (Example)

"Speech was estimated to be about 80% intelligible if context was known, and about 50% intelligible if context was not known."

Using a scale with equal-appearing intervals

Normal speech   1   2   3   4   5   6   Most severely disordered speech

*Categories taken from Fudala (1970)

Figure 8-1. Some indexes that describe the degree of deficit as reflected in intelligibility or severity ratings.

derstood in that environment. Or we may ask that person to estimate how limited the client is in her ability to communicate in daily living. The second type of listener judgment of disability is made by the clinician. It may be based on taped or face-to-face conversational samples. These judgments may use either numerical rating scales or categorical scales.

Global listener judgments, especially those made by parents or close associates of the client, have very high face validity because they are derived from the client's life and reflect her ability to communicate on a daily basis. A global judgment made by the clinician also has considerable validity, because it usually reflects how the client communicates with someone who has no previous acquaintance with her.

Incidentally, it is important to attend to a parent who tells you that no one, not even the parent, readily understands a child whom you are evaluating. Lack of intelligibility is one of the most important criteria used to determine how urgent it is that a child receive intervention services. Certainly, the child who is unintelligible and who cannot make her wants and needs known is seriously handicapped.

Ability to communicate in the everyday world

Quantitative Measures of Disability in Speech Sound Production

The speech-language pathologist has a number of ways to quantify intelligibility or severity of speech difficulty. Some of these measures are based on a recorded conversational speech sample. One measure that is often used to quantify intelligibility is the percentage of words that the transcriber can understand or figure out. A well-known measure used to quantify severity in children with phonological disorders is the percentage of consonants that are correct (Shriberg & Kwiatkowski, 1982). In the assessment of dysarthria caused by brain damage, you might want to use a multifactori-

Several ways to measure degree of disability

al index of the efficiency of communication that looks at both accuracy of consonants and rate of speech (Yorkston & Beukelman, 1981b).

There are other ways to quantify intelligibility and severity besides those based on taped conversational samples. For example, there are numerous published tests that the clinician can use to assess speech formally, such as the *Goldman-Fristoe Test of Articulation* (Goldman & Fristoe, 1986) or the *Assessment of Phonological Processes* (Hodson, 1986). Most formal tests require the client to name pictures or objects while the clinician transcribes the client's production of specific target phonemes in each word. Most such tests result in a total score or a standard score that can be compared to normative data (at least for children). The degree to which a child does not meet the norms for his age group is an index of severity of disability. In the assessment of adult dysarthria, there is a well-known procedure for presenting randomly chosen word lists and sentence frames for the client to produce (Yorkston & Beukelman, 1981a). Judges who do not know the specific words the client is producing then try to write down what the client said. The resulting score can then be compared with typical performance, which is ordinarily 100% intelligible.

The types of quantitative measures discussed here have less face validity than global listener judgments because they allow the clinician plenty of processing time, and because these measures usually are based on word-by-word transcriptions or glosses. However, these measures are used because they appear to be accurate measures of severity or intelligibility, because they appear to be related to the global measures, and because they are sensitive measures to use in evaluating change in a client's speech over time. Moreover, such measures can provide valuable information that cannot be obtained from global measures. For example, formal tests typically sample all the consonants in English, not just the consonants the client chooses to attempt in a conversational sample, so that the speech-language pathologist obtains a more complete picture of the client's sound system.

Determining the Components of Disability

Components of disability are aspects of spoken communication that contribute directly to disability. For example, in a preschool child, the presence of many error patterns may make a large contribution to unintelligibility. In an adult with dysarthria, labored speech with weak articulator contacts may be the primary contributor to perceived severity of the client's speech. Other components may not be related specifically to articulatory production but to voice, resonance, prosody, or fluency. Finally, language (content, form, and/or use) may contribute to disability. For example, an adolescent with phonological errors may also show pragmatic errors by shifting from topic to topic with little warning to the conversational partner. These abrupt shifts in topic contribute to the listener's judgment that intelligibility is reduced.

The ways in which we assess the components of disability vary, depending somewhat on the traditional diagnostic grouping in which our client fits. Sometimes we simply screen in one area by listening carefully to the client; for other clients we may need to do an extensive evaluation.

Screening in some areas, extensive evaluation in others

Nevertheless, every evaluation should include attention to the client's articulation or phonology (or both), prosody, voice, resonance, fluency, and language (content, form, and use).

Components of Disability: Articulation and Phonology

When a client is referred for evaluation because of poor intelligibility or because of obvious phonetic errors (distortions), we expect to evaluate this area extensively. If the client has many consonant substitutions, or if she appears to distort specific speech sounds, we may well administer one of the published tests of speech sound production and report the nature of the errors. We would also tape a conversational sample to determine the nature of the errors in conversation and to determine the frequency of occurrence of those errors.

When young children have poor speech intelligibility, we expect them to exhibit many of the phonological processes that we know are typical of unintelligible speech. We can think of these typical phonological processes as patterns of speech sound errors. For example, a child might omit all final consonants in words, or the child might produce most velar consonants as alveolars. For such children, we would use both formal tests of phonology and our analysis of a conversational sample. From these two kinds of observations, we can derive several inventories, generate a list of phonological processes the child uses, and determine whether any of the child's productions are unusual or idiosyncratic. (This approach is similar to the one outlined in Stoel-Gammon & Dunn, 1985, Chapters 4-6.)

The most important inventory is the phonetic inventory, which is a listing of all the different sounds a child uses in two or more positions in words, regardless of what the adult target sounds are. For example, Sammy, a child of 3 years, 1 month has the phonetic inventory shown in Table 8-1, which includes ɸ (this symbol is called *phi*, and it represents a voiceless bilabial fricative).

Sammy's phonetic inventory is extremely restricted and is comparable to that of a child of about 18 months. Sammy uses only one final consonant, no clusters, and very few fricatives, all of which should have been attempted by age 3, although these elements are not always correct at that age. It is obvious that Sammy has very little flexibility in attempting to say the words of his language, which contain a much greater variety of sounds.

Table 8-1. Sammy's phonetic inventory of consonants.

Initial		Final
w		
m	n	m
p	b	
t	d	
ɸ	f	

Note: ɸ is a voiceless bilabial fricative.

The second inventory we might construct is called a phonemic inventory, in which we examine what the child does for each adult phoneme target. A part of Sammy's phonemic inventory is shown in Table 8-2. Table 8-2 shows us that even in this small part of the phonemic inventory, Sammy collapses a number of adult distinctions. For example, he uses [t] for both adult /t/ and adult /k/. And he does not use most final consonants, so that there is the potential for many of his words to be homophones (words that sound the same). For example, his version of *bath* and *bat* would sound the same: [bæ].

Our third inventory is a listing of all the word shapes used by the child, using C to stand for consonants and V for vowels. In Sammy's case, the word shape inventory is extremely limited: V, CV, CVm, CVCV. In contrast, the English language has a much larger variety of word shapes, including clusters and multisyllabic words.

The last inventory in our analysis is the list of phonological processes the child is using. There are many ways to do this, including formal tests, formalized analyses of conversational speech, and computerized analyses. Typically, the speech-language pathologist looks for regularities in the pattern of errors. Many test forms and analysis systems are arranged to facilitate such a search. For example, in Figure 8-2 you can see portions of two formal tests that facilitate your search for patterns of errors. One of these, the SHAPE, also provides a computer-assisted procedure to determine phonological processes used.

Identifying phonological
processes

You can also determine phonological processes without using a formal test instrument — you can simply examine the phonemic inventory you have prepared. For example, even in the small portion of Sammy's phonetic inventory, shown in Table 8-2, it is possible to identify phonological processes very easily: Sammy is obviously using the processes of fronting

Table 8-2. A portion of Sammy's phonemic inventory.

Initial		Final	
Adult Target	Sammy's Version	Adult Target	Sammy's Version
w	w		
m	m	m	m ~ ø
n	n	n	ø
ŋ	ŋ	ŋ	ø
b	b	b	ø
t	t	t	ø
d	d	d	ø
k	t	k	ø
g	d	g	ø
f	Φ ~ f	f	ø
v	b	v	ø

Notes: Φ is a voiceless bilabial fricative, ø is the null (omission) symbol, and ~ means "alternates with."

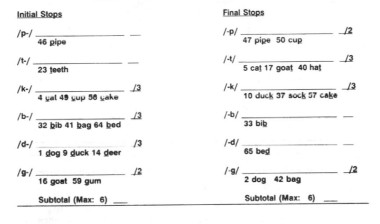

Bankson-Bernthal Test of Phonology

Phonological Process Inventory

Assimilation	Fronting	Final Consonant Deletion	Weak Syllable Deletion	Stopping	Gliding	Cluster Simplification	Depalatal-ization	Deaffrication	Vocalization
tæt tæ	tæ	kæ tæ							
det tet gek	de det	ge de							
	tʌp tʌ	kʌ tʌ							
	tændi					kæni kædi			
gɔg dɔd	dɔt	dɔ							
		be							
		bo							
dot do		go do							
gʌŋ	dʌn dʌ	gʌ dʌ							
	tau								
		kræ				twæb kwæb kæb tæb fræb			

Target Word/ Phonetic Transcription	Word Correct	Transcription of Child's Production	Modeled
1. cat kæt	☐	____	☐
2. gate get	☐	____	☐
3. cup kʌp	☐	____	☐
4. candy kændi	☐	____	☐
5. dog dɔg	☐	____	☐
6. bed bed	☐	____	☐
7. boat bot	☐	____	☐
8. goat got	☐	____	☐
9. gun gʌn	☐	____	☐
10. cow kaʊ	☐	____	☐
11. crab kræb	☐	____	☐

Smit-Hand Articulation and Phonology Evaluation

Initial Stops

/p-/ _____ —
   46 pipe

/t-/ _____ —
   23 teeth

/k-/ _____ /3
   4 cat 49 cup 56 cake

/b-/ _____ /3
   32 bib 41 bag 64 bed

/d-/ _____ /3
   1 dog 9 duck 14 deer

/g-/ _____ /2
   16 goat 59 gum

Subtotal (Max: 6) ___

Final Stops

/-p/ _____ /2
   47 pipe 50 cup

/-t/ _____ /3
   5 cat 17 goat 40 hat

/-k/ _____ /3
   10 duck 37 sock 57 cake

/-b/ _____ —
   33 bib

/-d/ _____ —
   65 bed

/-g/ _____ /2
   2 dog 42 bag

Subtotal (Max: 6) ___

Figure 8-2. Excerpts from two examples of formal tests that assist the clinician in determining which phonological processes the child uses. In the first example, the **BBTOP** (*Bankson-Bernthal Test of Phonology*, Bankson & Bernthal, 1990), each target word is placed next to a grid showing the kind of error that each relevant process would represent. In the second example, the **SHAPE** (*Smit-Hand Articulation and Phonology Evaluation*, Smit & Hand, in press) is an analysis form that helps the clinician arrange the data so that multiple examples of the same sound are together and so that members of the major sound classes are listed together. This facilitates the finding of patterns of errors.

(producing velars as alveolars) and final consonant deletion (omitting all final consonants except /m/).

    Our final step is to determine if any of the processes or characteristics of a child's production are unusual or idiosyncratic. For example, Sammy's use of [ɸ] as an alternate to [f] is quite unusual. We can assume that unusual phonetic or phonological processes persisting beyond a few weeks suggest that the child has taken a wrong turn on the path to adult-like phonology.

When we are assessing the speech of clients from diverse cultural and dialect groups, we need to be careful to sort out which aspects of communication are within normal limits for the client's dialect or language group, and which represent disorder or delay. For example, although /r/ is pronounced in Standard English everywhere it occurs, there are several dialects of English in which /r/ occurring at the end of a word can be pronounced as a vowel, as in /fɔə/ (*four*); these dialects include Vernacular Black English, Bostonian dialect, and Southern dialect. Furthermore, in the United States there are many people whose English is influenced by a first language, such as Spanish or Chinese. Like Vernacular Black English, these variants of English may differ from Standard English in quite systematic ways, especially with respect to consonant systems. Consequently, a characteristic that would be considered an error in Standard English may be typical of the language of the client's community.

On the other hand, we must be careful that we attribute only appropriate features of a client's speech to dialect or language background, so that we do not miss real delay or disorder. And for children, the whole picture is sometimes complicated by competing demands that the child's speech fit into the community mold for social reasons and into the "school" mode (closer to Standard English) for educational reasons. Needless to say, this area of practice can become politicized; nevertheless, the focus must remain on the communication needs of the client.

Components of Disability: Other Speech Factors

Problems with speech sound production often coexist with other speech or language deviations, and these other deviations can make their own contribution to a communication disability. Deviations in prosody (stress, rate, intonation, and use of pauses) often are present with speech sound disorders, especially in clients whom we suspect have a verbal apraxia (difficulty sequencing the movements of speech). At present there are standard ways to transcribe stress patterns of words and to determine rate of speech, but there are no commonly used ways to transcribe or evaluate sentence intonation contours. However, the clinician should pay attention to whether the client marks the ends of declarative clauses or sentences with downward inflection, whether intonation contours and pauses correspond to syntactic units and questions, and whether emphatic statements carry appropriate intonation contours.

Other components of communication disability include voice, resonance, fluency, and language ability. Each of these topics is discussed in detail elsewhere in this book. However, we need to be aware that each of these factors can contribute to perceived unintelligibility, perceived severity, or both.

Determination of Potentially Related Impairments

There are many factors that may be related to the presence of speech sound disorders in persons who do not have any obvious physical difficulties of the oral mechanism. Some of these variables may bear a causative relationship to speech sound disorders; others possibly predispose the client to develop a disorder if other factors are present. Potentially related variables include the status of the hearing mechanism; perceptual abilities; integrity of the respiratory, laryngeal, and oral systems; status of general cognitive abilities; and the general health of the client. Potentially related variables also include the presence or absence of behavioral difficulties and the developmental history of the individual, including any hospitalizations. Interestingly, language ability may represent not only a component of a perceived disability, but it may also represent a potentially related factor, because language difficulties suggest a general problem in symbol use.

As a speech-language pathologist you need to be aware that sometimes we are very limited in what we can deduce about how variables may be related to speech sound disorders. For example, if we attempt to assess speech perception and the client performs very well on the test we have chosen, it is appropriate to say the client's speech perception skills are excellent (assuming a valid test). However, if the client performs poorly, we must be more cautious in our statements, because tests of speech perception are notoriously subject to confounding variables. In such cases there is always the possibility that we have simply not been clever enough to find a way to let the client show us her skills.

Many impairments influence speech sound production

Potential Impairments: The Auditory Mechanism

Severe-to-profound hearing loss has an obvious causal relationship to speech difficulties of persons who are deaf. In addition, mild-to-moderate hearing loss, past or present, and a history of otitis media may predispose a child to develop phonological delay or disorder, but probably not to develop the well-known characteristics of "deaf speech." Some discussions of these groups are presented in Chapters 17 and 18.

Potential Impairments: The Oral Mechanism

Obvious defects in the oral mechanism, such as cleft palate, clearly are related to characteristic speech errors, such as nasal emission on consonants. Other structural deviations, such as a very high hard palate, are not known to be related to any speech difficulties.

More important than minor structural deviations is the neuromotor integrity of the speech mechanism. Recent evidence suggests that subtle deficiencies in oral strength and coordination may be related to developmental verbal apraxia, a severe-to-profound impairment of speech in children. It is certainly possible that mild oral-motor impairment may be related to less severe phonological difficulties as well. Finally, in both adults and children we would want to note the presence of any groping movements of the articulators, because of their known relationship to apraxia of speech. See Chapters 4, 9, and 14 for more information about these relationships.

Potential Impairments: Speech Perception

It is intuitively appealing to assume that a client's ability to discriminate speech and categorize speech sounds is critical to accurate speech production; however, this statement is probably true only for clients whose errors are not developmental. That is, current research findings suggest that in young children, speech perception and production skills may develop in parallel. Unfortunately, even in older clients, speech perception is notoriously difficult to test without interference from other variables. Consequently, as was indicated earlier, it is much more difficult to interpret errors in performance than it is to interpret good performance. For example, if you show children a set of four pictures, such as *bee, beet, bead*, and *bean*, and ask them to point to the one you say, even some children who say all these words accurately will make "perception" errors. Because these children do produce the words accurately, it is likely that some other variable influenced their errors in this little test.

On the other hand, there are clients who do very poorly on perception tasks and who truly do not say sounds accurately because they do not perceive them accurately. Consequently, if your client gives every indication of not being able to perceive differences in speech stimuli you present, then this client most likely will not make progress in remediation unless you provide perceptual training.

Potential Impairments: Cognitive Status

Relating phonological
development to cognitive
development

In children with developmental delay, the status of cognitive development may aid in the interpretation of the findings from your analysis of the child's phonology. For example, if Sammy's phonological status is that of an 18-month-old and his cognitive functioning is at a similar level, then Sammy may be doing as well as can be expected in phonological development. In other words, we peg phonological development to mental age rather than to chronological age.

We should note that, even if Sammy's cognitive development and phonological development are comparable, we still have obligations to Sammy (and to other children with developmental delay). First of all, we need to ensure that Sammy is communicating critical needs and wants in ways that his caregivers understand. Second, we need to counsel the caregivers to provide an environment that is rich in speech and language input, and ensure that the caregivers provide this stimulation in ways that Sammy can make use of (such as talking about the here and now, using short utterances, and using considerable repetition). Third, we need to monitor Sammy to make sure that subsequent phonological development keeps pace with other aspects of development.

Another possibility is that a child's phonological status is less developed than his cognitive status would suggest. In such cases, intervention is warranted because we assume that the child's phonology and ability to communicate can be brought up to a level commensurate with mental age.

In adults, cognitive status continues to be an important variable, whether we are dealing with developmental delay or with a cognitive deficit resulting from acquired neurological damage. In such clients, the importance of this variable lies in the area of prognosis and in determining what type of intervention we will recommend. Additional discussions of the importance of cognitive status are found in Chapters 5, 7, 13, and 16.

Potential Impairments: Language Abilities

Because a child's phonological system is one part of the larger linguistic system, we can expect interactions with other aspects of that system. For example, because there is a strong relationship between syntactic errors and severity of the phonological disorder, we expect to have to deal with both in our treatment although some studies suggest that treating just one area improves the other as well. Another language area of particular interest is the relative status of receptive versus expressive language. Many children with phonological disorders show deficits in expressive language (especially in grammar and in oral vocabulary), but they have receptive language that is within normal limits. When receptive language is better than expressive, we assume that with intervention the child eventually can achieve an expressive language and phonological level that is commensurate with her receptive language level.

Other language characteristics

On the other hand, the child with a phonological disorder who shows both receptive and expressive language delays poses a different problem. This child may be better served by making sure the child has functional communication through speech and by incorporating phonological intervention into a broader intervention for the general language deficit.

Potential Impairments: Psychosocial Factors

Both intrapersonal and interpersonal factors can have an impact on communication and on intervention. For example, clinical depression is relatively common in persons who have had a stroke affecting communication. One result of this depression is that the client may not be interested in putting forth his best effort at communication, or he may be unwilling to attempt certain diagnostic tasks.

Exploring psychosocial factors

Children with speech sound disorders only rarely show clinical depression, but other psychosocial variables are relevant to your assessment. For example, the child who is teased about speech or who experiences considerable parental pressure to speak correctly may become reticent and may be reluctant to experiment with new sounds. And, of course, a child who has experienced deprivation and abuse may show any number of behavioral consequences, including impaired communication.

Potential Impairments: The Client's History

The client's medical and developmental history help us to interpret our other findings. Premature birth, especially if the baby has a very low birth weight, may be associated with subsequent delays in development. Perinatal distress or adverse events at about the time of birth, such as anoxia, may be related to a specific neuromotor impairment, or they may produce an overall delay in speech and language. If a child is slow to achieve developmental milestones such as sitting unaided, walking, and producing the first word, this suggests an overall delay, and phonological development should be evaluated accordingly. Finally, a hospitalization or severe illness in childhood may have general delaying effects.

In the case of adult-onset speaking difficulties, the nature and the extent of neurological or other impairment will influence your findings. These factors also may be important in determining a prognosis. For example, if you are evaluating a client who has multiple sclerosis (MS), and if his speech shows primarily components of incoordination, you may recommend treatment focusing on rate and stress patterns rather than on strengthening the oral musculature. At the same time, the prognosis for improvement in the client with MS must be guarded, because MS is a progressive illness.

Estimates of Handicap

Handicap: interaction of
disability with environment

The limitations in ability to communicate that we have discussed usually constitute a handicapping condition in aspects of the client's life. For example, children with speech disorders may be regarded less favorably by their peers than are children without such disorders. Or adults with cerebral palsy may believe that they are stigmatized by their speech.

The person with a speech sound disorder sometimes experiences a handicap in education. For example, the child with a severe phonological disorder may volunteer to answer a question in class, but if the teacher expects that no one in the class will understand the child, the youngster is not likely to be called on. Or the adult with an obvious speech disorder may be counseled out of certain activities or experiences.

Finally, the client may experience a handicap in choosing or pursuing a vocation. For example, a man who is the foreman in a crew of electricians may not be able to return to his former position following a stroke that leaves him dysarthric. Sometimes even a mild degree of disability may have serious vocational consequences. A woman with a lateral lisp who wants to become a courtroom lawyer will find that the lateral lisp is an obstacle to achieving her goals, although the lateral lisp is a far less severe problem than a dysarthria.

Obviously, estimates of handicap are based to a considerable degree on the judgment of the speech-language pathologist. Often the very fact that a client has been referred by someone else for evaluation suggests that a handicap exists. Sometimes sensitive questioning of the client will reveal feelings of being stigmatized or devalued because of the speech disorder.

In the early days of our profession, one of the ways in which a communication disorder was defined was this: An individual has a communication disorder if either the person or anyone in his environment thinks that he has one. We tend to neglect this definition in most of the areas covered by speech-language pathologists, except for voice and fluency disorders. However, in the area of speech sound disorders we also need to pay attention to the opinions of the client and the client's caregivers or associates. After all, it is from the client's social interactions and the reactions and opinions of others that handicap arises.

You should be aware that investigating this area sometimes poses dilemmas for us. For example, we may feel overwhelmed by the seeming callousness with which a client has been treated, apparently on the basis of having a speech sound disorder. On the one hand, we try to find ways to improve the client's speech, but on the other hand, we may wonder if our time could be spent more profitably trying to change society's attitudes about handicap. Frequently, of course, we must do both.

Evaluating Prognostic Indicators

Prognostic indicators are characteristics or factors that can influence the client's progress over time in ability to communicate. Of course, stating a prognosis is always an educated guess on our part. And because of the ethical standards of our profession, the speech-language pathologist must be careful not to promise or to be seen as promising a specific outcome. Rather, we usually make statements that many clients with certain specified characteristics achieve the predicted level of functioning.

Predicting the results of intervention

You will notice that several prognostic variables were mentioned under other sections of the evaluation. It should not be surprising to find prognostic variables mentioned in both places. If a factor represents an impairment that is implicated in delayed development or has caused a deficit, then that factor can continue to exert a negative influence unless it is alleviated or removed.

When we discuss prognosis, we usually specify the predicted outcome assuming that intervention is provided. Alternatively, we may give two prognostic statements, one assuming intervention and another assuming no intervention. In the case of a child with a phonological disorder, we may develop a prognostic statement as follows:

> The prognosis for Jimmy to become intelligible to most listeners within a 2-year period, with treatment, is good. Without treatment the prognosis is fair-to-poor.

Prognostic Indicators: Severity

One of our first prognostic considerations is the severity of the speech sound disorder. When the disorder is severe, it can affect the prognosis in two ways. First, the eventual outcome may not be as positive as it would be in the case of a mild or moderate disorder. Second, the amount of time needed to reach a particular outcome may be longer. This is not to say that a mild disorder always has an excellent prognosis; probably every practicing speech-language pathologist has experienced the frustration of working with a client with a mild disorder who did not improve much in treatment. Rather, the degree of confidence with which we can predict a limited outcome is greater when the disorder is severe.

Prognostic Indicators: Characteristics of the Client

Several personal variables can influence a projected outcome. These include motivation, consistency, stimulability or response to trial intervention, and medical, developmental, and therapeutic history.

Motivation as a Prognostic Variable. The client's motivation, or the desire to make a change, appears to be a variable that is particularly important for adults and for children beyond about 9 or 10 years of age. For younger children, we typically supply the motivation in the form of positive reinforcement and activities that keep the client's interest. In older children and adults, motivation is important, but it is also a "slippery" variable, in part because it is very much influenced by the clinician's ability to structure the treatment to provide success for the client. Motivation is also "slippery" because it depends in part on other events and conditions in the client's life. For example, the adolescent client with distorted /s z ʃ tʃ dʒ/ may have difficulty attending to treatment because his parents are at the point of divorce.

Stimulability or Response to Trial Intervention. Stimulability is the ability to improve sound production under conditions of focused stimulation. Trial intervention is a short period of treatment when the client's ability and potential to make changes are assessed. In adults, both stimulability and improvement during trial intervention are positive prognostic indicators. In young children with phonological disorders, stimulability is considered a prognostic indicator for improvement, both with and without intervention.

Variation in Production. Inconsistency and contextual variation refer to two types of variability noted in the client's spontaneous speech production. Many clients exhibit little variation in the way they produce specific targets, and we say that their errors are "consistent." However, other clients show variability or "inconsistency" in their speech. For some of these clients, there is no apparent pattern to the inconsistency. For others, we can determine that there are particular phonetic contexts in which the client usually produces an accurate sound (contextual variation). The chief value of finding these occasional correct productions is that they can provide the starting point for treatment for that target. In other words, the existence of correct variants is a mildly positive prognostic indicator.

Variation in producing the target speech sounds

Medical, Developmental, and Therapeutic History. As we discussed earlier, medical and developmental history can be important for both children and adults. If earlier medical or developmental problems continue when we see a client, we may be skeptical about the probability of improvement. However, if the condition has been resolved, the prognosis is more positive. Medical history is especially important in cases of adult-onset neurological problems. For example, a client's history of one or more chronic, serious medical conditions would suggest a relatively poor prognosis.

Therapeutic history may also be an important variable in some cases. If a client has had several years of intervention for the same speech sound difficulties that you have documented in your evaluation and has made little progress, then the prognosis for improvement with more intervention is relatively poor. The exception might be if the type of intervention the client received appears to have been inappropriate for the types of speech sound difficulties you have documented.

Other Prognostic Variables

In addition to considerations of the status of the client, there are two other areas that we explore in determining a prognosis. The first is the existence of social or familial support for the client. Children who are candidates for treatment usually live with their families or are in a foster care situation. Ordinarily, there will be support and encouragement for the child's efforts and for changes the child will be making. However, in seriously stressed or dysfunctional families, you can expect that intervention for the child may have to take a back seat to the resolution of other major difficulties in the family's life. In fact, family counseling may be one of your recommendations in such cases, because the child will not be able to make progress in communication until the family's difficulties are resolved.

Adult clients may not have family nearby, but it is a positive prognostic sign when the client clearly has the support of a social group, whether or not that group is made up of family. On the other hand, clients without such a support group will have to rely on their own internal resources and on interactions with the speech-language pathologist to support them in the work of intervention.

A second consideration is the availability of resources for the client. Resources in this case refer to the availability of services and the financial support to pay for them. If a community offers a variety of services and makes sure that they are available to all, then the client's prognosis is relatively positive. If, on the other hand, the client lives in an area where services are few and far between, and the client will not be able to get to them, the prognosis is less positive. If financial support is not available to pay for services, the clinician may try to find support for the client or may refer the client to a social worker.

Need for social support and resources

THE COMPREHENSIVE DIAGNOSTIC STATEMENT

The goal of these assessments is the development of a comprehensive diagnostic statement about the client's communication difficulties, which will include statements of how the relevant variables contribute to the chosen index of conversational speech. A logical and recommended format for this statement is:

- General diagnostic statement, including the speech-language pathologist's overall severity rating

- Estimates of disability in speech communication

- Statement of the components of the disability

- Statement of potentially related impairments

- Estimate of degree of handicap imposed by the disability

- Statement of prognosis

Statements of this sort may be titled "clinical impressions" or "clinical summaries."

The recommendations that follow the statement should address the variables for which the speech-language pathologist can initiate change. For example, if the client is a dysarthric adult and one component of the disability is a weakened respiratory system, we may refer him for further medical examination and perhaps physical therapy.

An example of such a comprehensive diagnostic statement might be this statement about Russell, a 20-year-old college freshman with a history of treatment for speech sound disorders (phonological processes). You have determined that he exhibits mild weakness in the oral musculature, and you suspect a very mild form of cerebral palsy, although no such medical diagnosis appears in his records:

Russell exhibits difficulties in speech sound production that are moderate to severe for a person of his age. He exhibits phonological process use that is typical of much younger persons, complicated by very mild oral neuromotor weakness that may have been present since birth. (GENERAL DIAGNOSTIC STATEMENT)

Russell's conversational speech is judged by the clinician to be about 80% intelligible with careful listening, and his percentage of understandable words is 87% (in a sample of 100 different words). (INDICES OF DISABILITY)

The most important components of Russell's reduced intelligibility appear to be (a) frequent omissions of sounds (deletion of final and intervocalic nasals and obstruents) in connected speech, (b) weak articulation of the sounds that are produced, together with (c) vocal intensity that is frequently inadequate (COMPONENTS OF DISABILITY). Russell exhibits very mild weakness of the mandible, lip, and tongue musculature affecting primarily the tongue tip; he also reports that his mother told him that he had feeding difficulties in the first year of life. He reports no history of otitis media or of severe illness during childhood. Hearing was screened and found to be within normal limits. Russell reports that in his college classes that do not require a speaking component, he is getting grades of B and C. (POTENTIAL RELATED IMPAIRMENTS — ARTICULATORY MUSCULATURE, AUDITORY SYSTEM, MEDICAL HISTORY, LANGUAGE, AND COGNITION)

Russell was referred to this clinic by one of his classroom instructors, and Russell himself states his concern about the effects of his speech on his ability to make friends; consequently, it appears that Russell experiences both academic and social limitations because of his speech (ESTIMATES OF HANDICAP).

The prognosis for improvement with intervention is fair. One positive indicator is that Russell is readily stimulable for improved articulatory precision and for production of all deleted consonants. Another positive indicator is that although vocal intensity in conversation is often inadequate, Russell can generate increased intensity in conversational speech with little apparent effort and can sustain it for at least 30 seconds. On the other hand, the fact that Russell has already experienced extensive intervention but has not maintained the skills he needs for adequate oral communication is a poor prognostic indicator (PROGNOSTIC STATEMENTS).

Recommendations for Russell include the following:

1. A 3-month course of trial intervention focused on strengthening articulatory contacts and on intelligible production of utterances longer than 2–3 words.

2. During this period of trial intervention, the clinician should be in communication with Russell's instructors for both monitoring and counseling purposes.

3. Russell should consult with a neurologist to confirm that the oral motor weakness is not progressive.

EMPHASES IN DIFFERENT DIAGNOSTIC GROUPS

Although this chapter has focused on the common aspects of evaluation for speech sound disorders, you should expect to tailor your evaluation to the client's general diagnostic group, while maintaining the flexibility to alter those emphases, if necessary. And, of course, you will plan a very different evaluation for a child from the one you would plan for an adult.

When a child exhibits a phonological delay or disorder, you will pay close attention to the developmental history and to the caregiver's account of the dynamics in the home relating to the child. You will plan to elicit and analyze more than one speech sample, perhaps one from conversation during a play period and another from a formalized assessment instrument. You will probably do a screening examination of the oral mechanism, in part because it is difficult to elicit certain oral movements from very young children. And because phonological disorders often coexist with language disorders, you will assess language in several domains.

Different emphases in different diagnostic groups

If the client you are assessing makes phonetic errors, such as a lateral lisp, you may plan to use a formal, published test that elicits all the consonants of English. You will assess stimulability and document any inconsistency or contextual variation. You may evaluate speech discrimination abilities. You will consider if the current status of the child's dentition or dental occlusion plays a role in the phonetic errors. Finally, because clients with phonetic errors are often children of school age, you will consider issues of motivation and social support.

When your client appears to have a verbal apraxia, your evaluation will include an emphasis on detailed examination of the functioning of the oral mechanism, as well as on the characteristics of client's speech. You will carefully evaluate prosody. If the client uses gesture extensively, you will document that. In the case of children, you will want to know if the child has previously had treatment and what the results were.

If your client is dysarthric, you will concentrate on an appraisal of the speech and respiratory mechanisms, as well as the client's speech characteristics. Prosody is an important variable. Medical history is also very important, in part because it will document the location and extent of any brain damage, and in part because it is important in determining a prognosis.

SUMMARY

This chapter has provided you with a framework for your evaluations of persons who have speech sound disorders. The range of speech sound disorders is very large, perhaps the largest of any of the communication disorders that we study. Nevertheless, the same principles are appropriate for each: describe the disability and its components, estimate the extent to which the disability is handicapping, determine the components of that disability, investigate potentially related variables or impairments, determine a prognosis, and make appropriate recommendations. Now it is up to you, the speech-language pathologist, to flesh out the framework for your own evaluation of an individual client.

REFERENCES

Bankson, N. W., & Bernthal, J. E. (1990). *Bankson-Bernthal Test of Phonology.* San Antonio: Special Press.

Goldman, R., & Fristoe, M. (1986). *Goldman-Fristoe Test of Articulation.* Circle Pines, MN: American Guidance Service.

Fudala, J. B. (1970). *Arizona Articulation Proficiency Scale: Revised.* Los Angeles: Western Psychological Services.

Hodson, B. W. (1986). *Assessment of phonological processes — Revised.* Danville, IL: The Interstate Printers and Publishers.

Shriberg, L. D., & Kwiatkowski, J. (1982). Phonologic disorders III: A severity metric. *Journal of Speech and Hearing Disorders, 47,* 256–270.

Smit, A. B., & Hand, L. (in press). *Smit-Hand Articulation and Phonology Evaluation.* Los Angeles: Western Psychological Services.

Stoel-Gammon, C., & Dunn, C. (1985). *Normal and disordered phonology in children.* Austin, TX: Pro-Ed.

Yorkston, K. M., & Beukelman, D. R. (1981a). *Assessment of intelligibility of dysarthric speech.* Tigard, OR: C.C. Publications.

Yorkston, K. M., & Beukelman, D. R. (1981b). Communication efficiency of dysarthric speakers as measured by sentence intelligibility and speaking rate. *Journal of Speech and Hearing Disorders, 46,* 296–301.

RECOMMENDED READINGS

Yorkston, K. M., Beukelman, D. R., & Bell, K. R. (1988). *Clinical management of dysarthric speakers.* San Diego: College-Hill Press.

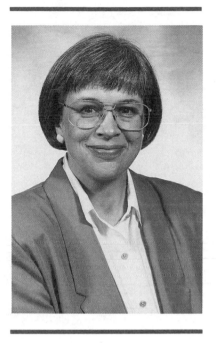

ANN BOSMA SMIT, Ph.D.

M.A. 1969, The University of Iowa
Ph.D. 1980, The University of Maryland

Dr. Smit is an associate professor at Kansas State University in
Manhattan, KS. Her interest in speech sound disorders developed at
the University of Iowa, where she earned the master's degree and
later served on the faculty, and at the University of Maryland, where
she earned her doctoral degree.

CHAPTER

9

Motor Speech Disorders

Linda Smith Jordan, Ph.D.

I am happy to have the opportunity to discuss motor speech disorders with you. I plan to present this material in a fashion that will allow you to see the similarities as well as the differences among the specific topics that fall within this classification.

Initially, it is necessary for us to differentiate speech from language. *Speech* is produced by shaping the vocal tract to produce sounds. Basic motor processes are involved in the production of speech. Although speech has been used by some as synonymous with "articulation," it is now widely recognized that production of speech requires appropriate use of respiration, phonation, resonance, and prosody in addition to articulation. Prosody is a term for the melody of the speech. Variations of prosody are produced by altering pitch, loudness, and rhythm. This chapter details assessment of the speech disturbances associated with lesions to the motor system. Throughout this discussion you may feel as though you are experiencing déjà vu — as though you are dealing with familiar words and suggestions. Many terms are also relevant in other chapters, but all your assessment skills will be called into play when working with a client with a motor speech disorder.

Language results from the combination of speech sounds into meaningful units, a code expressing concepts and thoughts. Language can be expressed through spoken, written, or gestural forms. It is received through auditory and visual modalities. Speech is the microscopic unit with which language is constructed.

This chapter focuses on two motor speech disorders associated with lesions of the nervous system. *Dysarthria* is any speech disorder from problems with muscular control that result from a single lesion, multiple lesions, or a diffuse lesion to the central or peripheral nervous systems. *Apraxia of speech* is a speech disorder resulting from a disruption of motor planning ability for speech production that occurs because of brain damage.

You will want to become familiar with the nervous system and the way it functions. A brief overview of the neural substrate of motor functions necessary for the execution of speech production and the programming of volitional units into speech sounds and sequences follows.

The most basic level of function is provided at the lower motor neuron level, which functions reflexively, as in the anterior horn cells of the spinal cord and the motor nuclei of the cranial nerves. A reflex is an involuntary response (such as a swallow, cough, or crossed knee jerk) to a stimulus.

Seven of the 12 cranial nerves have functions related to speech, swallowing, or hearing. Functions of the cranial nerve related to motor speech behavior are referred to as bulbar activity. The group of dysarthrias characterized only by problems with function of the lower motor neuron area are flaccid dysarthrias, those in which we also see weakness or paralysis.

At a higher level, the reticular formation of the brain stem regulates the reflex activity of the lower motor neurons. At a still higher level, the basal ganglia and related nuclear masses regulate automatic, subconscious aspects of motor performance. At the highest level, the upper motor neurons represent the cortical role in motor speech movements. The accuracy of the performances produced by the previous levels is controlled by the cerebellum. Finally the preprogramming of the movements of motor speech is also dependent on cortical function. Speech problems caused by disruption of the function of the nervous system at the reflex levels, the reticular formation, the basal ganglia and related nuclear masses, the upper motor neurons, the cerebellum, or combinations of those are classified as the *dysarthrias*.

Speech problems resulting from cortical damage, specifically left hemisphere damage, frequently fit the description of *apraxia of speech*, with individuals exhibiting speech production problems because of disruption of motor planning ability. It is also the case that some reported instances of apraxia of speech have resulted from subcortical lesions.

WHICH MOTOR SPEECH DISORDERS ARE CLASSIFIED AS DYSARTHRIA?

The most common motor speech disorder is labeled as *dysarthria*. Until relatively recently dysarthria was defined only as disruption of articulation, particularly by persons outside of the discipline of speech pathology. Actually there is a group of disorders, each a dysarthria, resulting from disturbances of muscular control with symptoms such as weakness, slowness of

> Your understanding of how speech is produced will help you to understand speech production disorders.

response, fatigue, or incoordination. Such impairments interfere with one or more of the basic processes necessary for speech production. Darley and associates describe impairments of the processes of respiration, phonation, resonance, articulation, and/or prosody as components in dysarthria (Darley, Aronson, & Brown, 1969a, 1969b, 1975). These processes are features helping describe variable characteristics of speech production.

Disturbances of muscular control are constant features of a neurologic disease or injury. The type of neurologic impairment determines the amount and type of motor performance loss. Motor speech errors are, therefore, *consistent* and predictable. In dysarthria, the articulation errors can primarily be described as omissions and distortions. A client may attempt a word twice and produce two identical articulation errors (for example, "tea," "tea," for "she"). Other characteristics of the speech produced by the client with dysarthria are caused by disruption of the processes of respiration, phonation, resonance, and prosody. Metter points out that these disruptions may be represented "along a hyperfunctional-hypofunctional continuum, with normality typically lying somewhere in the middle" (Metter, 1985, pp. 343–344). Depending on the process that is involved, and where the behavior falls on the hyperfunctional-hypofunctional continuum, your clients with dysarthria may exhibit breathiness, short phrases, monopitch, low pitch, hypernasality, variable nasality, harsh voice, breathy voice, strained or strangled voice, monoloudness, loudness control problems, inappropriate silences, or short rushes of speech, in addition to the articulation errors of imprecise consonants and distorted vowels.

> This example of errors illustrates substitution errors, one of the less common errors of speakers with dysarthria.

The classification of dysarthria includes the speech disorders of individuals with a variety of neurological diseases, such as Parkinson's disease, multiple sclerosis, ALS, and cerebral palsy. Some diseases progress in severity and a resulting speech disorder, which is a symptom of the disease, may increase in severity. In contrast, because some diseases can be expected to improve, with concomitant improved functions, speech production may also improve. Still other diseases are relatively stable from onset, and associated problems in speech production are likely to be relatively consistent over time.

WHICH MOTOR SPEECH DISORDERS ARE CLASSIFIED AS APRAXIA?

The motor speech disorder, *apraxia of speech*, is characterized by difficulty producing deliberate, volitional movements, even though there is no weakness, slowness, or incoordination resulting from muscular impairment. The muscles are capable of normal function, but the programming of the muscles by the brain is incorrect or imprecise. A cardinal feature of these errors is *inconsistency* and, therefore, unpredictability. To repeat, the underlying problem is one of motor programming not one of muscular control, the cardinal feature of dysarthria. Motor programming can vary from attempt to attempt and, as a consequence, three attempts can produce three very different results (for example, "tea," "see," "day," for "she"). The articulatory errors you will see in clients with dysarthria may be substitutions, repetitions, additions, prolongations, omissions, or distortions. You

The client with apraxia of speech is frequently as unprepared for and surprised by the errors he hears himself produce as you are.

will frequently observe that the errors are anticipatory; that is, the errors will be produced in anticipation of a correct production of a phoneme later in a word or phrase. Problems may also be perseveratory, continuing to be produced in error, even after a correct production. Prosody may appear to be interrupted because of the individual's use of compensatory behaviors (stopping and restarting, slowed rate). Occasionally, patients with apraxia of speech have difficulty initiating phonation.

The diagnosis of apraxia of speech is somewhat controversial within our profession. Some colleagues regard these error patterns as phonological or language problems (Dunlop & Marquardt, 1977; Martin, 1974). Defining the disorder as a motor programming disorder is useful to others by explaining the inconsistency of performance. The description is useful to a client and the family, especially in helping them understand the inconsistent nature of the problem.

WHAT KINDS OF CLIENTS HAVE MOTOR SPEECH DISORDERS?

The classification of motor speech disorders is applicable for both children with congenital or early onset disorders and for adults with acquired disorders. For children, the influence of the disorder on future development must always be considered. A child's inability to interact meaningfully with others in a verbal environment is likely to have a limiting effect on growth and maturation of intellectual as well as social concepts.

At times, information about the history of a child's speech and language development is particularly useful in helping confirm or justify a family's initial concerns about a child's overall performance. Your evaluation may be one of the early steps in seeking and confirming a diagnosis that supports a motor speech disorder.

ARE THERE WAYS TO CLASSIFY THE DIFFERENT TYPES OF DYSARTHRIA?

There are many different dysarthrias because there are many different lesions to the nervous system. In the marginal notes that follow I briefly introduce you to diseases which are likely to have dysarthria as a symptom.

A variety of systems have been used to classify the dysarthrias. You may find a particular scheme especially useful in helping you select assessment procedures. Another may be of use because it allows you to anticipate the progression of the disease and plan an effective remediation program. Darley and colleagues offer a number of classification systems for consideration:

> Dysarthrias can be classified according to age of onset (congenital, acquired); etiology (vascular, neoplastic, traumatic, inflammatory, toxic, metabolic, degenerative); neuroanatomic area of involvement (cerebral, cerebellar, brain stem, spinal or central, peripheral), cranial nerve involvement (V, VII, IX–X, XII); speech process involved (respiration, phonation, resonance, articulation, prosody); or disease entity (parkinsonism, myasthenia gravis, amyotrophic lateral sclerosis, etc.). (Darley et al., 1975, p. 12)

Note that these classifications are not exclusive. That is, a dysarthria may be described in a stroke patient as "acquired," "vascular," "cerebral," and/

or "involving respiratory and articulation processes." Following a motor vehicle accident, an individual might be described as having an "acquired," "traumatic," "brain stem lesion involving cranial nerves IX, X, and XII," which "affects articulation and phonatory processes."

You can classify dysarthria from such medical history information as age of onset, etiology, neuroanatomic area of involvement, or disease diagnosis. Determination of any speech process involved is your responsibility as a speech pathologist.

Darley et al. (1975) advanced our appreciation of dysarthria by their research about the differential clusters of speech characteristics associated with six types of dysarthria. The patterns are described by groupings determined by organization of the peripheral and central nervous systems. Each of the groups is characterized by different compositions of speech behaviors. On learning this system based on perceptual characteristics, you will be able to make judgments of specific causes for a client and the related probable disruption of the person's nervous system. This type of perceptual analysis requires extensive training, but it will expand your ability to communicate with others on the neurological team.

> Parkinsonism is a progressive disease characterized by rigidity, resting tremor, and slow movements. You will hear low volume levels, increased frequency of voicing errors (phonatory onset and offset errors), and changes of speech rate control.

WHAT IS THE GOAL IN ASSESSMENT OF MOTOR SPEECH DISORDERS?

The goal in working with the individual with dysarthria is to identify the motor functions that have become less than optimal. You can then attempt to identify the means and degree to which the performance can be enhanced or compensatory behaviors can be taught or provided. You will approach your assessment of a person with dysarthria with individualized questions, depending on the clinical orientation you develop.

Dysarthria or apraxia may occur in isolation from each other and other disorders. On the other hand, both dysarthria and apraxia of speech occasionally occur in conjunction with aphasia, a language disorder. Furthermore, dysarthria and apraxia of speech can also co-occur. It is always wise to attempt to differentiate the symptoms caused by each motor speech disorder from those produced by any other communication, learning/cognitive, psychiatric, or structural disorder. Many times this is a difficult task. The knowledge you have acquired about normal development of language, motor, and cognitive skills will help you with this effort.

> Myasthenia gravis is a neuromuscular disease characterized by rapid muscle fatigue and weakness. Articulation may be affected, but function of the velopharyngeal mechanism is particularly vulnerable.

A variety of approaches may be appropriate at this early stage in your professional development. An initial challenge that you face when attempting to assess the individual with a motor speech disorder is to identify and understand the causative factor. Sometimes you obtain information about the neuropathology from the medical history. For instance, your client may come to you with a documented cranial trauma, stroke, or diagnosed disease. When the individual comes to you with an already confirmed medical diagnosis, your knowledge of that disease may suggest a probable course of action for future assessment and/or treatment.

At this stage of training you are capable of observing, describing, and determining the replicability of behaviors. Observations of movement patterns during nonspeech motor activities, such as those described in Chap-

Amyotrophic lateral sclerosis (ALS) is a progressive degenerative disorder of the upper and lower motor neurons. There are different patterns of involvement. Degeneration of the swallowing and respiratory musculature result from bulbar involvement. You may hear flaccid and/or mixed dysarthria.

ter 4, provide insights about the predictable performance of the speech production mechanism in other contexts. The structures can be viewed in relatively more isolation than possible during speech production. Nonspeech tasks are less complex for your client, because performance of a nonspeech activity does not require coordination of such functions as breathing, voicing, and articulating speech sounds. Observations of movements of each of the oral structures, control of phonatory behaviors, and control of respiratory function, in the absence of the requirement that a verbal response be formulated, are important for you to make during your assessment of the individual with dysarthria or apraxia.

HOW CAN YOU DIFFERENTIATE THE MOTOR SPEECH DISORDERS?

You will want to make many observations to help with identification and assessment of motor speech disorders. As described, observations about the consistency of performance will help differentiate between dysarthria and apraxia of speech. Repeated attempts to produce the same speech unit will produce very similar efforts and results by the speaker with dysarthria. You will recognize that the speaker is attempting the same utterance on all attempts. On the other hand, the speaker with apraxia will not be able to produce exact replications of his efforts in all attempts to produce the same speech unit. You may not recognize the attempted target on many of his attempts, unless you are aware of the context or intent of the utterance of the speaker with apraxia of speech.

The individual with dysarthria produces speech that is predictable from one attempt to another and does not produce unexpected "islands" of error-free speech. By contrast, an individual who has speech production problems attributable to apraxia of speech may produce segments of accurate speech surrounded by speech attempts characterized by frequent, but not necessarily consistent, errors. The instances of error-free apraxic speech are not predictable, but a review of the contexts in which they occur for an individual may reveal patterns. Errors are more likely to occur in automatic, frequently rehearsed contexts, than in attempts to produce purposeful, deliberate communication.

Another way to review a speech sample is to compare spontaneous or emotional responses with the planned purposeful (volitional) efforts. For example, the individual with apraxia may be able to accurately speak when counting from 1 to 10, but may not be able to produce any one of those numbers with the same precision of production to answer questions of addition, subtraction, or time. At the same time, you may observe that the individual "knows" the accurate answer by the client's attempts to respond by gesture or written response. Reactive speech such as "hello," "I'm fine," and "thank you," also tend to be error-free. One time, I spent many minutes with Mrs. Jay, a patient I had diagnosed with apraxia of speech, employing phonetic placement techniques to elicit "hello." After repeated failures, I remembered the greeting I had received when I had entered her room. I said "Goodbye," and left, closing the door. Within minutes, I returned with a cheery "Hello" and was rewarded with a surprised and accurate "hello" and a laugh. We had to repeat this scenario several times before Mrs. Jay was able to produce the greeting each time she intended to do so, but she eventually did!

Phonetic complexity contributes to performance difficulty for the client with dysarthria. When he is not able to produce a phoneme in a simple context, he likely will not be able to produce it in a more complex, although more automatic, response. In contrast, although the patient with apraxia of speech may display similarly poorer articulation with increased phonetic complexity in a volitional effort, he may, in an emotional outburst, produce the same words that had been so problematic during the thoughtful attempt. I remember a client who had struggled with attempts to tell me which days he would not be able to make appointments the following week with the articulate observation, "This is *so* frustrating, just yesterday I could say Monday, Tuesday, Wednesday, Thursday, Friday, just *fine*." Such observations are of value in differentiating between the client with dysarthria and the client with apraxia of speech. The phonetic complexity of a target does not predict the success/failure of an attempt at production by your client with apraxia of speech.

You will never regret the time you spend learning and polishing your phonetic transcription skills. These skills are invaluable when attempting to document consistency between efforts to reproduce the same response. You will similarly be able to describe efforts to produce the same phoneme in different phonetic contexts. Your observations about the effects of different phonetic contexts will be of value, later, when developing strategies to be used in remediation activities.

Your examination of nonspeech as well as speech activities will help you appreciate motor behaviors in different contexts. Compare and contrast a client's performances, observing for evidence of weakness, asymmetry, or incoordination. When you have observed a performance that you consider to be adequate, introduce an alteration of requirements in an attempt to observe under what "stresses" performance begins to break down. Such stress might be achieved by calling for increased rate, increased volume, or the raising or lowering of pitch. There are a variety of "stresses" that can be introduced to a speaking task that will provide you with valuable observations about the function of motor speech production. You will want to observe the contribution of the stress of increased speaking rate to accuracy of speech produced. For an individual with dysarthria, increased rate may be problematic if it results in decreased opportunity to utilize compensatory strategies. In contrast, speech may improve as the speaking rate is increased for the client with apraxia. Given a constant requirement, the dysarthric individual will typically produce a constant effort. However, *increased* speaking rate changes the requirement. The requirements with which an individual must cope also change when an increased length of utterance (increased number of words or syllables) is demanded. Production of different volume levels places different requirements on the speech production system. A whisper differs from a shout. Variations of volume within a production require adjustment of essential variables within the total effort. Similarly, pitch changes, both between and within utterances, require fine adjustment of the speech production mechanism. In summary, you can vary the demands on the motor system by asking your

Multiple sclerosis is a progressive demyelinating disease. There is no pattern to this disease as the demyelinating process worsens and improves. Therefore, the symptoms vary widely. Darby (1985) estimates that 50% of the patients will exhibit a mixed form of dysarthria.

client to increase speaking rate, increase the length of utterance, increase or decrease volume, and/or change of pitch (either between or within utterances). As you vary the demands, you will observe changes in speech behavior that will give you clues to the type of motor problems with which you are dealing.

WHAT OTHER ADJUSTMENTS OF THE SPEECH PRODUCTION MECHANISM ARE IMPORTANT TO OBSERVE DURING THE ASSESSMENT OF MOTOR SPEECH?

All speech production uses the air supplied by the lungs to provide the power source for speech production. Neurological damage may be responsible for interfering with the contractions of the abdominal muscles or the diaphragm. As a result, the air supply that speech production is dependent on becomes limited. The speaker may no longer be able to use the phrasing patterns that are familiar to her, because she can no longer produce as many syllables on an exhalation. She may also have difficulty producing words at louder volume levels. Observe the effects on your client's speech by changing either of these variables.

The chapter on voice production discusses the way in which the air stream is put into vibration by the larynx. Neurological problems that affect the function of the laryngeal mechanism may result in voice changes. Most likely these changes will lead to breathiness and reduced loudness. Some patients may also have problems in control of the laryngeal muscles, producing a tremulous, unsteady feature to their voice. If the vocal folds don't meet normally during sound production, air may be lost on each attempt to produce vocalization. Attempt a temporary description of the voice quality of your client. As with all the other observations, be aware of consistency or lack of it.

The individual with dysarthria may have problems closing the palatopharyngeal port. As a result you may hear hypernasality, nasal emission, and inefficient use of the air supply during speech. In other words, the speaker may sound as though he is "talking through the nose," exhibiting nasal snorts, or having difficulty controlling the oral-nasal balance for speech. Such features contribute to imprecise speech sound production. These problems are physiologic and result either from inability to completely close the velopharyngeal port or to close it with proper timing. Observe an attempt at speech production with no intervention on your part. Then, occlude your client's nostrils and ask that the same speech effort be repeated. She may report a perception of a difference in the amount of effort necessary to produce speech with the nostrils occluded. Also, you may observe a difference in the number of syllables that she is able to produce on one breath of air.

The vibrating, resonating, airstream of sound production is shaped by contacts of relevant structures in the oral mechanism: the tongue, lips, teeth, and palate within the specific shape of the oral cavity. Neurological involvement affects the individual's ability to achieve appropriate shapes of the oral cavity, movements of the oral structures, and accuracy of desired oral contacts. As you review your transcriptions of your client's speech efforts, do you note a pattern to the errors produced? For instance, does she typically have difficulty producing sounds that require high intra-oral pressure (s, z, sh), sounds that require lip closure (m, p, b), or sounds that require elevation of the back of the tongue (e, k, g). Are some other patterns apparent?

The timing and coordination of all the aspects of speech production are responsible, at least in part, for the prosodic features achieved by the individual. Observation of the function of these aspects of speech production and, above all, the consistency of each function, is important in the evaluation of an individual with a motor speech disorder.

I have encouraged you to form hypotheses as you gather observations. I want also to urge you to test alternative explanations. For example, what you initially assume to be a problem with inadequate respiratory function may turn out to be a system taxed by inefficient valving (therefore, excessive air loss) at the level of the larynx or velopharyngeal mechanism.

IS WHAT WE HEAR, ALL WE KNOW?

Much of your assessment of the individual with dysarthria will be based on your perception of the acoustic event of the speech produced by the dysarthric client. In addition to the perceptual measures for describing motor speech disorders that have been the focus of this chapter there are a number of instrumental procedures providing analog data to help us understand our clinical findings. Technology may help us document consistency by allowing us to measure gradations that are too small to be heard or seen. Also, we may be helped in identifying underlying mechanisms that are not previously recognized. Among these instrumental procedures are ultrasound, cinefluoroscopy, cineradiography, and endoscopic evaluations. Such techniques permit observations of structures that are typically less accessible for visual observations, such as the tongue, velum, pharyngeal walls, and the larynx. Available instrumentation allows us to make objective measurements of oral strength, of endurance or resistance to fatigue, and of speed and latency of response. These measurements may seem a little overwhelming at this point, but you need to be aware of the names of a few of the tools that will be available to you in the future.

IS THERE ANOTHER WAY TO DESCRIBE A MOTOR SPEECH DISORDER?

An effective way of describing a speech disorder is to measure the intelligibility of the speaker. A variety of methods have been suggested as described by Yorkston and Beukelman (1978). Listener transcription of a speaker's utterance (word or sentence) is perhaps the most reliable measurement and has been developed into a formal assessment procedure by Yorkston and Beukelman (1984). Transcription is especially revealing when the listener is given no knowledge of the speaker's subject. Hammen, Yorkston, & Dowden (1991) demonstrated that a listener's knowledge of context provided a "strong and consistent" enhancement of intelligibility.

Such knowledge facilitates the listener's attempts to understand the speaker with dysarthria.

Measurements of intelligibility can be used to assess change in performance as a result of a change in instructions, a response to treatment, or as a measure of the impairment, disability, or handicap. It provides a measure of speech from a functional point of view.

IS IT POSSIBLE TO "ASSIST" A CLIENT WHO HAS POOR INTELLIGIBILITY?

When dealing with a client with a motor speech disorder with premorbid use of language, it may be possible to assist communication by relying on what he *can* do! In some situations, he may retain his premorbid (before brain damage) reading abilities and, if his visual-motor coordination is good enough, he may be able to point accurately to a selected item in a graphic display. Unfortunately, some clients may not exhibit these skills because of vision problems, loss or paralysis of upper limbs, or cognitive disabilities.

If the client has retained spelling abilities and is able to point efficiently, a spelling board can provide him as much power of communication as exists in a dictionary. If he is not able to point manually, directed gaze may be employed to indicate selections. As his listener, you must help him keep track of progress in his spelling attempts.

If he cannot spell or read, encourage him to look at a selection of pictures or pictograms and indicate his selections in some fashion for communicating desires or answers to questions. Again, help him remember where he is in a communication attempt.

When your client is able to read and point efficiently, you may offer a menu of frequently selected words, phrases, and sentences. Such material may be offered on an oaktag board or through computer assistance. There is computer capability to offer material to the listener as spoken presentations.

There are a number of good resource materials for assistive or augmentative communication for use with individuals with speech impairment. Representative reviews may be found in Beukelman, Yorkston, and Dowden (1985); Church and Glennen (1991); and Munson, Nordquist, and Thuma-Rew, (1987).

This chapter has, in general, covered motor speech disorders that develop in individuals who have previously developed what, at least for them, were normal communication skills. Another very important part of an adult caseload includes individuals who sustained motor problems of the speech production mechanism at birth. These individuals will have had cerebral palsy or motor speech problems that developed after birth, but before speech and language development had been completed. Such conditions present a different kind of challenge for speech-language pathologists. Diagnosis must account for neurologic impairment that led to speech-language assessment based on the client's speech and language developmental status at the time of motor insult. Individuals with such histories require special study. They comprise another group who will profit from your expertise in devising and providing appropriate assistive communica-

Jamie's mother had measles during the first trimester of her pregnancy with him. He has spastic cerebral palsy. Cerebral palsy is a term for the group of neurological disorders with motor function problems which have their onset in infancy.

tion techniques during the assessment process. When you have difficulty understanding your client, you will be helping yourself when you help your client communicate more effectively.

HONESTY DEMONSTRATES THE MOST RESPECT

Clinicians, as well as families and friends, sometimes pretend that they understand a dysarthric speaker when they do not. Therefore, the listener's responses are inappropriate or vague. The listener loses the speaker's confidence in the sincerity of the interaction. The speaker is likely to question the listener's interest in the speaker as a person. The speaker loses the motivation to attempt to communicate, at least in that environment. In an attempt to keep things "pleasant," you may undermine your primary intent — to enhance communication. I have found it more effective to be honest and state, "I didn't understand; did you say . . . ?" and then offer some alternative communication technique to assure more success on future efforts.

SUMMARY

This chapter has summarized motor speech disorders. Speech is the production of sound requiring the appropriate use of respiration, phonation, resonance, articulation, and prosody. *Dysarthria* is a problem of muscular control resulting from a single, multiple, or diffuse lesion to the central or peripheral nervous system. Several approaches have been used for describing and classifying dysarthria. *Apraxia of speech* is a disruption of motor planning ability for speech production because of brain damage. A variety of observations are helpful in assessing the motor speech disorders. These are useful when attempting to differentiate the motor speech disorders.

You will find your work with clients with motor speech disorders to consist of rewarding partnerships between you and your clients. The clients frequently voice the complaint that their bodies have "betrayed" them. With the insights gained from your assessment, you can help them understand the specific ways in which they can control the speech and language functions that they have retained and communicate with maximum efficiency. The goal *may* be oral communication, although possibly altered from a client's pretrauma manner. The goal *may* be development and use of the most efficient alternative communication techniques possible. It *will* be to preserve the power afforded your client by communication through whatever means possible. A broad knowledge of speech-language pathology science is important in planning assessment and remediation for the client with a disorder of motor speech.

Best wishes for your future work in the field of motor speech disorders.

REFERENCES

Beukelman, D. R., Yorkston, K. M., & Dowden, P. A. (1985). *Communication augmentation: A casebook of clinical management.* Austin, TX: Pro-Ed.

Church, G., & Glennen, S. (1991). *The handbook of assistive technology.* San Diego: Singular Publishing Group.

Darby, J. (1985). Epidemiology of neurologic disease that produce communicative disorders. In J. Darby, M.D. (Ed.), *Speech and language evaluation in neurology: Adult disorders* (pp. 29–41). Orlando, FL: Grune & Stratton.

Darley, F., Aronson, A., & Brown, J. (1969a). Clusters of deviant diagnostic patterns of dysarthria. *Journal of Speech and Hearing Research, 12,* 462–496.

Darley, F., Aronson, A., & Brown, J. (1969b). Differential diagnostic patterns of dysarthria. *Journal of Speech and Hearing Research, 12,* 246–269.

Darley, F. L., Aronson, A. E., & Brown, J. R. (1975). *Motor speech disorders.* Philadelphia: W.B. Saunders.

Dunlop, J. M., & Marquardt, T. P. (1977). Linguistic and articulatory aspects of single word production in apraxia of speech. *Cortex, 13,* 17–29.

Hammen, V. L., Yorkston, K. M., & Dowden, P. (1991). Index of contextual intelligibility: Impact of context in dysarthria. In C. A. Moore, K. M. Yorkston, & D. R. Beukelman (Eds.), *Dysarthria and apraxia of speech* (pp. 43–53). Baltimore, MD: Paul H. Brookes.

Martin, A. D. (1974). Some objections to the term "apraxia of speech." *Journal of Speech and Hearing Disorders, 39,* 53–64.

Metter, E. J. (1985). Motor speech production and assessment: Neurologic perspective. In J. K. Darby, M.D. (Ed.), *Speech and language evaluation in neurology: Adult disorders* (pp. 343–362). Orlando, FL: Grune & Stratton.

Munson, J. H., Nordquist, C. L., & Thuma-Rew, S. L. (1987). *Communication systems for persons with severe neuromotor impairment: An Iowa interdisciplinary approach.* Iowa City, IA: The University of Iowa (Division of Developmental Disabilities).

Yorkston, K. M., & Beukelman, D. R. (1978). A comparison of techniques for measuring intelligibility of dysarthric speech. *Journal of Communication Disorders, 11,* 499–512.

Yorkston, K. M., & Beukelman, D. R. (1984). *Assessment of intelligibility of speech.* Austin, TX: Pro-Ed.

RECOMMENDED READINGS

Dworkin, J. P. (1991). *Motor speech disorders: A treatment guide.* St. Louis: Mosby-Year Book.

Hardy, J. (1967). Suggestions for physiological research in dysarthria. *Cortex, 3,* 128–156.

Johns, D. F. (Ed.). (1985). *Clinical management of neurogenic communicative disorders* (2nd ed.). Boston: Little, Brown.

Love, R. J. (1992). *Childhood motor speech disability.* Columbus, OH: Merrill/Macmillan.

McNeil, M. R., & Kennedy, J. G. (1984). Measuring the effects of treatment for dysarthria: Knowing when to change or terminate. *Seminars in Speech and Language, 4*(4), 337–358.

Netsell, R. K. (1986). *A neurologic view of speech production and the dysarthrias.* San Diego: College-Hill Press.

Rosenbek, J., & LaPointe, L. (1985). The dysarthrias: Description, diagnosis and treatment. In D. Johns (Ed.), *Clinical management of neurogenic communicative disorders* (pp. 97–152). Boston: Little, Brown.

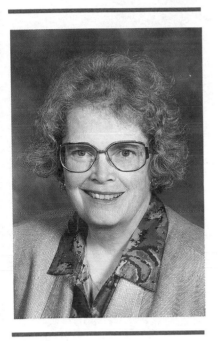

LINDA SMITH JORDAN, Ph.D.

M.A. 1964, The University of Iowa
Ph.D. 1972, The University of Iowa

Dr. Jordan is a Senior Speech Pathologist in the Department
of Neurology and Adjunct Professor in the Department of
Speech Pathology and Audiology, The University of Iowa. She has
special interests in the evaluation and treatment of patients with
communication problems related to neurogenic problems and shares
these interests through supervision of students in the clinical M.A.
program. In 1989, in recognition of her clinical skills, she was the
Iowa nominee for the Louis B. DiCarlo Award.

CHAPTER

10

Stuttering

Patricia M. Zebrowski, Ph.D.

As a student clinician and as a professional in the field you will most likely see children and adults who have been referred to you for "stuttering." Your specialized training in speech-language pathology will make you uniquely qualified to help these individuals. You will no doubt find your work with them to be interesting and sometimes perplexing, but almost always challenging and rewarding as well. The main reason clinicians encounter such a wide variety of experiences in treating this population is that stuttering is one of the most intricate and least understood of all speech disorders. It is believed to have multiple causes and that it perpetuates through a complex interaction among general communications skills, learning, the reactions and responses of listeners to stuttering, and the speaker's response to listener reactions. Therefore, speech-language pathologists must know how to diagnose and treat not only the *observable* speech behaviors associated with stuttering, but also the *unobservable* thoughts, attitudes, and feelings about stuttering reflected by the client and his significant others.

In this chapter, you will learn how to diagnose stuttering and its associated speech and nonspeech behaviors. But, as you will see, analyzing the speech behaviors that characterize stuttering is only part of the story. In addition, you will learn how to evaluate the important relationships existing between stuttering and the speaker's beliefs and attitudes about stuttering, listener reactions to stuttering, and the speaker's responses to those reactions. Hopefully, you will gain an appreciation for the uniqueness of these interrelationships — that is, correlations between different aspects of the problem of stuttering may vary in degree and kind among people who stutter.

We begin with a discussion of how to differentiate "stuttering" from "disfluency," as well as how to examine the behaviors associated with each to determine both the need for and initial focus of therapy. To start, we'll need to consider disfluency *type* and the ways in which judgments of disfluency and stuttering relate to the combined effects of type of disfluency and listener perceptions of type.

UNDERSTANDING "STUTTERING" WITHIN THE CONTEXT OF DISFLUENCY AND FLUENCY

When is disfluency "stuttering"?

Stuttering is a disorder of speech *fluency*. Speech fluency can be described as the forward-moving flow of ongoing speech (see Conture, 1990a, 1990b; Williams, 1978). It is the way in which a speaker "connects" the sequential sounds, syllables, words, sentences, and phrases produced as he is talking. When a person moves from one sound to the next or "connects" one word or sentence to the next in a relatively smooth, undisturbed fashion, his speech sounds "fluent." On the other hand, when a person disrupts or interrupts these smooth sound-to-sound or word-to-word connections, his speech can be described as "disfluent" (the prefix *dis* means *without*). Most speakers produce disfluent speech from time to time. Therefore, disfluency itself is not abnormal or unusual. However, there is a *type* of disfluent speech, which when produced in (relatively) frequent amounts, is considered to represent "stuttering," and not the disfluent speech of normal talkers.

DISFLUENCY TYPES: PRODUCTION AND PERCEPTION

Are there different types of disfluency?

As previously discussed, it is extremely important for you to be able to describe and measure disfluent speech objectively, both for diagnostic reasons (Is he stuttering or is he *normally* disfluent?) as well as to provide yourself with a map for how to design treatment (What is he doing when he stutters, and what does he need to do to speak more easily?). To accomplish this, it is helpful to consider a scheme for classifying the different types of speech disfluencies people have been observed to produce. The following section offers such a scheme.

The speech disfluencies that people produce can be classified into two broad categories: within-word and between-word disfluencies. Figure 10-1 provides examples of both disfluency types.

Within-word speech disfluencies are produced when the speaker disrupts a connection or "transition" between sounds *within* a word. This can be accomplished in three ways. In the first way, the person repeats a sound or a syllable in a word more than once and so does not smoothly move away from that sound and into the subsequent one. This disfluency type is referred to as a *sound/syllable repetition*. The second way that a person in-

Disfluency Type	Examples
Within-word speech disfluencies	
a. Sound/syllable repetition	"He is ruh-ruh-running home."
b. Audible sound prolongation	"Mmmmore cake, please."
c. Inaudible sound prolongation	(lips closed, no accompanying voice) "Buy some milk, please."
Between-word speech disfluencies	
a. Monosyllabic whole-word repetition	"I-I-I can't do that." "He-he-he is a big boy."
b. Multisyllabic whole-word repetition	"She really-really is here."
c. Phrase repetition	"I was-I was going to invite them." "They are-they are fun people."
d. Interjection	"I will, you know, be late."
e. Revision	"She is-she was here." "Please stay-please go."

Figure 10-1. Examples of various types of speech disfluencies. After Conture, 1990b and Williams et al., 1968.

terferes with the fluent production of a word is to hold, draw out, or prolong an individual sound within a word for an abnormally long time. As with sound/syllable repetitions, when a person produces *sound prolongations*, the smooth sound-to-sound movement which characterizes normally fluent speech is disrupted. When voicing and/or turbulent noise (as in production of /s/, for example) is produced, the prolongation has an auditory correlate (can be heard), and therefore is described as an *audible sound prolongation*. When no voicing or noise is produced, the disfluency is referred to as an *inaudible sound prolongation*. An example of an inaudible sound prolongation can be observed when a speaker produces the appropriate articulatory shape for a certain speech sound (for example, tongue tip touching alveolar ridge for /l/) and holds that posture stationary with no accompanying voice or release of air.

Between-word disfluencies are those in which the smooth transition between words is in some way disrupted. In general, there are more readily observable examples of between-word than within-word disfluencies in speech. One way people interfere with the linking of words is to repeat an entire word in a particular phrase or sentence more than once. This is referred to as a *whole-word repetition*, either *monosyllabic* or *polysyllabic* (depending on whether the repeated word has one [mono] or several [poly] syllables). *Phrase repetitions* are similar, except that an entire phrase is repeated more than once, rather than a single word. In addition, speakers sometimes insert individual syllables or routine, nonmeaningful words or phrases *between* adjacent words in a sentence. These are called *interjections*. Frequently used interjections include "uh," "um," and "ah," as well as "like" and "you know" ("I want to find out how to, you know, evaluate speech fluency!"). Finally, *revisions* are produced when a person says the first few words or beginning phrase of a sentence, but in some way changes the structure or topic before completing it. When the speaker does not complete the message in any way, this disfluency type is referred to as an *incomplete phrase* or *sentence*.

Disfluencies Produced by People Who Stutter

The majority of people who stutter begin doing so during their preschool years (Bloodstein, 1987). An important research focus has been to describe and compare the speech disfluencies produced by children who stutter and those who do not. Much of what we know about the disfluent and stuttered speech of children has been obtained through either parents' answers to interview questions or their written responses on questionnaires. In addition, several investigators have collected and analyzed speech samples from stuttering and nonstuttering children.

Results from these studies have essentially shown that the speech disfluencies of stuttering and nonstuttering children are similar in *kind*, but different in *degree* or frequency. Specifically, both groups of children produce *all* types of disfluencies, both within- and between-word. As a group, however, children who stutter produce *more* disfluencies in general (are more disfluent), and specifically produce *more* within-word disfluencies than nonstuttering peers. Later in this chapter, this consistent observation will be used, along with other available information, to help in decision-making about which children are *most likely* stuttering or at-risk for stuttering and which are not.

Listener Judgments of Disfluent Speech

One of the earliest theories of stuttering onset (what causes a young child to begin producing stuttered speech) described stuttering as a speech problem essentially "created" by listeners. In his "diagnosogenic" theory of the onset of stuttering, Wendell Johnson proposed that stuttering in children was the result of listeners' (and specifically, parents') negative evaluations of a child's *normal* disfluencies (Johnson, 1959). Although the basic premises of the "diagnosogenic" theory have been challenged by numerous clinicians and researchers, part of this theory's significance is that it highlighted the importance of listener contributions to the problem of stuttering. As a result, numerous studies have been conducted to examine the ways in which people perceive and judge various characteristics of disfluent speech.

Results from these investigations have shown that listeners tend to use *frequency* and *type* of speech disfluency to make judgments about (1) whether a disfluency is "stuttered," "not stuttered," or "normal" and (2) whether a speaker is "stuttering," a "stutterer," or "normally speaking." Further, listeners use the same characteristics to make judgments about the *severity* of stuttering.

1. Usually observed during preschool yrs. Similar to nondisflu but differing in frequency/amount

As one might expect, the more instances of disfluency a speaker produces, the more likely listeners are to judge that person to be "stuttering" or a "stutterer." In addition, the higher the frequency of disfluency, the more listeners tend to judge the individual's disfluent speech as "severe." Studies that have examined the relationship between disfluency type and listener judgment have shown that listeners most frequently judge *within-word* speech disfluencies to represent stuttered speech or stuttering, with *between-word disfluencies* most frequently regarded as not stuttered or "normal." For the most part, *repetitions* of sounds, syllables and, to some extent words, are the disfluency type most often labeled as stuttering. Sound prolongations are also generally regarded as "stuttering," but less frequently so. Finally, between-word disfluencies (interjections and revisions) are typically judged to be "not stuttered" or "normal" by listeners.

[handwritten margin note: Rep. of sounds, syll, and some extent words are often labelled stuttering]

Production and Perception: Putting It Together

Children and adults diagnosed to be stuttering produce *more* disfluencies and more within-word speech disfluencies than nonstuttering speakers, and listeners tend to judge those persons' speech to be stuttered. That is, although some bias or stereotyped view of speech and speech disfluency may influence judgments, it is most likely that listeners judge disfluencies based on their familiarity and exposure to what people who stutter do when they talk.

Taken together, results from studies of production and perception tell us that the *type* of disfluency a person produces (within-word), along with frequency of disfluency, are two objective indicators of who is stuttering and who is not. Further, this *interrelationship* between the characteristics of the speech of children who stutter and listener judgments of their speech most likely holds important consequences for the development of stuttering. For example, if a child produces a relatively high frequency of sound/syllable repetition, it is likely that his parents or other significant others will consider him to be "stuttering" or "a stutterer." As a result of this judgment, parents may give the child negative feedback about his speech. Finally, as a response to adverse reactions to repetitions of sounds and syllables, the child might develop the habitual use of inappropriate speech production strategies to attempt to change or keep from producing these repetitions (Conture, 1990b; Zebrowski & Conture, 1989). This proposed relationship between stuttered speech and listener reactions to stuttering, as well as the speaker's responses to both, suggests that these factors should be examined during an evaluation.

Summary

Speech disfluency refers to disruption in the typically smooth transition or movement between sounds and words in speech. This disruption can be produced either within or between words. Within-word speech disfluencies include sound/syllable repetitions and (in)audible sound prolongations. Between-word disfluencies include whole-word repetitions, interjections, revisions, phrase repetitions, and incomplete phrases or sentences. Research findings as well as clinical observations have shown that children and adults who stutter produce more disfluencies, in general, and specifically more within-word speech disfluencies than nonstuttering speakers. Further, listeners are far more likely to judge within-word, rather than between-word disfluencies to be stuttered. Stuttering, then, can be defined as a disruption in the smooth transition between sounds and words, characterized by a high proportion of within-word disfluencies. Finally, the relationship between stuttering, listener reactions to stuttering, and the speaker's responses to those reactions needs to be evaluated.

STUTTERING ASSESSMENT IN CHILDREN

The assessment of any speech and language problem, including stuttering, is the first step toward solving the larger problem of how to provide treatment. When we are dealing with children, the first goal of our assessment procedures usually is to determine whether or not a problem exists. In this way, the evaluation goals for children are importantly different from those we might set for adults. Specifically, because the problem of stuttering begins in childhood (typically during the preschool years), it is likely that the main concern for children is to determine whether they are stuttering, at-risk for stuttering, or are normally disfluent. On the other hand, adults referred for a stuttering evaluation are probably not wondering whether or not they stutter, but are most likely looking for information about the nature, severity, and extent of their problem and the likelihood that they can be helped. Of course, you want to address these same issues when evaluating a child's speech, but for many young children these are secondary concerns stemming from the main question of differential diagnosis.

How can we tell whether a child exhibits a fluency problem?

Figure 10-2 is a schematic representation of the three main goals or "questions" that need to be answered in the assessment of stuttering in children, along with subgoals for achieving each. That is, before you can answer the most important questions of (1) Is this child stuttering or at-risk for developing a stuttering problem? (2) Is treatment needed and recommended? and finally, (3) What should be the focus of therapy, or the kind of treatment approach taken? We need to gather information on several different fronts.

Question 1: Is the child stuttering or at-risk? You can answer this question during your diagnostic evaluation by meeting subgoals 1 through 4, as depicted in Figure 10-2. Specifically, you need to (1) describe and measure speech (dis)fluency through focused observation of the child's conversational speech as well as administration and scoring of formalized "techniques," procedures, and rating scales, (2) talk with the child when appropriate to find out his beliefs and attitudes about talking and speech disfluency, as well as any thoughts about his own speech, (3) interview the parents or primary caregivers to determine their concerns, attitudes, and beliefs about disfluency and stuttering, both in general and specific to their child, and (4) determine the parents' or caregivers' verbal and nonverbal reactions and responses to the child's disfluent speech.

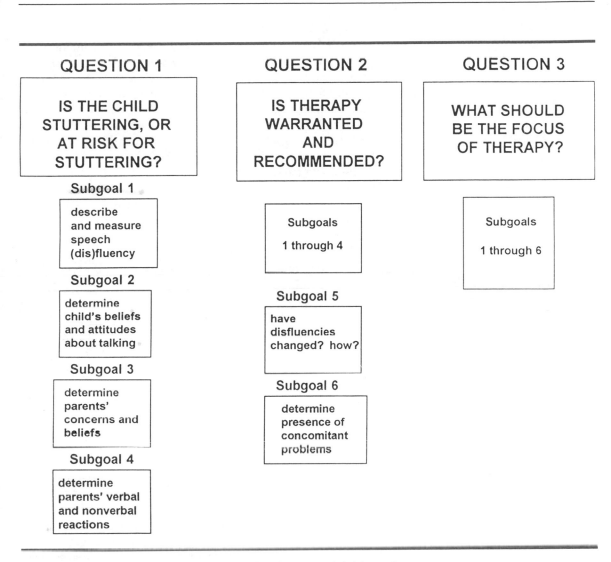

Figure 10-2. Questions to be addressed in the diagnosis of children who stutter.

Question 2: Is therapy warranted and recommended? The second question, once you've answered the first, is to decide on the appropriateness of therapy. To answer this question you will need the information obtained for question 1. However, you will also need to *compare* the results from your observation of the child's *present* speech (dis)fluency characteristics (subgoal 1), with parental report of those characteristics at the time the problem was first noted (subgoal 5). Further, you will need to determine the presence or absence of coexisting speech, language, hearing, or speech-related neuromuscular problems through observation and administration of standardized and informal tests (subgoal 6). The importance of subgoal 5 is that it allows you to speculate about the *rate* of progression or change of the child's disfluency problem. How much and how fast have the frequency and type of speech disfluency changed since the problem first began?

Question 3: What should be the focus of therapy? Finally, the third question in assessment is that *if* therapy is recommended (Question 2), what should be the focus? In other words, what are the skills, behaviors, or issues that should first be addressed in treatment? Your decision will be based on careful consideration of *all* of the subgoals (1 through 6). It is important to realize that the primary purposes of an evaluation are to attain goals 1 and 2 (Is there a problem and does it require treatment?), and that your intent in accomplishing this third goal is to offer some suggestions, or "guidelines," for the initial focus of therapy. For example, if based on your observations and interviews, you conclude that the parents believe that their child stutters as the result of some deep-seated psychological problem, then you would probably suggest that the first few therapy sessions focus on counseling and information-sharing with the parents. Or, if the client is a preschool child exhibiting concomitant stuttering and articulation problems, you might suggest that therapy employ *indirect* methods for simultaneously treating both. You would not provide specific therapy plans, but rather make some broad suggestions for the direction treatment should take.

Question 1: Is the Child Stuttering or At-risk?

This section covers the "nuts and bolts" of answering the three questions for assessing children's stuttering just discussed. Let's begin with how you can determine whether or not the child is stuttering or at-risk for stuttering. As Figure 10–2 shows, you first need to describe and measure the child's speech (dis)fluency.

Subgoal 1: Describing and Measuring Speech Disfluencies

There are a number of measures to help you to describe not only the extent of a child's disfluent speech, but also its characteristics. Currently, there are no standardized tests that will help you to decide which children are stuttering and which are normally disfluent. Therefore, you need to base your decision partially on objective measures taken from the speech of the children being assessed, considered along with results from some commercially available assessment "techniques," procedures, and rating scales.

Collecting a Sample of the Child's Speech.   The first measures discussed are usually obtained from samples of the child's conversational speech. To acquire a representative sample of the child's spontaneous speech and language, you will need to ask the parents or caregivers to engage in conversation with the child, which you either audiotape, videotape, or while you watch behind a one-way mirror in an adjoining observation room.

Make sure to provide age-appropriate materials for the parents to use as conversational "props." These can include small toys, Playdough, puzzles, Colorforms, and the like. Books and drawing materials don't work well, because often the parents end up reading to the child or encouraging the child to read, or the child draws and colors silently. Similarly, large or "noisy" toys (this latter category includes Legos and blocks), as well as puppets, don't work well because they can either obscure the child's face or can potentially be used by the child to make noise, (for example, banging on a table with Legos), which makes listening to speech difficult. More importantly, puppets can result in the child employing a way of talking other than his typical mode, one that may be fluency-enhancing. You can tell parents that they do not have to talk about the provided materials; in fact, you can encourage them to talk about anything they want. However, if the materials are appropriate for the child's age, as well as interesting to him, the chances are high that the play materials will be useful in stimulating the child to talk.

As you watch the parents and child talk, attempt to collect several types of information. Although the size of the speech sample you collect and analyze can and will vary, Conture (1990b) has suggested that a 300-word sample of conversational speech is a sufficient size for observing a range of performance. Obviously, the larger the sample, the more opportunity you will have to make observations and measures of speech disfluency. Further, your measures will most likely be more reliable. Although you should simultaneously videotape and audiotape the parent-child interaction so you can reliably make measures, you should also attempt to make preliminary measures "on-line" while observing the child and his parent(s).

The Importance of On-line Analysis.   The ability to analyze the child's speech (dis)fluency *as it is being produced* is an important skill to develop. When you assess a child's speech, it is important to give immediate feedback to the parents or client before they go home. In this situation, most parents want your opinion if their child is stuttering before the examination is concluded. Even though measures made from video- and/or audiotaped samples (with the luxury of reviewing segments several or many times) will likely be the most accurate, you need to quantify behavior on line to make your diagnosis and provide the parent(s) with information and recommendations.

Frequency of Speech Disfluency.   Once the child and parents are engaged in conversation, you should attempt to describe the child's speech by making a variety of measures. The first, frequency of speech disfluency, reflects the *amount* of speech disfluency the child produces, regardless of type (within- or between-word). It is an important diagnostic measure, by partially telling you the extent to which the child disrupts the flow of speech and communication. In addition, overall frequency of disfluency is the measure clinicians typically use to document *broad* improvement in therapy.

Usually, you report an average and a range of disfluency, so that you can form an impression about the variability of disfluent speech. Frequency is expressed in percentage, and can be measured by either counting the number of disfluent syllables per total syllables produced in a sample or by counting the number of disfluent words per total words produced. The unit of measure (either syllables or words) is not as important as the consistency with which it is used; that is, if you express frequency in percentage of disfluent syllables, you need to do so consistently when describing the client's speech throughout subsequent evaluations and treatment of that client.

During your evaluation, you can calculate frequency as the average number of disfluent words in 100 words spoken, expressed as a percentage. It is recommended that you count the number of disfluent words in *at least one* 300-word sample, and compute the average and range of disfluency produced (Conture, 1990b). Results from studies of the speech of young stuttering and nonstuttering children have shown that, in general, children who stutter produce *more* speech disfluencies overall than children not diagnosed to be stuttering.

Types of Speech Disfluency and Their Distribution. In recent years, the proportion of different disfluency types produced has been considered a more sensitive indicator than frequency in differentiating children who stutter from those who are normally disfluent. Further, analyzing the type(s) of disfluencies a child most frequently produces can help you to understand what the child *is doing* to interfere with talking, how the child's disfluencies have changed over time, and how these changes might be related to coping or "compensatory" speech production strategies the child has developed. Here, we discuss type as it might help you to answer the question, "Is the child stuttering, or at-risk?"

Studies comparing the disfluent speech of young stuttering and normally disfluent children have shown that children who stutter produce more *within-word* speech disfluencies (sound/syllable repetitions and sound prolongations) than their nonstuttering peers (Johnson, 1959; Kelly & Conture, 1992; Yairi & Ambrose, 1992; Yairi & Lewis, 1984; Zebrowski, 1991). This holds true regardless of age, even for preschool children who are very close to stuttering onset. That is not to say, however, that nonstuttering children do not produce repetitions of sounds and syllables or sound prolongations in their speech. The consistent observation has been that, in general, stuttering and nonstuttering children produce the same *kinds* or *types* of speech disfluencies but in different proportions with the children who stutter producing more within-word speech disfluencies. Further, studies have shown that children who stutter typically produce *at least* three within-word speech disfluencies in 100 words of conversational speech, while nonstuttering children produce *fewer* than three in 100 words.

These research findings, along with our own and others' clinical experiences have led us to consider children who produce three or more within-word speech disfluencies in 100 words of conversational speech to be either stuttering or at-risk for developing stuttering. Obviously, this observation plays an important role in your diagnosis, but it is only one piece of the puzzle. Further, the likelihood or probability that a child is stuttering or at-risk increases with increased proportion of within-word disfluencies (above three) per 100 words produced or parent(s)' or primary caregiver(s)' concern that the child is stuttering or a "stutterer."

You need to document the types and proportions of speech disfluencies the child demonstrates through analysis of the same 300-word sample from which you've measured frequency. Individual proportions are determined by dividing the number of instances of a specific disfluency type (for example, sound prolongation) by the total number of disfluencies produced in the sample and are expressed as percentages of the total. As with frequency of disfluency, you will need to make on-line observations of dis-

There are many pieces in the diagnostic puzzle.

Within-word disfluencies are one piece of the puzzle.

fluency types and distributions to be able to make a diagnosis at the time of the evaluation. Then, before writing your diagnostic report, you can review the video- and/or audiotaped recording of the same conversational sample and make the measures again.

Sound Prolongation Index (SPI).   The Sound Prolongation Index, or SPI, is a measure of disfluency type. It is the proportion of all disfluencies that are sound prolongations (either audible or inaudible). The SPI was introduced by Schwartz and Conture (1988) as one measure for distinguishing among children who stutter. It has since been used in several studies as a way to form subgroups of stuttering children or to describe the disfluencies produced by these children. They concluded that children exhibiting SPIs of 25% or more (25% or more of the child's total disfluencies are sound prolongations) are likely to require direct intervention for their stuttering.

The Sound Prolongation Index is another piece.

SPI
S proportion of all sound prolongations either audible or inaudible

Duration of Within-Word Speech Disfluencies (Stutterings).   The duration of individual moments or instances of within-word disfluencies has long been considered a diagnostic indicator of the presence and severity of stuttering. Recent work, however, has shown that there is little, if any, difference in the duration of sound/syllable repetitions or sound prolongations produced by very young children who stutter and those who do not (Kelly & Conture, 1992; Zebrowski, 1991). In addition, it appears that there is no relationship between stuttering duration and either a child's age, the length of time the stuttering problem has existed, or the overall frequency of speech disfluency the child produces (Louko, Edwards, & Conture, 1990; Schwartz, Zebrowski, & Conture, 1990; Zebrowski & Raszkowski, 1993). In general, children who stutter produce sound/syllable repetitions and sound prolongations averaging one-half second or so in duration (500 ms), ranging from one-quarter of a second (250 ms) or less to approximately one-and-one-half seconds (1,500 ms).

Let's consider disfluency and stuttering as reflecting the child's difficulty in making smooth transitions or connections between sounds, syllables, and words. If we do so, then the average range of stuttering duration, along with how often (frequency) and how (type) the child stutters can provide a detailed description of the degree and variability of difficulty displayed by an individual child. For example, a child who averages 40% disfluent (40 disfluent words in 100 words spoken) who also exhibits a high proportion of sound prolongations (SPI greater than 25%) of relatively long duration (greater than 500 ms) is possibly using more "fixed" speech production strategies to move between sounds and words.

Stuttering duration is another piece.

Duration should be measured, then, as another way to describe, or characterize, the ways in which the child disrupts the smooth, forward flow of speech. Further, clinical observations indicate that a decrease in the duration of instances of stuttering is often the earliest sign of progress in therapy (Conture, 1990b; Conture & Caruso, 1987). During your evaluation, you can use a digital stopwatch to make on-line measures of *at least* 10 within-word speech disfluencies. By measuring 10 stutterings, you will be able to obtain a mean duration and a range from low to high. You can use these duration measures to further describe the problem but, as we'll discuss later, you can also use them in determining stuttering severity through conventional rating scales and instruments.

Speaking Rate.   There is clear evidence that, for the rate of their *fluent speech only*, children who stutter do not speak significantly faster or slower than nonstuttering children (Kelly & Conture, 1992). We have found, however, that the measurement of *overall* speech rate (that is, the rate of speech when all pauses and disfluencies are included) is helpful for a number of reasons. First, there is an *inverse* relationship between overall speech rate and both stuttering frequency and duration. That is, the more disfluent or stuttered speech the child produces or the longer the duration of stutterings, the fewer words per minute he will be able to produce, therefore, speech rate will be slower. You can measure speech rate, then, to gain a better understanding of how disfluencies and stuttering are affecting the *amount* of speech output a child is able to produce and, thus, are interfering with communication. Second, you can compare this measure with a later rate measure obtained when and if the child receives therapy. One might speculate that speech rate will increase as a child either becomes more fluent or shows a decrease in duration of stutterings.

There are several ways to measure speech rate in the clinic and laboratory, some regarded as more accurate and precise than others. You can sample the child's speech rate by counting the number of words produced in 10 separate, randomly selected 10-second intervals. Overall rate can be calculated for each sample by dividing the number of words by the time in seconds (10 in this case) and multiplying by 60 (seconds) yielding the number of words produced in 1-minute's time. You can then compute the average rate and range in words per minute of all 10 samples.

Overall speech rate is another piece.

Associated Speech and Nonspeech Behaviors.   Often, a child shows visible or audible physical behaviors while he is repeating or prolonging sounds or syllables. These are called **associated behaviors**, and are also sometimes referred to as **secondary behaviors**. Associated behaviors can take many forms and some children and adults who stutter develop highly complex and idiosyncratic ones!

The most common *nonspeech*-related associated behaviors include eye movement (lateral, up-down and blinking, closing or widening), head movement, and torso and limb movement. Some typical *speech*-related associated behaviors are audible exhalations or inhalations immediately before an instance of stuttering; pitch rises during the production of a stuttered disfluency; visible physical tension in the lip, cheek, jaw, or neck muscles; and nostril flaring. Even the youngest children who stutter and those who are within weeks or months of stuttering onset have been observed to produce associated behaviors.

Associated behaviors are thought to reflect a child's *awareness* at some level that he is doing something "different" when he stutters. At most, the behaviors are thought to be associated with the child's attempts to cope with, compensate for, or in some way change speech disfluencies. (See Conture & Kelly, 1991 for a discussion of why young stuttering children might produce associated behaviors.) An additional view might be that as-

Associated behavior is another piece.

sociated behaviors are related to the things a child does to try to "keep from stuttering" (Williams, 1979).

During your evaluation, you should document the number and variety of associated behaviors produced by the child. For some children, the appearance of associated behaviors is the first indication of a beginning awareness of the problem. Further, associated behaviors are sometimes the only evidence of awareness you will be able to observe, especially in young children who are unable or unwilling to talk to you about their speech and their concerns about disfluency. Finally, normally disfluent children typically *do not* produce associated behaviors when they are disfluent, so the presence of associated behaviors can help to differentiate stuttering from nonstuttering children.

Severity. Severity is a dimension of stuttering that is often described. It is also the most familiar way in which speech-language pathologists and listeners, in general, characterize stuttering (Bloodstein, 1987). You can talk about a child's stuttering in terms of its frequency of occurrence, type, and duration, but almost always parents and other professionals will ask, "Yes, but how *severe* is the problem?" Thus, even though severity is not as useful in *clinical* terms for describing the nature and characteristics of a child's individual stuttering problem, it is *very* useful in that it helps you to communicate about stuttering in terms familiar to most.

Severity involves making a global judgment of the *degree* of the child's stuttering problem, and describing this degree with the terms "mild," "moderate," or "severe" (or a combination of terms when a problem is thought to border on a category; for example, "mild-moderate"). Listeners use the frequency, type, and duration of disfluency, along with the appearance of associated behaviors to make severity judgments.

Because severity is a subjective dimension, one problem in using it has been its reliability within and between clinicians and clinics. That is, a stuttering problem judged to be "moderate" in severity, might be judged as "severe" by another clinician in another setting. One way to make the measure of severity more objective is to use commercially available or published rating scales. Both the *Iowa Scale for Rating Severity of Stuttering* (Johnson, Darley, & Spriestersbach, 1978) and the *Stuttering Severity Instrument for Children and Adults* (SSI) (Riley, 1980) are severity rating instruments that you can include as part of your diagnostic protocol. Both instruments will allow you to assign either a number or a numerical score to a composite profile of the child's disfluent speech (based on either observations or direct measures of frequency, type, duration, and associated behaviors). The numerical ranking (as in the case of the "Iowa Scale") or score (as in the SSI) is associated with a level or degree of severity ranging from "no stuttering" to "severe" and "very severe stuttering."

As reported by Ludlow (1990), Riley (1972) demonstrated a high rank correlation (.89) between severity ratings obtained through the "Iowa Scale" and the "SSI." In addition, in a study examining the diagnostic records of 100 children who stutter, Conture, LaSalle, and Yaruss (1990) observed significant correlations between measures of stuttering frequency and scores on both the Iowa Scale and the SSI. Although not without prob-

[handwritten margin note: For some children 1st signs of assoc beh is beginning awareness of problem]

lems, the convenience, ease of use, and concurrent validity of both the Iowa Scale and the SSI make them useful parts of an assessment battery.

Adaptation and Consistency of Stuttering.   Adaptation and consistency of stuttering are two well-known phenomena that have been observed in both adults and children who stutter. **Adaptation**, or the **adaptation effect**, is the tendency for the frequency of disfluency to *decrease* during successive *oral* readings or speakings of the same material. **Consistency**, or the **consistency effect**, refers to the tendency for disfluencies to be produced on the *same words* during successive oral readings or speakings of the same material. Both "effects" are exhibited by people who stutter *as a group*; that is, some adults and children who stutter do not show either adaptation or consistency when reading the same passage several times in a row.

Adaptation and consistency are other pieces.

Adaptation and consistency should be measured for a number of reasons. First, if a child adapts or is consistent, such information can provide you with additional evidence that he is performing similar to other children who have been diagnosed to be stuttering; that is, his stuttering behavior is predictable. In addition, you can use the results of adaptation and consistency tasks to answer the third diagnostic question: What should be the focus of therapy? For example, if the child consistently stutters on bilabial sounds (/m/, /p/, and /b/), perhaps an early focus for treatment would be to teach the child appropriate strategies for smoothly moving into or away from those sounds at the single word level. If a child does not adapt or is not consistent, you might view this as an indication that he is not like other stuttering children as a group, but instead may be either at-risk for stuttering or normally disfluent. A second, and related possibility, is that the child will be essentially fluent while successively reading or speaking the test passage or sentences. This might suggest that it is fairly simple to elicit fluent speech from the child or that he has not yet come to "expect" to stutter on particular sounds or words.

You can measure both adaptation and consistency by asking a child to read or repeat a short passage or series of sentences five times in succession (with no pauses or conversation in between repetitions). For school-aged children, age-appropriate passages of about 50 words or so are fine. For younger children, you can use sentences developed specifically for this procedure by Neelly and Timmons (1967). If the child can read, instruct him to read the entire set of sentences from top to bottom "over and over" until told to stop. If reading the sentences is difficult for the child or he is a nonreader, instruct him to, "Say these sentences just like I do," to elicit repetitions from him.

Adaptation is calculated by subtracting the number of disfluencies in the fifth reading (or repetition) from the number of disfluencies in the first reading and dividing by the number of disfluencies in the first reading. The degree of adaptation is expressed in percentage. An adaptation measure of 50% or higher indicates that the child exhibits the adaptation effect; the higher the percentage, the more adaptation has been demonstrated. Conversely, a score below 50% indicates that the child has not significantly reduced the frequency of disfluency over five readings or repetitions.

Consistency is calculated by comparing the disfluencies produced in the first three readings or repetitions only. Three **consistency indexes**

(Johnson et al., 1978) are calculated: 1–2 (comparison of reading one and two), 1–3 (comparison of reading one and three), and 2–3 (comparison of reading 2–3). The index for each comparison is computed by dividing the proportion of disfluently produced words in one reading that are also produced in a second reading by the number of disfluently produced words in the second reading. So, the equation for the 1–2 comparison (readings 1 and 2) would be the percentage of disfluent words in reading 1 also in 2, divided by the number of disfluencies in reading 2. If an index is 1.0 or higher, the child is consistent in the location of disfluencies within the passage or sentence. The higher the index (> 1.0), the more consistency the child exhibits.

Stuttering and Communicative Demand.   The Stocker Probe Technique (Stocker, 1980) is a formal procedure allowing you to observe the child's disfluent speech in relationship to increasing levels of communicative demand or responsibility. In this procedure, the child is asked 5 questions about each of 10 different common objects. The questions range from low to high in the demands for creativity, intelligibility, and fluency that the child needs to use to respond successfully. The assumption is that for children who stutter, there is a strong relationship between these demands and fluency; that is, the higher the demand, the less fluent the response. Such a relationship has not been observed in normally disfluent children (Stocker & Usprich, 1976; Weiss & Zebrowski, 1992). You can use the Stocker Probe primarily to see if such a relationship exists for a child; if so, then this observation is one more piece of evidence that the child is stuttering or at-risk. In addition, the way the child responds to the varying levels of demand can indicate where to start in therapy. If the child is essentially fluent when responding to relatively low level probes such as answers to questions ("Who would you buy it for?"), but is consistently disfluent for higher level probes ("Make up your own story about it."), then you might start teaching fluency strategies within these less demanding contexts, therefore increasing the probability for success

> Communication demand is another piece.

Subgoal 2: Determine a Child's Beliefs and Attitudes About Stuttering

In addition to measuring and describing the child's speech (dis)fluencies, you need to find out something about the child's level of awareness and concern about his disfluent speech. As previously discussed, young children who are unable or unwilling to "talk about talking," require that you look for associated behaviors to provide some indication of awareness. You will need to do the same for older, school-aged children, but you should also spend some time during evaluations talking with the child about his speech. Williams (1985) and Zebrowski and Schum (1993) provide detailed descriptions of how to talk with children who stutter and their parents.

The main purposes of your discussion with the child during the diagnostic are to find out (1) what he believes "stuttering" is, (2) any reason the child has for talking this way, (3) what, if anything, he does to help himself when he talks, and finally, (4) is he worried or bothered about talking in any way? The best way to start the discussion is by asking the child, "Why do you think you came here today?" and letting his response point the way for additional probing. For example, if the child says, "I don't know," then you can *gently* ask him if he can think of "any reason" for the visit that day. Do not lead the child or put words in his mouth. If he continues to say, "I don't know," then an alternative line of questioning should be used, beginning with the instruction to "Tell me about your talking," followed by specific questions such as "Are you a good talker?" "What do you like about your talking?" and "What would you like to change about your talking?"

If the child does not respond to your questions or prompts, then the discussion should end. If, on the other hand, the child reports knowing a particular reason for the visit ("I don't talk well," "I stutter," and so on), then the next question should be something like, "What does that (stuttering, kind of talking, speech) sound like? Why don't you show me?" From there, the conversation should move to a discussion of why he thinks or believes he talks this way, what he does to help himself, and what bothers him the most about his speech.

You need to be careful at this point to avoid commenting on the correctness or incorrectness of the child's thoughts and beliefs. This discussion is primarily to help you gather information and form impressions about the child's beliefs — not to provide the child with a tutorial on the problem of stuttering! When and if the child begins therapy, you can be a source of information. During the evaluation, however, you should be an active listener, letting the child talk and making sure you frequently check your understanding by repeating to the child what was said. In our experience, children who stutter, even younger ones, often form beliefs and possess attitudes about their stuttering that may lead to the development of speech behaviors produced in an attempt to either suppress or change their disfluencies.

Recently, Brutten (1985) has developed, and De Nil and Brutten (1991) have obtained norms for, a test to assess the attitudes children who stutter possess about talking and stuttering: *Children's Attitudes About Talking — Revised* (CAT). The CAT contains 32 statements about talking that a child reads and decides are either "true" or "false," based on how closely each statement represents the way he feels. The clinician can then compare the child's responses to those of a group of 70 stuttering and 271 nonstuttering children ranging from 7 to 11 years of age. For school-aged children, using the CAT helps to gauge a child's attitudes and beliefs when he is unwilling or unable to discuss them. In addition, the test statements included in the CAT can be used as guidelines for interview questions or discussion topics when probing for information about a child's attitudes, beliefs, and concerns about his speech.

The speaker's attitudes about talking is another.

Subgoal 3: Determining the Parent(s)' Concerns and Beliefs

When evaluating stuttering in children, it is essential to interview the parent(s) or primary caregiver(s). The main purposes of the parent interview are to obtain a history of the child's speech (dis)fluency, as well as to find out the parent(s)' major concerns and beliefs about the child's disfluent or stuttered speech. Just as children themselves frequently develop "theories" about why they stutter, so do their parent(s) possess beliefs and hypotheses either about what caused or maintains the child's disfluent speech.

The interview should be similar to any you might conduct with parents. That is, background information about the child's overall development should be obtained, as well as the child's speech and language, health, educational, and social-emotional history. In addition, a specific history of the presenting problem should be obtained. For details about obtaining and reporting case histories, refer to Chapter 3 in this text.

You should ask the parent(s) when the problem was first noticed, by whom, and the manner and degree in which it has changed since it began. It is important that parent(s) *describe* what the child's speech disfluencies looked and sounded like both at the time first noticed and at present; however, it is even more helpful if the parent(s) *show* you examples of the child's disfluencies at both points in time. From the parental model, you can obtain a clearer picture of whether or not the child's disfluencies have changed over time in frequency or type, as well as gauge the parent(s)' willingness to produce disfluent speech. A parent who is unwilling to produce disfluent speech is likely to be very uncomfortable with disfluencies. In addition, you can compare the parental model to your clinical observations of the child's speech disfluencies. A large discrepancy (for example, the parents imitate effortful sound prolongations with many associated behaviors, although you observe the child producing mainly "easy" sound/ syllable repetitions) often indicates that the parental perceptions and the child's productions may be "out of sync," a situation that might contribute to the perpetuation of the problem and points to the need for the speech-language pathologist to provide parent counseling.

Parental beliefs and concerns about the *cause* of the child's stuttering often take one of three forms: (1) there is something physically (but as yet undetected) wrong with the child, (2) there is something psychologically or intellectually (again, undetected) wrong with the child, or (3) the parents have done or failed to do something that, in turn, caused the stuttering (see Zebrowski & Schum, 1993, for a detailed discussion). Of course, any or all of these variables might be related to a particular child's stuttering to some extent, but if so, these aspects are most likely related to the continued perpetuation, development, or exacerbation of the problem and not necessarily its origin. That is, the variables are likely *contributing*, but not *causal* factors. The presence of such parental beliefs about the cause of stuttering emergence can influence the ways in which the parent(s) interact with the child, and, therefore, need to be identified and addressed by the clinician.

Parental behavior may be a piece.

Subgoal 4: Determining the Parental (Non)Verbal Reactions to Stuttering

Finally, during the evaluation you need to observe the ways in which parents react and respond to the child's instances of disfluency and stuttering. Some of this information can be obtained from the interview by directly asking the parents what they do when their child is disfluent, why they do it, and whether or not it seems to help. In addition, it is helpful to observe the child and his parent(s) talking together, as a way of examining both parental reactions to stuttering, as well as the general style of the parent-child verbal interaction.

As described earlier, during the first 10–15 minutes of the evaluation, you should collect a sample of the child's speech while he talks with his parents. During this time, you should also watch the interaction between the child and his parent(s), paying particular attention to the parents' rate of speech and the duration of their turn-switching pauses (the length of time the parents wait before responding after the child has finished an utterance), as well as their nonverbal and verbal behaviors during and after the child produces a disfluency (overtly commenting about the child's speech, providing directions for "how to" talk, eye contact and facial expression, body movement and positioning). You should also observe the *quantity* and *quality* of the speech and language the parents use while talking with the child, along with the amount of interruptions produced by both the child and the parents.

As discussed earlier, although there is no evidence that any of these parent (or child) behaviors *cause* children to begin stuttering, it has been speculated that these factors might *contribute* to either the continued development of stuttering in children or their recovery from a stuttering problem. You should make observations about parent behavior to help you further identify children at-risk for stuttering. For example, a child who produces slightly more than three within-word disfluencies in 100 words, with few to no associated behaviors or observable awareness, but whose parents persist in correcting instances of disfluency, talking to him at accelerated speech rates, and reacting to his disfluencies with facial expressions indicating worry, concern, or disapproval, may be at-risk for developing a stuttering problem. You can use the information obtained from your observation to determine both the need and the issues for parent counseling.

Summary

To determine whether or not a child is stuttering or at-risk for stuttering, you will need to make a number of objective measures of speech (dis)fluency from a conversational speech sample. These measures include: overall frequency of speech disfluency, types of disfluencies and relative proportion, duration of within-word (stuttered) disfluencies, speech rate and associated (non)speech behaviors. In addition, you need to make judgments about the severity of the problem based on the above measures and results from formalized instruments, such as the SSI. You will need to examine variability in the distribution of the child's disfluent and stuttered speech through the Stocker Probe Technique, as well as by measuring adaptation and consistency. While you are collecting a sample of the child's conversational speech for analysis, you need to observe parental verbal and nonverbal reactions to the child's disfluent speech. Finally, you should interview the parents and, when appropriate, the child, to determine everyone's attitudes and beliefs about stuttering.

Question 2: Is Therapy Warranted and Recommended?

If the answer to our first question is "yes;" that is, that the child is either stuttering or at-risk, then you will need to answer the second question: Is therapy warranted and recommended? As shown in Figure 10–2, you can develop an answer to this question by considering the information provided when you meet subgoals 1 through 4, along with additional information concerning if and how the child's disfluencies have changed over time, and whether the child exhibits coexisting speech, language, or related problems.

If the child produces *at least* 3 within-word disfluencies in 100 words *and* the parents are concerned about the child's "stuttering," or believe he is a "stutterer," you should most likely recommend treatment. The case for this recommendation becomes even stronger if the child also conveys self-concern about speech. This treatment might take the form of direct parent counseling with indirect treatment for the child, participation in a parent-child fluency group (Kelly & Conture, 1992), parent counseling only, or direct stuttering therapy for the child, in which you explicitly address the differences between fluency and stuttering and teach the child strategies for producing fluent speech. In addition, for some children the information obtained through subgoals 5 and 6 is important in your decision to recommend intervention.

When shall we recommend treatment for a child?

Subgoal 5: Determining Change in Speech Disfluencies Over Time

You will need to form an impression of the ways in which the child's speech disfluencies have changed since first noticed by the parents or if speech has changed at all. Such changes can be observed in overall frequency (the child is more or less disfluent in general), proportions of different types, duration (instances of stuttering have increased or decreased in duration), presence or absence of associated behaviors, the child's reported awareness and concern about disfluency and stuttering, and the variability of disfluency (for example, is the child's overall frequency of disfluency stable over time or are "peaks and valleys" shown such that he follows 2 weeks of highly disfluent speech with 3 weeks of essentially fluent talking?).

You can determine *type* of change in two ways. First, during the parent interview, ask the parents to describe any changes they have noted in their child's disfluent speech since the problem first began. Second, ask the parents to *demonstrate* to you what the child's disfluencies were like when first noticed and then demonstrate to you what disfluencies are like at the present time. As previously discussed, if the parents can't or won't imitate their child's disfluent speech, a description will suffice. Then compare these two examples, as well as the parents' example or description of the child's beginning disfluencies with your observations of the child's disfluent speech during the evaluation. You can attempt to determine *rate* of change by considering these descriptions and observations of change in light of the amount of time the child has been stuttering.

Based on this assessment of type and rate of change, recommend therapy if the child's speech disfluencies have increased in frequency or duration, have shown decreased variability, or the child has increased the proportion of sound prolongations he produces since the problem first began. In addition, if these changes have occurred over a relatively short period of time, a stuttering problem might be developing at a fast rate.

Subgoal 6: Determine the Presence of Concomitant Problems

It has been well-documented that a subgroup of children who stutter exhibit coexisting speech and language problems (Louko et al., 1990). Presently, it is unclear how these problems might interact, or whether a child's speech and language problem "causes" the child's stuttering or vice versa. In particular, some children who stutter also display concomitant articulation problems, and it has been speculated that these children might take longer to show progress in stuttering therapy or might not show as much progress as children without additional problems. In some cases, the child's articulation or language problems interfere more with communication than the child's stuttering and, therefore, take precedence for treatment. In other cases, both stuttering and articulation (or language) need to be the simultaneous focus of therapy.

You should routinely assess the child's other speech, language, and related behaviors during your stuttering evaluation. Chapters 5 and 8 provide detailed descriptions of how to assess these behaviors and you are directed to look there for guidance. Although you should not necessarily conduct a full-scale articulation or language assessment early in the diagnostic process, you should carefully select one or two methods or tests for sampling these communicative behaviors to form a general impression of the child's abilities in areas other than fluency. In addition, you should conduct an oral-peripheral examination to assess structure and function of the speech mechanism. Chapter 4 provides a protocol for conducting such assessment.

If you determine that the child is stuttering or at-risk, and also has concomitant problems, you might not recommend stuttering therapy. For example, you might suggest that the child receive *indirect* articulation therapy (if warranted) that does *not* focus on correct, precise or physically tense articulator "placement," accomplished through drill procedures. Or you might recommend that the child receive language-based stuttering therapy, focusing on simultaneous treatment of oral language and fluency skills.

Summary

For some children, recommending the appropriateness of therapy for stuttering depends on your observations of type and rate of changes in speech disfluency and your analysis of concomitant problems. Through interviews with the parent(s) and observation of the child, you can determine whether or not the child's stuttering has increased in frequency, duration, or proportion of sound prolongation and/or decreased in variability. Through the same procedures you can attempt to discern how rapidly these changes have occurred since the problem of stuttering was first noticed. Finally, it is important to assess the type and degree of any concomitant speech, language, or related problem to determine both the appropriateness of treatment focusing primarily on stuttering and the probability of success in therapy.

Question 3: What Should Be the Focus of Therapy?

As previously discussed, it is important to provide some guidelines for initial therapy focus once you've decided to recommend treatment. Doing so certainly helps you if you are to be the clinician providing therapy. In addition, providing suggestions for treatment emphasis to another clinician (if that is the case) is an important professional courtesy, in that it is not only helpful, but also shows the receiving clinician that we have thought about a particular case beyond the "does he or doesn't he" stage.

As shown in Figure 10-2, you should use *all* the information obtained during the evaluation (subgoals 1 through 6) to develop such guidelines or suggestions. As an example, suppose you evaluate a 5-year-old boy who is producing a relatively high proportion of sound prolongations with many associated behaviors and exhibiting a concomitant articulation problem. Suppose as well, that during the interview the parents of this child expressed the belief that the child stutters because he was the only one of their four children born at home and "the stress was too much for everyone." Finally, when the parents and the child engage in conversation, the parents frequently interrupt and talk simultaneously with the child.

In this case, your recommendations for initial therapy focus might include parent counseling and information sharing, particularly on what is known and not known about the "causes" of stuttering in children and the difference between "causal" and "contributing" factors in the problem of childhood stuttering. In addition, you might want to discuss with the parents the various ways in which they can modify their verbal interactions with their child. Further, you might recommend indirect treatment for the child, focusing simultaneously on articulation and fluency-enhancing strategies.

The preceding is one example of some possible recommendations. A general rule of thumb for developing suggestions for treatment is to consider all the behaviors and comments produced by both the child and his parents and determine which interfere the most with communication, which need to be addressed before others can be targeted, or both.

STUTTERING ASSESSMENT FOR ADULTS

As previously discussed, when an adult is referred to a speech-language pathologist for "stuttering," the purpose of assessment is seldom to answer the question, "Is this person stuttering or at-risk for stuttering?" as it usually is for a child. Most adults who stutter have been doing so since they were young children and have been diagnosed as stuttering in the past. That is not to say that these same adults have received consistent therapy or any therapy, for that matter, but the question of "stuttering or not stuttering" has been answered. For this reason, the main question of assessment changes from "does or doesn't he?" to "*how* does he?" or what are the characteristics of the person's disfluent and stuttered speech as well as the stuttering problem?

Figure 10-3 is a schematic representation of the three main questions for the assessment of stuttering in adults, along with subgoals. As you can see, the second and third "main" questions are the same as those for children and it is only the first that differs. In addition, the subgoals are different from those set for children; that is, you want to answer most of the same questions but you seek different information to do so.

How is stuttering in the child and the adult different?

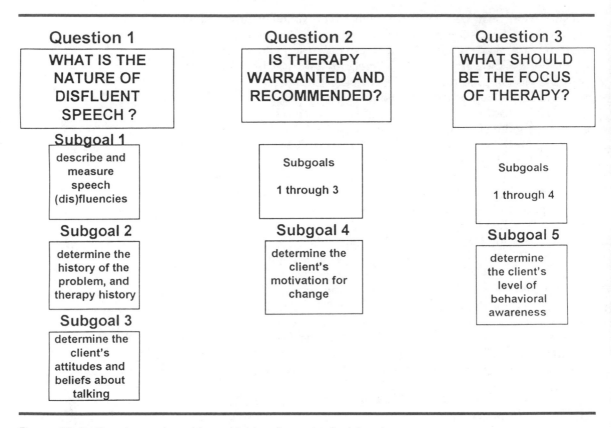

Figure 10-3. Questions to be addressed in the diagnosis of adults who stutter.

Question 1: What is the nature of disfluent and stuttered speech? As shown in Figure 10-3, your first goal is to determine the characteristics of the disfluent and stuttered speech the person produces. This question can be answered by achieving subgoals 1 through 3, as indicated in Figure 10-3. You need to describe and measure speech (dis)fluency through observation of conversational speech as well as through the administration and scoring of formalized procedures and rating scales or techniques. In addition, you will need to interview the client to determine the history of the problem, therapy history, and to learn attitudes and beliefs about both speaking and stuttering, as well as a self-description and demonstration of the things he does to help himself when he stutters.

Question 2: Is therapy warranted and recommended? Once you've answered the first question, you need to use the information obtained (subgoals 1 through 3) to determine if treatment is needed and whether or not we are going to recommend it. To help you decide whether to recommend therapy, you should try to assess the client's level of motivation (subgoal 4). It's important to consider that sometimes speech-language pathologists do *not* recommend therapy, even though they conclude from diagnostic information that a client's communication problem warrants intervention. For example, an adult who stutters may seek professional help at the insistence of another person, such as a spouse or a supervisor. He may not want to enroll in therapy, but attempts to do so to placate or please others. Certainly he may *need* therapy to learn how to talk more fluently, but if the speech-language pathologist determines that the client either does not *want* to change the way he speaks, or does not want to invest the necessary time and effort needed for therapy, then treatment may not be recommended.

Question 3: What should be the focus of adult therapy? Finally, as with children who stutter, if you recommend therapy as a result of your evaluation, you want to be able to provide some guidelines for treatment emphasis. You can develop appropriate suggestions for the initial focus of therapy when you achieve subgoals 1 through 3. As shown in Figure 10–3, there is an additional subgoal that will help you determine an appropriate place to start in therapy. This fourth subgoal is to assess, to the extent possible, the client's behavioral self-awareness of his instances of stuttering. Is he able to identify *when* he produces a stuttered disruption, and *what* he does when instances of stuttering are produced? You will obtain some information about the client's level of awareness during the interview when you ask him to describe and to show examples of what concerns him the most about his speech. Similarly, when you ask questions about the situations or conversational partners that are the *most* and *least* difficult for the client, you can make some judgments about the degree of self-awareness and concern he exhibits about his speech. Although the client's verbal descriptions of his speech and related issues provide you with insight into his *cognitive* awareness of speech and stuttering, an important factor for success in treatment is the extent to which he is aware of the *physical* feeling of both stuttering and fluency. For this reason, as part of your evaluation, you need to examine the client's ability to *identify* his instances of stuttering after, during, and, if possible, *before* he produces them.

Question 1: What Is the Nature of Disfluent and Stuttered Speech?

The remainder of this chapter will focus on the questions that need to be answered during a stuttering evaluation for adults. As shown in Figure 10–3, these questions are qualitatively different from the ones you ask when you assess stuttering in children. Specifically, your initial question for adults often is not *if* they are disfluent or stutter, but *how* they do it. Although the first question of interest is different, as shown in Figure 10–3 the information necessary to answer it is similar for both children and adults.

Subgoal 1: Describing and Measuring Speech (Dis)Fluency

You need to make essentially the same measures of speech (dis)fluency for adults as you would for children. That is, from a 300-word sample of spontaneous speech, as well as several formal assessment instruments, you need to measure (1) frequency of disfluency, (2) type of speech disfluency and proportion of each, (3) duration of within-word or "stuttered" disfluencies, (4) number and variety of associated behaviors, (5) severity, (6) speaking rate, and (7) adaptation and consistency of stuttering.

You can collect a speech sample for analysis while you engage the client in conversation during the first few minutes of the evaluation. You can also use portions of the client interview, if necessary, to provide you with samples of spontaneous speech. As with children, simultaneously audio- and videotape the evaluation to increase the accuracy and reliability of your measures; however, the importance of on-line analysis needs to be emphasized here.

When talking with the adult who stutters, you need to attend simultaneously to *what* the client is saying, as well as analyze *how* he is saying it. This is a difficult task and will require a conscious effort on your part. With practice and experience, however, it is a skill that can be mastered. One model helpful for such "analytical listening" has been described by Adams (1974). It involves using the processes associated with fluent speech production as reference points against which to compare stuttered speech. The basic premise is that to speak fluently, a person needs to control the flow of air from the lungs into the vocal tract, as well as to coordinate this airflow with both vocal fold vibration and articulator movement and positioning. When a person produces a sound/syllable repetition or a sound prolongation (stuttering), you will need to make a hypothesis about what this individual *is doing* with his speech production system to produce the disruption in speech. Once the "hypothesis" of what the person is doing to interfere with fluent talking is made, you will need to develop therapeutic strategies for helping the individual initiate and maintain speech fluently.

For example, suppose during your evaluation you observe that 60% of the client's disfluencies are inaudible sound prolongations. Because these are in the category of within-word disfluencies, it is highly probable that they represent "stuttering." Further, suppose you also observe that this client is producing these inaudible sound prolongations by holding his articulators stationary in a particular position, with no accompanying voice or airflow. To initiate fluent speech, the client will need to initiate airflow and voicing smoothly while simultaneously moving his articulators to form sounds and transitions between sounds. It is your job as a speech-language pathologist to teach the client how to accomplish this.

Subgoal 2: Determine History of the Problem and Therapy History

As with any referral, it is important to obtain a history of the individual's problem. Again, refer to Figure 10-3 for guidelines on how best to accomplish this. For adults who stutter, it is important to know when they first started to stutter and who first noticed it. In addition, you will want to know what the client remembers about the reactions of significant others to his stuttering (usually parents, relatives, teachers, and childhood friends). You will also want to know how, if at all, the client's stuttering has influenced decisions or choices he has made earlier in his life (for example, career choices). Finally, you will need to find out what the client's perception is of how his stuttering has changed over time. All of this information will help you to form an impression about both the significance stuttering has in the client's life and his motivation to change.

During the interview, you will also want to find out the history of any therapy the client may have received. Specifically, it is helpful to know how

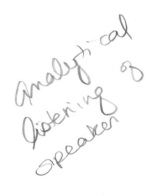

often treatment was received, for how long, and what type. If a client has received a good deal of previous therapy, with either little progress or maintenance, you will need to think about possible reasons for this situation. Of course, the best way to begin developing possible explanations for the client's lack of sustained fluency is to ask why he thinks his efforts have not been successful! Conversely, if the client has reached adulthood and has received little to no therapy for stuttering, then you will most likely have to spend a good deal of time in counseling and information-sharing about the nature of stuttering (what we know and don't know). Further, it might be that this client's stuttering is more habituated than for someone who has stuttered for the same amount of time, but who has a history of therapy (even if sporadic).

Subgoal 3: Determine the Client's Attitudes and Beliefs

When you interview an adult who stutters, you ask why he *thinks* he stutters, as well as why he *believes* that he does. You should differentiate between thinking and believing, because many times the client has had previous therapy and so has discussed what is known and not known about the cause(s) of stuttering with a previous clinician. That often contributes to his *thinking* about why he stutters. However, what a person thinks and what he feels or believes are often not the same. For example, if a client believes that stuttering is caused by some deep-seated psychological problem, even though intellectually he knows this is not the case, this belief might negatively influence his confidence in his ability to be helped and your ability to help him.

Assessing his attitudes and feelings about his stuttering is sometimes not easy.

Related to the client's beliefs about what stuttering is and why he stutters are the attitudes he possesses about talking. That is, does he generally like to speak and feels confident in his abilities to communicate, or does he view talking as unenjoyable and himself as a poor speaker? Research with adults who stutter shows that their attitudes about talking are better predictors of long-term improvements in speech fluency than their overall frequency of pretherapy stuttering (Guitar, 1976; Guitar & Bass, 1978).

Presently, there are several questionnaires available that help to assess the client's attitudes about talking and stuttering. A modified version of the *Erickson Scale of Communication Attitudes* (Andrews & Cutler, 1974) is available, which you can ask the client to fill out either at the beginning or end of the evaluation. The *Erickson Scale*, similar to the CAT for children, contains a series of statements about communication that the client indicates as either "true" or "false." Norms are available for both stuttering and nonstuttering adults, as well as for stuttering adults posttherapy, so it is possible to compare the client's score with these groups.

Question 2: Is Therapy Warranted and Recommended?

You will use all the information obtained by subgoals 1 through 3 to decide whether or not to recommend treatment for adults. In addition, as shown in Figure 10–3, you should also try to determine whether or not the client is motivated to change, and the degree of motivation.

Subgoal 4: Determine the Client's Motivation for Change

During the interview, ask why the client has come for an evaluation at that time; in other words, "Why now?" Many times, the reason is related to concerns others may have about his speech; for example, the spouse or employer. Or, the client has either made or is attempting to make other life changes, for example, a new job or enrolling in college. In such cases, the client may feel that success in new endeavors hinges on his ability to speak more fluently. Finally, the client may report that he has "had enough" of his stuttering or has "hit bottom" and is ready to work toward improving his speech. The person who is motivated to change his speech *for himself* rather than for another person or because he thinks disfluent speech will interfere with attaining a career or personal goal, may be more likely to maintain his motivation for remaining on the long road ahead in therapy.

A major challenge: to encourage the client to be forthright about motivation for change.

Question 3: What Should Be the Focus of Therapy?

As with children who stutter, if you recommend therapy for adults, you should try to make some suggestions for initial treatment focus in the recommendations section of your report. By using all of the information obtained throughout the evaluation, you will be able to make these suggestions. For example, perhaps the client needs to obtain information about the problem of stuttering and what we know about its etiology. Or, he may need some additional counseling for related concerns. Further, at the Wendell Johnson Speech and Hearing Clinic (University of Iowa), we use either a "stuttering modification" approach or an integration of both "speak more fluently" and stuttering modification approaches. Therefore, we try to assess the client's level of *behavioral* awareness of when stuttered speech is produced and what is done to produce it. This behavioral awareness by the client of *what he is doing*, both while speaking fluently and while stuttering, is necessary for his success in treatment.

Subgoal 5: Determine the Client's Level of Behavioral Awareness of Stuttering

When talking to the client about his stuttering, ask him to show you what he does when he talks which concerns him, or what he does when he considers himself to be stuttering. Sometimes the client will be unable or unwilling to show you, but will instead describe the behavior. Similar to the parents of stuttering children, who cannot or will not *show* you what their child does while speaking, an adult client who states that he can't or won't imitate stuttering might have difficulty objectively self-analyzing his speech. Further, he may possess such strong negative emotions about stuttering that he is unwilling to produce an example of stuttered speech for any reason. Finally, he might be relatively unaware of the specific characteristics of his stuttering, such that he really can't show you; rather, he might be vaguely aware on an emotional level that "something is happening somewhere" when he speaks and stutters, but he is unable to determine what he is doing while talking and when he is doing it.

One way of determining the client's behavioral self-awareness of his stuttering is to use a technique that Conture (1990b) has described as "on-line" identification. It is easy to do this during the evaluation, and it is helpful in obtaining some impression of the client's awareness of "when" he stutters. Ask the client either to read a short passage or describe a picture to you and either raise his finger or tap the table *as soon as he feels himself using stuttered speech*. Make sure to make the distinction between "hearing" and "feeling" explicit, and between "emotional feeling" ("butterflies-in-the-stomach") and "physical feeling" (kinesthetic or proprioceptive awareness) for the client. Some clients will identify their moments of stuttering *after* they have produced them, some will identify *during* their production, some immediately *before*, and some not at all. Of course, the most helpful "time" to identify stuttering is immediately before or while producing it. Observe the client's performance to make recommendations about where to start in the identification process during the initial stages of treatment.

Summary

This final section has provided guidelines for the assessment of stuttering in adults. You will use many of the same measures described for children to evaluate the fluent and disfluent speech of adults. In addition, you should attempt to form clinical impressions of those related behaviors most likely to influence therapy outcome. These include the client's beliefs and attitudes about talking and stuttering, his level of motivation for making changes in his speech, and the extent to which he is behaviorally aware of when and how he produces stuttered speech.

SUMMARY

Presented here are the components of a comprehensive stuttering assessment for children and adults. In addition to analyzing the speech and non-speech behaviors characterizing disfluency and stuttering, it is important also to evaluate the relationship between stuttering and the speaker's beliefs and attitudes about stuttering. Definitions and descriptions of speech fluency, disfluency, and stuttering were provided, along with a discussion of how to differentiate the latter two.

The goal of assessment for children is to obtain information which allows you to answer the questions: (1) Is a child stuttering or at-risk? (2) Is therapy warranted and recommended? and (3) What should be the focus of therapy? To address these questions, you will need to describe and measure the child's speech (dis)fluencies along several dimensions, begin to uncover the child's and parents' beliefs and attitudes about stuttering, observe the parents' responses to the child's stuttering, determine change in the child's speech disfluencies since they were first noticed, and assess the presence of concomitant speech, language, or related problems in the child. For adults who stutter, the information you obtain during the evaluation should help to answer the questions: (1) What is the nature of disfluent and stuttered speech? (2) Is therapy warranted and recommended? and (3) What should be the focus of therapy? Similar to children, to answer these questions for adults who stutter you need to describe and measure the client's speech disfluencies. Further, you will need to carefully interview the client to determine both the history of the problem and therapy history, attitudes and beliefs about talking and stuttering, and his levels of both motivation for participating in therapy and behavioral awareness of what he does when he stutters.

REFERENCES

Adams, M. R. (1974). A physiologic and aerodynamic interpretation of fluent and stuttered speech. *Journal of Fluency Disorders, 1*, 35–47.

Andrews, G., & Cutler, J. (1974). Stuttering therapy: The relation between changes in symptom level and attitudes. *Journal of Speech and Hearing Disorders, 39*, 312–319.

Bloodstein, O. (1987). *A handbook on stuttering* (4th ed.). Chicago: National Easter Seal Society.

Brutten, G. J. (1985). *Communication Attitude Test*. Unpublished manuscript, Southern Illinois University, Carbondale.

Conture, E. G. (1990a). Childhood stuttering: What is it and who does it? *ASHA Reports, 18*, 2–14.

Conture, E. G. (1990b). *Stuttering*. Englewood Cliffs, NJ: Prentice-Hall.

Conture, E. G., & Caruso, A. J. (1987). Assessment and diagnosis of childhood disfluency. In L. Rustin, H. Purser, & D. Rowley (Eds.), *Progress in the treatment of fluency disorders* (pp. 84–104). London: Taylor & Francis.

Conture, E. G., & Kelly, E. M. (1991). Young stutterers' nonspeech behaviors during stuttering. *Journal of Speech and Hearing Research, 34*, 1041–1056.

Conture, E. G., LaSalle, L. R., & Yaruss, S. (1990). One hundred young stutterers: Making sense of their clinical records. A miniseminar presented to *The Annual Meeting of the American Speech-Language-Hearing Association*, Seattle, WA.

De Nil, L., & Brutten G. (1991). Speech associated attitudes of stuttering and nonstuttering children. *Journal of Speech and Hearing Research, 34*, 60–66.

Guitar, B. (1976). Pretreatment factors associated with the outcome of stuttering therapy. *Journal of Speech and Hearing Research, 19*, 590–600.

Guitar, B., & Bass, C. (1978). Stuttering therapy: The relation between attitude change and long-term outcome. *Journal of Speech and Hearing Disorders, 43*, 392–400.

Johnson, W. (1959). *The onset of stuttering*. Minneapolis, MN: University of Minnesota Press.

Johnson, W., Darley, F., & Spriestersbach, D. (1978). *Diagnostic methods in speech pathology*. New York: Harper & Row.

Kelly, E. M., & Conture, E. G. (1992). Speaking rates, response time latencies, and interrupting behaviors of young stutterers, nonstutterers, and their mothers. *Journal of Speech and Hearing Research, 35*, 1256–1267.

Louko, L. J., Edwards, M. L., & Conture, E. G. (1990). Phonological characteristics of young stutterers and their normally fluent peers: Preliminary observations. *Journal of Fluency Disorders, 15*, 191–211.

Ludlow, C. (1990). Research procedures for measuring stuttering severity. In J. Cooper (Ed.), *Research needs in stuttering: Roadblocks and future directions*. *ASHA Reports, 18*, 26–33.

Neely, N., & Timmons, R. (1967). Adaptation and consistency in the disfluent speech behavior of young stutterers and nonstutterers. *Journal of Speech and Hearing Research, 10*, 250-256.

Riley, G. D. (1972). A stuttering severity instrument for children and adults. *Journal of Speech and Hearing Disorders, 37*, 314-320.

Riley, G. D. (1980). *Stuttering severity instrument for children and adults.* Tigaard, OR: C.C. Publications.

Schwartz, H. D., & Conture, E. G. (1988). Subgrouping young stutterers: Preliminary behavioral perspectives. *Journal of Speech and Hearing Research, 31*, 62-71.

Schwartz, H. D., Zebrowski, P. M., & Conture, E. G. (1990). Behaviors at the onset of stuttering. *Journal of Fluency Disorders, 15*, 77-86.

Stocker, B. (1980). *Stocker Probe Technique for the Diagnosis and Treatment of Stuttering in Young Children.* Tulsa, OK: Modern Educational Corp.

Stocker, B., & Usprich, C. (1976). Stuttering in young children and level of demand. *Journal of Fluency Disorders, 1*, 116-131.

Weiss, A., & Zebrowski, P. (1992). Disfluencies in the conversations of young children who stutter: Some answers about questions. *Journal of Speech and Hearing Research, 35*, 1230-1238.

Williams, D. E., Silverman, F. H., & Kools, J. A. (1968). Disfluency behavior of elementary-school stutterers and nonstutterers: The adaptation effect. *Journal of Speech and Hearing Research, 11*, 622-630.

Williams, D. E. (1978). Differential diagnosis of disorders of fluency. In F. Darley & D. Spriestersbach (Eds.), *Diagnostic methods in speech pathology* (2nd ed.). New York: Harper and Row.

Williams, D. E. (1979). A perspective on approaches to stuttering therapy. In H. Gregory (Ed.), *Controversies about stuttering therapy.* Baltimore: University Park Press.

Williams, D. E. (1985). Talking with children who stutter. In J. Fraser (Ed.), *Counseling stutterers.* Memphis: Stuttering Foundation of America.

Yairi, E., & Ambrose, N. (1992). A longitudinal study of stuttering in children: A preliminary report. *Journal of Speech and Hearing Research, 35*, 755-760.

Yairi, E., & Lewis, B. (1984). Disfluencies at the onset of stuttering. *Journal of Speech and Hearing Research, 27*, 154-159.

Zebrowski, P. M. (1991). Duration of the speech disfluencies of beginning stutterers. *Journal of Speech and Hearing Research, 34*, 483-491.

Zebrowski, P., & Conture, E. (1989). Judgments of disfluency by mothers of stuttering and normally fluent children. *Journal of Speech and Hearing Research, 32*, 625-634.

Zebrowski, P. M., & Raszkowski, L. M. (1993). *A preliminary study of stuttering duration in children.* Unpublished manuscript. University of Iowa, Iowa City.

Zebrowski, P., & Schum, R. (1993). Counseling the parents of children who stutter. *American Journal of Speech-Language Pathology*, 65-73.

RECOMMENDED READINGS

Stuttering Assessment Issues and Methods

Costello, J. M., & Ingham, R. J. (1984). Assessment strategies for child and adult stutterers. In W. Perkins & R. Curlee (Eds.), *Nature and treatment of stuttering: New directions.* San Diego: College-Hill Press.

Characteristics of the Fluent and Stuttered Speech of People Who Stutter

Bloodstein, O. (1970). Stuttering and normal nonfluency — A continuity hypothesis. *British Journal of Disordered Communication, 5,* 30–39.

Johnson, W., & Knott, J. (1937). Studies in the psychology of stuttering: I. The distribution of moments of stuttering in successive readings of the same material. *Journal of Speech and Hearing Disorders, 2,* 17–19.

LaSalle, L., & Conture, E. (1991). Eye contact between young stutterers and their mothers. *Journal of Fluency Disorders, 16,* 173–200.

Van Riper, C. (1982). *The nature of stuttering.* Englewood Cliffs, NJ: Prentice-Hall.

Williams, D. E., Silverman, F. H., & Kools, J. A. (1968). Disfluency behavior of elementary-school stutterers and nonstutterers: The adaptation effect. *Journal of Speech and Hearing Research, 11,* 622–630.

Williams, D. E., Silverman, F. H., & Kools, J. A. (1969). Disfluency behavior of elementary-school stutterers and nonstutterers: The consistency effect. *Journal of Speech and Hearing Research, 12,* 301–307.

Yairi, E. H. (1983). The onset of stuttering in two- and three-year old children: A preliminary report. *Journal of Speech and Hearing Disorders, 48,* 171–178.

Zebrowski, P., Conture, E., & Cudahy, E. (1985). Acoustic analysis of young stutterers' fluency. *Journal of Fluency Disorders, 10,* 173–192.

Related Speech and Language Behaviors of Children Who Stutter

Walker, J., Archibald, L., Cherniak, S., & Fish, V. (1992). Articulation rate in 3- and 5-year old children. *Journal of Speech and Hearing Research, 35,* 4–13.

Attitudes of Children and Adults Who Stutter

De Nil, L. F., & Brutten, G. J. (1991). Speech-associated attitudes of stuttering and nonstuttering children. *Journal of Speech and Hearing Research, 34,* 60–66.

Tests and Measures of Stuttering

Conture, E. G., & Caruso, A. J. (1978). A review of the Stocker Probe Technique for diagnosis and treatment of stuttering in young children. *Journal of Fluency Disorders, 3,* 297–198.

Parents' Judgments of Disfluent Speech

Glasner, P., & Rosenthal, D. (1957). Parental diagnosis of stuttering in young children. *Journal of Speech and Hearing Disorders, 22,* 288–295.

Stuttering Treatment

Peters, T., & Guitar, B. (1991). *Stuttering: An integrated approach to its nature and treatment.* Baltimore: Williams & Wilkins.

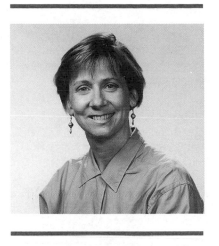

PATRICIA M. ZEBROWSKI, Ph.D.

Ph.D. 1987, Syracuse University

Dr. Zebrowski is an Assistant Professor in the Department of Speech
Pathology and Audiology at the University of Iowa. Her research
interests are in the area of stuttering, with special emphasis
on childhood stuttering. She teaches courses in stuttering and
intervention and supervises master's level students in diagnostic and
therapy practicum with children and adults who stutter.

C H A P T E R

11

Voice Disorders

Katherine Verdolini, Ph.D.

WHAT IS A VOICE DISORDER?

At the simplest level, a voice disorder is a persistent abnormality in the sound of the voice. As obvious as this definition may seem, it poses a number of questions. For example, what is the point of reference for "normal," that determines the boundaries of abnormality? Is it the quality of voice that can be expected from a lesion-free, disease-free system, or is it the quality of voice that is most typically encountered within the subject's usual cultural environment? Who is responsible for determining the presence or absence of an "abnormality"? Is it a speech/language pathologist (SLP) or other practitioner, or does the speaker determine abnormality? What about conditions that result in a voice that falls well within normal limits for lesion-free, disease-free individuals, and for the subject's general cultural milieu, but that fails to function well for some social, work, or other purpose? Finally, what about conditions in which the sound of the voice is satisfactory in all regards, but is physically uncomfortable?

There are several ways to define a voice disorder.

These questions raise important issues about the definition of a voice disorder and point out how the definition might not be as obvious as may appear. In this chapter we define a voice disorder as a condition in which voice functioning is unacceptable to the user in social, professional, or other contexts, and for which the SLP or other practitioner generally finds some corroborative evidence. By this definition, voice disorders would include situations in which the actual voice output is acceptable, but in which voicing is uncomfortable. The discussion is limited to phonation disorders, excluding disorders that primarily involve resonance problems, considered elsewhere in this book.

In this chapter, I will discuss how common voice disorders are, why they are important, what conditions cause them, and how to assess them clinically. To facilitate your reading, scholarly citations are mostly excluded within the text itself. Further readings are listed at the end of the chapter, organized by topic.

HOW COMMON ARE VOICE DISORDERS, AND WHAT IS THEIR FUNCTIONAL IMPACT?

There are not many data about how common voice disorders are, using any single definition, and none that we know of about how common they are from the speaker's perspective. In most studies on hoarseness in children, about 6% to 9% of children seem to be hoarse at a given moment in time and from about 3% to 6.5% of adults seem to be hoarse. The percentages are quite probably higher among persons who use their voices heavily for professional reasons. According to some of our own informal estimates, as many as one-third of some groups of professional voice users (including public school music teachers and singing voice teachers) may complain of voice problems and/or have some abnormality in the larynx at any given time.

A change in voice is sometimes an early symptom of throat cancer, seen generally in middle-aged and older adults. In other cases, a change in voice may signal the presence of another significant disease process, such as Parkinson's disease. However, voice problems in younger age groups most commonly do not signal a life-threatening condition or a serious disease process. But, voice disorders can produce functional consequences that are quite dramatic and significant to the patient. According to some estimates, about 50%–60% of clinical patients with voice disorders complained of moderately severe or severe disruptions in quality of life in professional, social, communicative, physical, and psychological domains as a result of the disorder. These findings corroborate our impression that persons with voice disorders often have significant functional impairments and distress because of the disorder and, thus, deserve our professional attention.

WHAT ARE THE CAUSES OF VOICE DISORDERS?

Voice disorders are caused by a number of factors, some physical (organic) and some not strictly physical (nonorganic). A discussion of the causes can be organized in several ways. The scheme in this chapter is particularly relevant for assessment. According to this system, voice disorders can be categorized as (a) those caused by discrete mass lesions of the vocal folds, (b) those caused by distributed vocal fold tissue changes, (c) those caused by organically based movement disorders, and (d) nonorganically based disorders. (See Figure 11-1 for a review of the major structures of the larynx, including the vocal folds.) Each condition will be briefly described, because it is important for you to understand them to understand the assess-

Have you ever had a voice problem? Do you know others that have?

The physician who specializes in disorders and diseases of the throat is an otolaryngologist.

Many factors can lead to a voice problem.

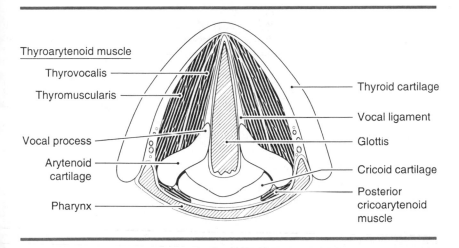

Figure 11-1. Schematic view of the larynx. The thyrovocalis and thyromuscularis form the muscular part of the "membranous" vocal cords.

ment procedure described later in the chapter. The discussion is summarized in Figure 11-2. You should extend your reading for more complete information (see for example, Colton & Casper, 1990).

A final comment before proceeding regards the relationship between laryngeal conditions and voice disorders. The relationship is not perfect (one-to-one). In particular, although various conditions may result in voice changes, the changes will vary for different people. This is an important principle to remember in considering the complexity of the relationship between structure and function in voice disorders.

Discrete Mass Lesions of the Vocal Folds

Discrete or circumscribed mass lesions of the vocal folds are a frequent basis for a voice disorder. These lesions are described in the following section, and include nodules, polyps, cysts, papilloma, keratosis and leukoplakia, contact ulcers, granuloma (benign tumors), and laryngeal cancer (malignant tumors).

These diagnoses are made by examinations by the otolaryngologist.

Lesions of the Membranous Folds

Description and causes.   Nodules, polyps, cysts, papilloma, keratosis and leukoplakia, and laryngeal cancer can all affect the membranous vocal folds, that is, the part of the vocal folds that vibrates to produce voice. Nodules and polyps are discrete lesions that develop at about the midpoint of the membranous folds (or the juncture of the anterior one-third and the posterior two-thirds of the entire length of the vocal folds). These lesions may appear on one or both vocal folds (that is, they may be unilateral or bilateral). Nodules involve fluid accumulation (edema) in early stages and a build-up of hardened tissues (proteinous, or collagen fibers) in later stages. As

Most people understand that a voice problem can result from a problem "in the throat."

Category	Description	Presumed Primary Cause and Possible Contributors	Primary Effect on Voice
Discrete Mass Lesions			
Membranous Folds			
Nodules	Protrusions at midpoint of membranous folds; edematous and/or collagenous	High vocal fold impact force High vocal fold tissue viscosity	Hoarseness
Polyps	Protrusions at midpoint of membranous folds; edematous, possibly vascularized	High vocal fold impact force High vocal fold tissue viscosity	Hoarseness
Cysts	Protrusions along membranous folds, often at midpoint; fluid-filled sacs of epithelium	Glandular blockage	Hoarseness
Papilloma	Laryngeal warts	Virus (presence of vaginal warts in mother, and vaginal delivery)	Hoarseness
Keratosis leukoplakia	White, plaque-like lesions	Irritants (smoke)	Hoarseness
Cancer	White, grainy lesions	Smoke and alcohol	Hoarseness
Posterior glottis			
Contact ulcers	Protrusions on medial, surface of arytenoids, possibly with contralateral concavity	Gastric reflux "Pressed" phonation Low pitch	Phonatory effort
Distributed Tissue Changes			
Reinke's edema	Distributed edema along membranous folds	Irritants (smoke)	Low pitch in speech
Laryngitis	Distributed inflammation	Bacteria, virus	Hoarseness
Bowing	Persistent bowing of folds (muscular deformation?)	Chronic heavy voice use Elderly age	Weak voice
Sulcus vocalis	Groove parallel to vocal fold margin	Congenital, developmental Heavy voice use	Weak voice
Trauma	(Appearance depends on type of trauma)	Mechanical, thermal, or chemical trauma	Variable
Organic Movement Disorders			
Peripheral paralyses	Limited (medial) movement of affected fold	Local trauma (including surgery) Virus Heart disease	Weak voice
Central paralyses	Resistance to movement	Cerebral cortex lesions (stroke)	"Tight" voice

(continued)

Figure 11-2. Summary of voice disorder categories.

Category	Description	Presumed Primary Cause and Possible Contributors	Primary Effect on Voice
Organic Movement Disorders (continued)			
Extrapyramidal disease (e.g., Parkinson's disease)	Small range of motion	Dopamine deficiency	Monotone voice in speech Weak voice
Nerve–muscle junction dysfunctions (myasthenia gravis)	Rapid fatigue in function	Rapid depletion of chemicals sustaining vocal fold contraction	Rapid voice fatigue
Spasmodic dysphonia	Abrupt adductions during speech (adductory); Abrupt abductions during speech (abductory)	Undetermined	Spasmodic voice
Non-Organic Disorders			
Mutational falsetto	Persistent high pitch in postpubertal male, with normal-appearing larynx	Psychological conflict Learned behavior	High pitch (falsetto)
Ventricular phonation	False (ventricular) vocal folds vibrate and produce sound	Sometimes compensation for poorly functioning true vocal folds	Gravelly voice
Conversion aphonia/dysphonia	Lack of voice (aphonia) or hoarse voice (dysphonia), with normal-appearing larynx	Psychological	No voice or hoarse voice
Muscular tension dysphonia	Persistent posterior glottal gap during phonation, and complaints of voice problems	Simultaneous contraction of laryngeal adductors and abductors	Breathy voice Phonatory effort

Figure 11-2 (continued)

such, mature nodules are like laryngeal "callouses." Polyps are typically described as more fluid-based and more bloody (vascular) than nodules. Polyps may be attached to the vocal fold margin (sessile) or may hang from the margin (peduncular).

The primary cause of both nodules and polyps appears to be trauma to the vocal fold margins. Trauma, in turn, is caused by high impact forces in that area of contact between the folds during phonation. Relevant for both assessment and for therapy, high impact forces may be caused by loud voice and, more specifically, loud voice that is produced with a pressing together of the vocal folds, or "pressed voice."[1]

Some physical changes in the vocal folds are caused by vocal strain. Others are not.

[1] Many clinicians talk about "voice abuse" and "voice misuse" as the cause of nodules and polyps. Voice abuse mainly refers to loud voice, screaming, and strong throat clearing. Voice misuse refers to physiologically "inefficient" voice use. We prefer the use of other, more neutral terms (for example, "pressed voice," or even "screaming"), because "abuse" and "misuse" may be perceived by the patient as having negative moral connotations and, as such, could be harmful to the therapeutic process.

In addition to the way the voice is used, other factors may increase the risk of nodules and polyps. These are mainly factors that lead to dry vocal fold tissue or that make it sticky. The theoretical and empirical bases for this argument are provided in readings in the reference list. For our purposes, the point is that smoke, alcohol, caffeine, diuretics, drying nasal sprays, dry air, and certain (drying) medications may dry vocal fold tissue and upper respiratory tract infections may make the tissue sticky. In either case, the risk of nodules and polyps may be increased.

Laryngeal cysts are fluid-filled sacs of epithelium[2] that usually develop on one vocal fold in about the same place as nodules and polyps. Cysts are apparently caused by a glandular block, so that mucous builds up within the sac that is formed by the intruded epithelium. When a cyst is present on one vocal fold, a nodule may appear on the other one, probably as a result of the cyst hitting against this other fold. Often, a cyst can be distinguished from a nodule only after it has been excised and is examined under a microscope (that is, by histological examination).

Papilloma are laryngeal warts. They develop in the epithelium of the vocal folds and can appear anywhere along the membranous folds, as well as elsewhere in the larynx. The most common cause apparently is genital warts in the mother during a vaginal delivery.

Keratosis and leukoplakia are white, flat, plaque-like lesions that also develop in the laryngeal epithelium, generally along the membranous folds, and are considered precancerous. The most common cause of these lesions appears to be chronic exposure to irritants, such as smoke.

Laryngeal cancer, or malignant tumors, are white, grainy lesions. They can develop at any point along the vocal folds or above or below them. Considerable clinical evidence points to a role of smoking as a primary cause of laryngeal cancer. However, recent research findings suggest that cigarette smoking alone may not be a strong causative factor but might be, in combination with heavy alcohol consumption.

Throat cancer is always a concern for middle-aged and older adults who are hoarse.

Primary effects on voice. All types of discrete mass lesions of the membranous folds tend to produce similar types of effects on the voice, although there are exceptions. With these lesions, the vocal folds usually do not close completely during phonation. Thus, considerable air may escape through the vocal folds during phonation, without being transformed into sound. This air gives the voice a "breathy" quality. Further, because of uneven mass distributions within the vocal folds with these lesions, vocal fold vibratory patterns may be irregular. The overall result is a "hoarse-sounding" voice. Patients with discrete mass lesions also usually have difficulty producing high-pitched and quiet sounds, because of the presence of the added mass. Patients also often complain that voicing is "effortful."

Can you imitate a breathy voice?

Lesions of the Posterior Glottis

Description and causes. Some discrete mass lesions typically affect the back of the larynx (the posterior larynx), rather than the membranous folds.

---

[2] The epithelium is the surface layer of the vocal folds. In the case of a cyst, the epithelium intrudes into lower layers of vocal fold tissue, forming a sac with fluid inside it.

By far the most common examples are contact ulcers and granuloma. The term "contact ulcer" refers to an ulceration of the inside (medial) arytenoid surface. There is often a protrusion on the other arytenoid, yielding a characteristic "cup and saucer" appearance. "Granuloma" refers to grainy, vascularized tissue, also on the medial arytenoid surface, on one or both sides. In many cases, the difference between "contact ulcers" and "granuloma" reflects a difference in how physicians prefer to use the terms rather than an actual difference in lesions.

Quite a bit of evidence suggests that gastric reflux contributes to the development of contact ulcers and granuloma in some cases. Gastric reflux is a condition in which the sphincter connecting the lower esophagus to the stomach functions incompletely. In this case, stomach (or gastric) juices may spill up through the esophagus and into the posterior airway over the arytenoids, particularly while a person is sleeping in the prone position. The person may awaken at night with regurgitation and with an acid taste in his mouth. Over time, the gastric juices may produce ulcerative tissue changes. In other cases, granuloma may be caused by intubation during surgery, that is, by the introduction of a "breathing tube" put between the vocal folds for the administration of anesthesia. Finally, voice use may contribute to the development of contact ulcers and granuloma. In particular, there has been speculation that a chronically low pitch during speech may contribute to these lesions because the arytenoids tend to "rock" at low frequencies, possibly because of a resonant frequency phenomenon. Finally, it is intuitive to think that if a person speaks with pressed (or hyperadducted) arytenoids, the risk of contact ulcers and granuloma may increase.

Primary effects on voice.   If contact ulcers and granuloma do not affect the membranous folds, as they generally do not, the actual voice output may be relatively unaffected. Voice quality may be normal or near-normal. The patient may mainly complain that phonation is effortful and that there is a distinct local pain in the throat. (Patients will often point to the arytenoid area.) The pain may be continuous (chronic) or it may occur only during phonation or swallowing. In some cases, patients may also complain of a pain in the ear on the same side as the laryngeal lesion. This is called "referred pain," because it is "referred" from cranial nerve X in the larynx, through the same nerve up to the ear.

Throat discomfort during talking is a matter for concern.

Distributed Vocal Fold Tissue Changes

Distributed vocal fold tissue changes represent a less cohesive set of conditions, as compared to discrete mass lesions. This brings us to a discussion of Reinke's edema, laryngitis, vocal fold bowing, sulcus vocalis, and tissue changes from laryngeal trauma.

Reinke's Edema

Description and causes.   Reinke's edema involves a widespread accumulation of fluid, or swelling (edema), usually in both vocal folds, in the layer of tissue right below the vocal fold epithelium ("Reinke's space"). Some clinicians refer to this condition as "polypoid degeneration." The causes are not entirely clear. However, some clinicians think that chronic exposure to irritants such as smoke may play a role in the development of this condition.

Primary effects on voice.   The most obvious effect of Reinke's edema on voice typically is an extremely low speaking pitch and the loss of an ability to produce high notes. The reason is probably related to the increased vocal fold mass with this condition. The voice is also often described as "raspy." If the vocal fold swelling is more or less evenly distributed along the entire length of both membranous folds, as is often the case, the characteristic "breathiness" that accompanies discrete mass lesions may not be present. This is because the vocal folds close more or less completely during phonation.

Laryngitis

Description and causes.   Laryngitis is a distributed inflammation of the larynx. The vocal folds may appear reddened and swollen. As a medical condition, laryngitis is caused by bacterial or viral agents. It may appear in conjunction with a more global upper respiratory tract infection or in isolation.

Laryngitis is a common voice problem.

Primary effects on voice.   The typical effect of laryngitis on voice is a dramatic, although usually temporary, compromise in most voice functions. That is, the voice is markedly hoarse and weak or altogether lacking. When present, phonation is intermittent and patients have great difficulty producing high notes, if they can produce them at all. The mechanisms underlying voice changes with laryngitis are not entirely clear. However, they may be partly caused by a combination of irregular masses together with unusual stiffness within the membranous folds.

Vocal Fold Bowing

Description and causes.   Vocal fold bowing involves an incomplete closure of the anterior vocal folds during phonation, producing a characteristic "bowed" appearance. This condition is most often encountered in elderly males. However, it may also be found in younger adult males with a history of long-term shouting. The laryngeal appearance implies a weakness in the adductory action in the membranous vocal folds themselves (but not in arytenoid adduction) and, possibly, a slight deformation in membranous vocal fold tissue.

Primary effects on voice.   The cardinal effect of vocal fold bowing is weak voice. The reason is that voice intensity (and loudness) depends on the degree of vocal fold closure during phonation and closure is incomplete along the membranous folds with bowing. The spontaneous speaking pitch may also be high. Both younger and older male patients sometimes complain that they are mistaken as female on the telephone. This effect may be due to a relative shortening of the vibratory portion of the membranous folds caused by a strong, compensatory adduction of the posterior vocal folds. Patients also often cannot produce very high or very low pitches.

Sulcus Vocalis

Description and causes.   A sulcus vocalis is a groove in vocal fold tissue, parallel to the vocal fold margin. A sulcus may be observed only in one vocal fold or sulci may be observed in both folds. The causes of this condition are not well understood. Some clinicians think that it may be determined at birth or may develop because of genetic factors, or that certain voice use patterns may cause it. However, the specific types of voice use patterns that may be involved, and how they may result in the development of sulci remain unclear.

Primary effects on voice.   There are limited data about the effects of sulcus vocalis on voice. In our experience, a primary effect is weak voice, possibly because the vocal folds do not adduct well along their entire length during phonation. Patients also typically complain of effortful phonation and of difficulty making high pitches.

Laryngeal Trauma

Description and causes.   A blow to the larynx can affect the vocal apparatus in different ways, depending on the location and the strength of the blow. In general, traumatic influences can be mechanical (for example, from a blow to the larynx across a steering wheel in a motor vehicle accident), thermal (as with smoke inhalation from a fire), or chemical (as with exposure to potent concentrations of ammonia, paint solvents, or other chemicals).

Physical injury to the throat requires immediate medical attention.

Primary effects on voice.   The specific effects of trauma on voice depend on the nature of the trauma. In fact, so many different types of trauma are possible that no general statement about specific effects can be made.

A series of physical (organic) conditions can produce movement disorders in the larynx and, sometimes, also elsewhere. These conditions include peripheral vocal fold paralyses and pareses, cortically based paralyses and pareses affecting the vocal folds, extra pyramidal disease processes, and nerve-muscle junction dysfunctions. Although the origin of another movement disorder, spasmodic dysphonia, is not actually known, some evidence points to a physical basis. Therefore, spasmodic dysphonia will be discussed in this section as well.

Diagnosis of these laryngeal movement disorders is made after examination by an otolaryngologist.

Peripheral Vocal Fold Paralyses and Pareses

Description and causes.   Peripheral paralyses are the result of a severe failure of nerve impulse conduction to muscle tissue, with subsequent loss of voluntary movement. Paresis is a relatively lesser degree of nerve impulse failure. In the larynx, peripheral paralyses and pareses usually affect only one vocal fold. Sometimes, these conditions are caused by local trauma from accidents or from neck or heart surgery, by viral processes (such as a cold), or by heart disease. (The relation to heart disease is that the same nerve that partially innervates the heart also innervates the left side of the larynx.) However, sometimes paralyses and pareses are an isolated disorder, with no discoverable connection to any other physical disorder or disease. They could theoretically affect any of the laryngeal muscles. However, by far the most commonly encountered cases involve a compromise in the adductory muscles, if not in other muscles as well. Assuming that a paralysis occurs with the affected vocal fold in the abducted position, the ability to bring that fold to the middle of the glottis is impaired. Over time function may return, although no data are presently available about how often spontaneous recovery is observed. Usually, the unaffected vocal fold compensates to some degree by crossing the midline of the glottal space during phonation.

Primary effects on voice. The major effects of peripheral paralyses and pareses on voice are breathiness, weakness (quiet voice), and a reduced phonation time during speech or singing (i.e. reduced ability to prolong sounds for a long time). These effects are caused by incomplete vocal fold closure during phonation.

Cortical Paralyses and Pareses

Description and causes. Lesions to the brain surface, or the *cerebral cortex*, can also result in vocal fold paralyses and pareses. A common cause for these conditions is stroke (cerebrovascular accident, or CVA).

Primary effects on voice. The primary effect on voice is a perceptually "tight" and "weak" (quiet) sound. The reason for these effects is increased resistance to movement in laryngeal muscles that occurs with cortical lesions.

Extrapyramidal Disease Processes

Description and causes. Disease processes affecting another part of the brain, the extrapyramidal region, can also affect voice. One of the most common examples is Parkinson's disease. In this condition, chemical deficiencies in the extrapyramidal system (specifically, a lack of dopamine, a chemical message transmitter) produce a generalized movement disorder characterized by small movements (*hypokinesia*) and slow movements (*bradykinesia*) that can affect the voice and speech as well as other functions. The laryngeal examination may reveal grossly normal-appearing vocal structures or the vocal folds may appear somewhat bowed.

Primary effects on voice. The effects of Parkinson's disease on voice are variable, and depend, among other things, on how advanced the disease is and on the types of medications the patient is taking. Perhaps the most characteristic effect is a quiet voice during spontaneous speech and minimal pitch and loudness variations ("monotone" voice). These effects are related to the limited range of vocal fold movement during speech. Specific testing often reveals an ability to produce greater pitch and loudness variations than the patient produces spontaneously.

Nerve-Muscle Junction Dysfunctions

Description and causes.   A condition called myasthenia gravis is characterized by a rapid fatigue in muscular contraction once contraction has been initiated. The dysfunction is related to a rapid depletion of chemical transmission from nerves to the muscles normally innervated.

Primary effects on voice.   The classic effect of myasthenia gravis on voice and on other physical functions is a rapid deterioration of function within a few seconds. For example, at the beginning of a phrase the patient may have a normally loud voice. However, within a few seconds the voice may be barely audible.

Spasmodic Dysphonia

Description and causes.   Adductory spasmodic dysphonia (SD) is characterized by intermittent interruptions in voicing from abrupt vocal fold closures during speech. Especially in the past, arguments were made for a psychogenic (psychological) cause. However, arguments have also been made for a physical basis. The organic (physical) explanation for the disorder probably prevails currently, adductory SD generally improves with injection of botulinum toxin that "relaxes" the spasticity by temporarily paralyzing one or both vocal folds. A less common form of SD is abductory, in which the "spasticity" results in uncontrolled and sudden *abductions* in the vocal folds during phonation (the opposite from adductory SD). Treatment by botulinum toxin appears less successful for abductory SD than for adductory SD.

Primary effects on voice.   The most obvious effect of SD on voice is the sudden shutting off of voice, sometimes described as "strangled voice" (adductory SD) or the sudden "giving way" of voice (abductory SD) during speech. Spasmodic effects are primarily observed during running speech (particularly following consonants) and may not be observed during sustained vowel phonation.

Nonorganically Based Disorders

Mutational Falsetto

Description and causes.   Mutational falsetto is the continued use of a high-pitched (falsetto) voice by a postpubertal male, without any apparent physical basis. For some patients, psychological conflict is implied as a basis for the disorder. In other patients, the disorder may simply reflect a learned pattern that is treated relatively easily with voice therapy.

Primary effects on voice.   By definition, the primary effect on voice is a high-pitched, falsetto voice during spontaneous speech, but an ability to produce lower, more age-appropriate pitches on stimulation.

Ventricular Phonation

Description and causes.   Ventricular phonation involves the use of the false vocal folds (the ventricular folds that lie immediately above the true vocal folds) as a sound source for voice. Most often, this type of phonation develops when the true vocal folds are injured in some way or are unavailable as a sound source, for example following laryngeal surgeries for cancer.

Primary effects on voice.   The primary effect is a low-pitched, gravelly voice, which is attributable to the large mass of the false vocal folds. By way of example, the late jazz trumpeter and vocalist, Louis Armstrong, had a characteristic singing style that may have involved ventricular phonation.

Conversion Dysphonia/Aphonia

Description and causes.   Conversion disorders affecting the voice involve a marked hoarseness (dysphonia) or lack of phonation altogether (aphonia) without any apparent organic cause. These conditions are strongly implied not only when the larynx appears normal, but also when normal voice can be elicited during vegetative functions such as gargling or coughing, and then sustained during speech. Usually, the patient reports a sudden onset, possibly in conjunction with an upper respiratory tract infection, and a highly consistent disorder subsequently. The condition often resolves entirely or almost entirely, within an hour or less of targeted voice therapy. Psychological causes are quite clearly implied. However, the exact psychological mechanisms that lead to conversion disorders are not well understood (Butcher, Elias, & Raven, 1993).

Sudden loss of the voice requires attention by the otolaryngologist and the speech pathologist.

Primary effects on voice.   As already noted, the primary effect is a severe, highly consistent dysphonia or aphonia with sudden onset. Also as noted, the disorder often resolves quite quickly with voice therapy.

Muscular Tension Dysphonia

Description and causes.   Muscular tension dysphonia (MTD), which some clinicians might call "vocal strain," is a condition in which the posterior vocal folds fail to close during phonation. Incomplete posterior vocal fold closure is quite common, particularly in females. However, MTD is distinguished from normal posterior vocal fold gaps because with MTD, patients complain of discomfort during phonation, whereas with simpler gaps, they generally do not. MTD appears to be caused by a simultaneous contraction of both vocal fold adductors and vocal fold abductors during phonation. Some clinicians contend that MTD may increase the risk of nodules.

Have you ever experienced vocal strain?

Primary effects on voice.   The effects of MTD on voice are variable. In some cases, the voice may simply be breathy and the patient may complain that voicing is effortful. In other cases, the voice may be quite hoarse and the patient may have great difficulty producing high notes. Formal assessment may reveal a better ability to produce high notes than occurs spontaneously.

Section Summary

In this section, we have discussed different conditions that lead to voice disorders and their causes as the basis for the following discussion on voice assessment. By being familiar with these conditions and their likely effects on voice, you should begin to have a good idea of what to look for during a voice assessment. You also should be prepared to interpret many of the results that you obtain.

WHAT IS THE ROLE OF THE SPEECH/LANGUAGE PATHOLOGIST IN THE CLINICAL ASSESSMENT OF VOICE?

In the clinical assessment of voice, your objective is to answer critical clinical questions. The ones we focus on are shown in Figure 11-3: (1) Is there a voice disorder? (2) If there is a voice disorder, how severe is it? (3) What specific voice functions are impaired (and to what degree are they impaired), reflecting the diagnostic condition? (4) What factors likely contributed to the onset of the disorder and what are maintaining factors? (5) What is the patient's motivational level to improve the voice disorder? (6) What are behavioral treatment recommendations? (7) What is the prognosis for improvement with the treatment plan recommended? An added objective is to ensure appropriate medical consideration of any physical dis-

Questions	Part of Assessment That Addresses Questions
1. Is there a voice disorder?	Case history
2. If so, how severe is it?	Case history Voice measures
3. What specific voice functions are impaired?	Otolaryngological report Voice measures
4. What factors likely contributed to the onset of the disorder and what are maintaining factors?	Case history Voice measures
5. What is the patient's motivational level to improve the disorder?	Case history
6. What are behavioral treatment recommendations?	Recommendations
7. What is the prognosis for improvement with the treatment plan recommended?	Prognosis

Figure 11-3. Critical clinical questions.

order and disease related to the voice problem, if such consideration has not already occurred.

As indicated in Figure 11-3, the answers to your questions will come from a variety of sources. These sources include medical reports (primarily from an otolaryngologist), your case history, and the specific voice measures that you make. We will describe the case history and the voice measures in detail shortly. However, first we discuss the clinical questions a bit further, with emphasis on aspects of the assessment procedure that address them.

Is There a Voice Disorder?

Of course, the first critical question is if there is a voice disorder! Consistent with our definition of a "voice disorder," we think that, ultimately, the answer to this question depends on the patient's perspective. As such, the answer emerges during the case history from the patient's self-descriptions of her voice and voice-related complaints.

Bottom lines: is the voice satisfactory to the patient's needs? Does the patient regard her voice as normal or "a problem"? Are there any indications of disease?

Most often, the patient's identification of a voice problem will coincide with yours. However, sometimes it will not. For example, the patient might be severely hoarse to your ears and may perform abnormally on a series of voice tests. However, he may report little or no negative impact on his quality of life as a result of voice functioning. In this case we would consider that there is no "voice disorder," strictly speaking. Hoarseness may even be considered a desirable attribute. We all can identify several professional entertainers who have "hoarse" or "husky" voices that not only seem not to be a problem to them, but may even assist their career because of ready voice identification. On the other hand, another patient may have a clear voice to your ears, with normal or even superior performance on formal voice tests, and yet describe phonatory discomfort or other voice dysfunctions that negatively impact on her quality of life. Patients such as this do have a voice disorder. For example, a patient may experience throat fatigue after business or social activities that require a lot of talking. Another patient may be a trained singer who experiences a vague "glitch" between high G-sharp and A. The point is that the patient's perspective is the key to determining whether there is a voice disorder.

If There Is a Voice Disorder, How Severe Is It?

The answer to this question is provided by the patient's complaints (case history) and by your direct observations of voice (voice measures). Using the combined information, you will identify a global severity level, against which you will assess subsequent progress (or lack thereof) with treatment.

What Specific Voice Functions Are Impaired (and to what degree are they impaired), Reflecting the Diagnostic Condition?

Your voice measures should provide you with an indication of the specific voice functions that are impaired, consistent with the diagnostic condition, and the degree to which functions are impaired. This information is important because it provides you with baseline measures of the *particular* disturbances for that patient, which will hopefully improve with treatment.

Usually, the voice measures that you make will be consistent with the diagnostic condition described by the physician. In rare cases, there may be a discrepancy. Such cases are interesting and provide an opportunity for you to interact with the physician, leading to more subtle diagnostic statements than might have been otherwise possible.

What Are Factors That Likely Contributed to the Onset of the Disorder, and What Are Maintaining Factors?

The answer to these questions will be important in planning therapy, because they will partially direct what will be done in therapy. For example, if you find that a patient with contact ulcers has a low speaking pitch, you might decide to help him increase the pitch during speech, because the low pitch might be part of what is maintaining the ulcers. You will not directly observe many etiologic factors during the voice assessment, but you will discern many of them from the case history and/or the medical report.

What Is the Patient's Motivational Level To Improve the Disorder?

During the case history or some other part of the assessment, you will want to establish how motivated the patient is to address a voice disorder. You will consider the motivational level in planning therapy.

What Are Treatment Recommendations?

The physician may make recommendations about pharmaceutical or surgical intervention. You will make recommendations about behavioral intervention (voice therapy). Ideally, a coordinated treatment package will be formulated by both of you. In making the recommendations, you will consider past clinical experience and information from empirical studies. You will also consider the patient's motivational level.

What Is the Prognosis For Improvement With the Treatment Plan Recommended?

With some experience, you can usually make prognostic statements on the basis of the combined medical and speech pathology assessment. Such statements are important for the team working with the patient and especially for the patient himself. Prognostic statements may also be required by third-party reimbursers (insurance companies).

Obviously, prognosis depends not only on the diagnostic profile, but also on the patient's motivational level. A high motivation level to improve the voice disorder generally improves the prognosis for most diagnostic profiles. The converse is also true.

Section Summary

This section has discussed general questions that you will probably want to answer in a voice assessment, along with the parts of the assessment procedure that address the questions. Next is a discussion of some of the important concepts behind a voice disorder, in general, and, finally, a discussion of assessment specifics.

ASSESSMENT PROCEDURE

What Are Important Concepts Underlying a Voice Assessment?

We need to identify the important conceptual foundations of a voice assessment, in general, no matter what the details. This issue is probably most easily addressed historically. Until not too long ago, a complaint was that voice assessment procedures often provided little solid information. One reason was that relatively few assessment procedures had been systematically developed. During the past two decades, considerable attention has been given to the theoretical and practical development of numerous voice measurement procedures. This trend has led to important changes in the way we practice our profession.

In the process of developing the various voice measures, new and sophisticated technologies have evolved. These technologies provide exciting possibilities for gaining a microscopic view of voice functioning that afford subtle insights about processes underlying voice disorders. However, sources of discouragement persist. As you might expect, none of the available measures (technologically supported or not) provides, by itself, comprehensive information about the voice. Further, none of the measures is without interpretive problems. Finally, many clinicians do not have access to sophisticated equipment.

Despite these considerations there is an approach that makes sense. This approach is based on two related tenets: (a) even more important than sophisticated measurement equipment, the most fundamental tools for a good voice assessment are a solid understanding of basic voice science and voice disorders and good analytic thinking skills, and (b) assuming this knowledge and skills, the clinician can use a *series of measures together* (rather than a single measure) to draw reasonable conclusions about voice. The key factors are knowledge about the rationale for and the limitations of each measure, knowledge about how each measure is properly elicited, and a practice of looking for converging evidence (or "profiles") across all the measures. (The principle of converging evidence or "profiles" will be illustrated at the end of the chapter in "Case Examples.") Ideally, a minimal number of measures will be used to answer the most number of questions.

The examination described here has several components.

With these considerations in mind, here are a series of common measures that can be used together to answer important clinical questions. Because this text is targeted for the SLP in practice without access to expensive equipment, the measures focused on here can be made with a minimal initial monetary outlay. However, similar principles can be applied to more sophisticated situations. For the measures presented here the required equipment can be purchased for about $50–$200, and includes: (a) a stopwatch, for timed trials (cost is approximately $10); (b) a Db meter for voice intensity measurements (cost is approximately $30 for a simple Db meter purchased at an electronics store); and (c) a pitch pipe (about $15) or a portable electronic keyboard (about $150) for pitch extractions. An audiotape recorder (preferably with a VU meter and counter) and audio tapes are also preferred (starting at about $50). The only "software" that is required is a list of normative data provided in appendices to this chapter (Appendix 11-A and Appendices 11-C–11-F).

PARTS OF THE ASSESSMENT

Standard parts of the voice assessment are indicated in Figure 11–4. They are: (1) The case history, (2) The clinician's observations of voice (voice measures), (3) Impressions, (4) Recommendations, and (5) Prognosis.

Case History

Typical parts of the case history are shown in Figure 11–4. As we have already noted, the case history generally provides information about what may have originally caused the voice disorder and what the maintaining factors are. The case history also provides you with information about the patient's self-perceptions of his voice (presence/absence of a voice disorder, specific functional impact, and severity). Finally, the case history provides you with information about how the patient needs to use his voice at that time and in the future, and about the motivational level to improve a voice disorder. Critical aspects of the case history are discussed next.

> The patient will provide valuable information about the nature and extent of the problem. Listen carefully.

Identifying Information

You will start the case history by noting the patient's age, sex, and occupation or usual activities.

Referral Information

You should note who referred the patient to your clinic and the referring diagnosis.

Patient's Complaints (Symptoms)

The patient's complaints are considered "symptoms" (as distinguished from "signs," which are the clinician's observations). You should ask the

CASE HISTORY

Identifying information (Age, sex, occupation, or usual activities)

Referral information and diagnosis (e.g., referring physician or other; referring diagnosis

Patient's complaints
    Open-ended questions
    Ratings of functional impact of voice disorder
        Professional (work) impairment
        Social impairment
        Communication impairment
        Physical impairment
        Psychological impairment
    Phonatory effort scaling (speech, singing)

Onset and course
    Onset: When?
    Circumstances surrounding onset
    Course since onset

Previous voice and speech history
    Previous voice/speech problems
    Previous treatment
    Previous voice/speech training

Medical information
    Otolaryngological
        Current (conditions, treatment)
        Past (conditions, treatment)
    General medical
        Current (conditions, treatment)
        Past (conditions, treatment, including major diseases, surgery, gastric reflux)

Behavioral and environmental factors that may affect vocal fold tissue
    Smoke (number of cigarettes per day; number of years smoked)
    Alcohol (number and type of drinks per week; number of years)
    Caffeine (number of beverages per day)
    Exposure to dry air
    Exposure to chemical irritants

Typical voice use patterns
    Social (past, present, future)
    Family (past, present, future)
    Professional (past, present, future)

Importance of resolving voice problem (1 = not important; 10 = extremely important)

(continued)

Figure 11-4. Parts of the Voice Assessment.

DATA COLLECTION SHEET

Patient's Name: _____   Date: _____

Diagnosis: _____   Clinician: _____

General Voice Index

    Functional Impairment
        Professional   _____
        Social   _____
        Communicative   _____
        Physical   _____
        Psychological   _____
    Phonatory Effort
        Speech   _____
        Singing   _____
    Auditory-perceptual Status
        Voice Quality   _____
        Severity   _____

Acoustic Index

    Average f_0 in speech _____ pitch _____
    Semitone pitch range from _____ to _____ (_____ semitones)

Physiological Index

    Membranous VF closure
        MPT trial 1 _____ trial 2 _____ trial 3 _____
        S.Z ratio
            /s/ trial 1 _____ trial 2 _____ (trial 3 _____)*
            /z/ trial 1 _____ trial 2 _____ (trial 3 _____)*
            ratio _____
        High-quiet singing 1 2 3 4 5 6 7 8 9 10
            dB _____
    Neural control
        L-DDK rate   _____
        L-DDK strength   _____
        L-DDK consistency _____

Impressions

    Description of voice; severity
    Diagnosis
    Factors that may have contributed to onset and maintenance

Recommendations

    Is voice therapy recommended?
    If so, how often, for what duration each session, for how long?
    What will the focus of therapy be?

Prognosis

*ages 5, 7, and 9 only

Figure 11-4 *(continued)*

patient to describe her complaints about voice. There are various ways to do this.

Open-ended questions.   The most obvious way for you to elicit information about symptoms is to simply ask the patient to self-describe complaints about voice. ("What is bothering you about your voice?")

Questions about the functional impact of voice.   You can also obtain information about symptoms by asking the patient to indicate to what degree the voice problem causes functional impairments. This information can be an aspect of establishing the severity of the disorder. The simplest way to obtain this information is to ask the patient to describe or to rate the disruption to her everyday functions, as they relate to voice. For example, you might ask: "How much does your voice interfere with your job performance? How much does your voice interfere with your social life? How much does your voice problem make it difficult for people to understand you or for you to express yourself? How much does your voice hurt or cause you discomfort? How much does your voice cause you emotional distress?" The answers to these questions reflect the degree of functional impairment from the voice disorder in professional, social, communicative, physical, and psychological domains. You can ask the patient to rate the answers on an ordinal scale from "1" (no impairment) to "5" (severe impairment). If you prefer a more structured format, you can use a questionnaire. (See Smith et al., 1993.)

Scaling of phonatory effort.   A third way to obtain information about symptoms is to ask the patient to indicate how effortful it is to talk and/or sing. The results may provide an important measure of severity of a voice disorder, because for many or most patients with voice disorders phonatory effort is a primary complaint. We prefer a direct magnitude estimation method. The general idea of phonatory effort scaling is appealing because phonatory effort is related to a physiological variable (subglottal pressure during phonation) and to acoustic variables (frequency and intensity of phonation). In our clinic, we provide patients with a reference of "100" to describe a "comfortable amount of effort" during phonation. We ask the patient to indicate how effortful it is to talk (and sing) relative to this number. A value of "200" would indicate twice as much effort as comfortable ("very effortful") and a value of "50" would indicate half as much effort as comfortable ("very easy"). Note that values exceeding "200" are possible, as are values of less than "50."

Onset and Course of the Problem

You need as much information as possible about the onset and course of the voice problem. This information generally provides insights about the factors that caused the condition and about factors that maintain it.

Regarding onset, you should ask the patient when symptoms were first noted, and what the surrounding circumstances were. ("When did you first notice problems? Were there unusual circumstances? For example, were you using your voice more than usual or in a different way? Did you have an illness at the same time?") Long-standing symptoms signal a *chronic* disorder. Recently emerged symptoms may imply an *acute* disorder, assuming the patient is an accurate historian. If onset corresponded to an increase in the amount of voice use or to a change in voice-use patterns, then voice-use patterns would seem to have played a role in the development of the disorder. If onset corresponded to a specific illness, then the illness might be relevant. In the absence of remarkable voice use patterns or an identifiable illness, a sudden onset may signal a nonphysical disorder, particularly if the disorder is aphonia.

Regarding the course of the symptoms, you should ask about fluctuations in the symptoms and the apparent cause of the fluctuations. Again, variations in voice related to voice-use patterns imply a role of these patterns in the maintenance of the disorder. Variations in voice related to illnesses imply a role of medical factors.

Voice and Speech History

You should obtain information about previous voice problems and about voice therapy or training. If the patient had previous voice problems, perhaps the previous problems were never entirely resolved and the current difficulties represent a reexacerbation. An example would be a patient who was hoarse in elementary school and who received voice therapy for treatment of vocal nodules then. The recurrence of hoarseness and nodules as an adult might signal an unresolved susceptibility. If the patient had prior voice training (for the singing or speaking voice), the training might be something to build on in the current treatment program. In other cases, previous training might be a problem to consider in planning therapy, if the training appears to have contributed to voice problems.

Medical Information

You need to obtain information about medical status for all patients. This information is especially important for hoarse patients who are in the age range for throat cancer or other significant laryngeal conditions and diseases. This information is also important in understanding the basis for a voice disorder and possible contributory causes. You will obtain medical information from reports made by the otolaryngologist; except in rare cases, word-of-mouth from the patient or family is not satisfactory. Nor are laryngeal examination findings from another medical specialist (not an otolaryngologist) satisfactory, because special training and expertise are required for such diagnosis.

Obviously, the speech pathologist depends on important assistance from the otolaryngologist.

As shown in Figure 11-4, you should obtain information about past and present otolaryngological status, other past and present medical or surgical conditions, medication history, and, in the case of suspected or known contact ulcers, gastric reflux symptoms (burning and choking sensations, especially during sleep; acid taste in mouth on awakening).

Behavioral and Environmental Factors That May Affect Vocal Fold Tissue Viscosity or Otherwise Affect Vocal Fold Status

As we discussed in an earlier section, certain nonphonatory behavioral and environmental factors may produce dry or sticky vocal fold tissue and, as such, may predispose vocal fold tissue to nodules or polyps. (See previous section on causes of discrete mass lesions.) These factors include alcohol and caffeine consumption, smoking, exposure to dry environments, and the use of drying nasal sprays and drying psychotropic medications. You should obtain information about these factors. You should obtain as precise answers as possible. For example, you should ask what is the number of cigarettes smoked per day and for how many years?

In addition to these factors, it may be useful to obtain information about exposure to chemical agents, such as ammonia-based cleaning fluids, paint solvents, and so on. Although these are not commonly relevant in causing a voice disorder, in at least two instances in our clinical caseload a voice disorder could be directly traced to exposure to chemical agents and not to any other factors that we could identify.

Patient's Typical Voice Use Patterns

You should get information about the patient's typical voice-use patterns and predicted future voice needs for two reasons. First, information about past and present voice-use patterns might point to causative factors for the voice disorder to be addressed in therapy. For example, a physical education teacher who complains of hoarseness may use her voice loudly for several hours a day in a gymnasium or even outdoors. It is easy to think that such voice-use patterns may have contributed to the development and maintenance of nodules (for example), and you will want to address these voice patterns in therapy. A second reason to obtain this information is that you need to keep the patient's present and future needs for voice use in mind in planning ecologically valid therapy.[3] For example, a patient with spasmodic dysphonia may need to use her voice daily as a telephone operator. Particularly if she depends on this work activity for income, you may want to plan as quick an intervention program as possible. Another example is a patient with a laryngeal paralysis who is the primary caretaker for an elderly, hearing-impaired person. The level of improvement in loudness required for this patient may be greater than for some other patients.

In gathering information about voice-use patterns, we generally ask about past, present, and future demands on the voice in social, family, and work settings (Figure 11–4). This type of questioning generally yields more complete information than a less structured approach.

Importance of Resolving the Voice Problem

The importance that the patient assigns to improving the voice disorder signals the probable motivational level for therapy, which will likely affect the prognosis for improvement. You might ask the patient to rate on a 10-

---

[3] Ecologically valid therapy refers to therapy that takes into consideration the demands on voice in the patient's particular work or social environment.

point scale: How important is it to you to resolve your voice problems? (1 = not important at all, 10 = the most important thing in the world.)

Direct Observations of Voice (Voice Measures or "Signs")

The primary reason for making direct observations of voice (voice measures) is to establish baseline measures of severity and to describe the specific ways that voice is disrupted. In some cases, etiologic factors may also emerge.

There are three general important points for the measures that follow. First, you should compare all the measures that you make with norms, if at all possible. To do this, you should elicit the measures using the same or similar procedures as were used for the development of the normative data that you are using. For each measure described here, norms are provided (Appendices 11-A, 11-C-11-F), as well as the appropriate data collection procedures (same Appendices). You may want to use other measures. If you do, you should compare them to normative data and follow the same data collection procedures as employed in the normative data studies.

Second, in comparing your measures to norms, you should calculate z-scores, wherever possible. A z-score is a unitless, standardized measure of how different a person's performance is from the norm on a given test. We generally consider z-scores equal to or exceeding a value of $\pm$ 1 (i.e., one standard deviation above or below the norm) as indications of abnormality. The abnormality could be in the direction of impaired functioning or in the direction of superior functioning, depending on the measure and the sign of the z-score. When you cannot calculate a z-score, either because the data are unamenable to it (as for categorical and ordinal data) or because normative values and/or standard deviations are not available, you should make some other summary statement about your patient's performance for that measure ("normal" or "mild, moderate, moderately severe, or severe impairment").

The third important point is that, whether you use the specific measures outlined in this chapter or other measures, you should select measures based on the clinical questions that you want to answer. The alternative, that seems to occur far too often, is that clinicians make measures simply because the tools are available. This leads to spending a lot of time making measures and then not being quite sure what to do with the answers.

If you wish, you can use a "Data Collection Sheet" such as the one in Figure 11-4 to collect your voice measures. This sheet gives you a place to write down your patient's raw scores. To summarize the data and to indicate z-scores or other summary statements, you might find the form in Figure 11-5 useful (Data Summary, or "Profile" Sheet). This particular form organizes the findings into (a) a General Voice Index (including measures of functional impairment, phonatory effort, and auditory-perceptual status), (b) an Acoustic Index (including fundamental frequency and intensity during speech), and (c) a Physiological Index, subdivided into measures thought to reflect membranous vocal fold closure patterns (Maximum Phonation Time or MPT, the S:Z ratio, and high-quiet singing) and measures that may reflect neural control of the larynx (laryngeal diadochoki-

The objective is to estimate how the patient's performance compares with that of normal speakers.

Patient's Name: _____ Date: _____

Diagnosis: _____ Clinician: _____

POORER THAN NORMAL					NORMAL			SUPERIOR			
General Voice Index (raw data)											
Functional Impairment											
Professional	5	4	3	2	1						
Social	5	4	3	2	1						
Communicative	5	4	3	2	1						
Physical	5	4	3	2	1						
Psychological	5	4	3	2	1						
Phonatory Effort											
Speech	200	175	150	125	100			75	50		
Singing	200	175	150	125	100			75	50		
Auditory-Perceptual Status *	**	***	****								
Speech	*	**	***	****	*****			******			
Singing	*	**	***	****	*****			******			
Acoustic Index											
X̄ fo speech (z-score)			±1.0		0						
X̄ I speech (raw data)	50		55		60	65	70				
Physiological Index											
Membranous VF closure											
MPT (z-score)	-2.5	-2.0	-1.5	-1.0	0			+1.0	+1.5	+2.0	+2.5
S:Z (z-score)	+2.5	+2.0	+1.5	+1.0	0						
High-quiet (raw data) 1 2 3 4	5	6	7		8	9	10				
Neural Control											
L-DDK rate (z-score) -2.5	-2.0	-1.5	-1.0		0			+1.0	+1.5	+2.0	+2.5
L-DDK strength	*	**	***	****	*****						
L-DDK consistency	*	**	***	****	*****						
Respiratory Status (z-score)	-2.5	-2.0	-1.5	-1.0	0			+1.0	+1.5	+2.0	+2.5

* severe
** moderately severe
*** moderate
**** mild
***** normal
****** superior

Figure 11-5. Data Summary ("Profile") Sheet.

netic[4] (or L-DDK) rate, strength, and consistency). All these measures will be detailed in the following sections. For now, the point is that, by using this or another data organization sheet to summarize your findings, with some experience you will be able to get a "feel" for the overall voice condition of your patient by glancing at a summary sheet. Another advantage is that you can compare your patient's pre- and posttreatment status on one sheet of paper that is graphically organized. An example for one patient is given in Table 11-1.

A method for graphic display of diagnostic findings is useful.

We will use the three indices as an organizational framework in the discussion of voice measures that follow.

General Voice Index

The first set of important measures compose what is called the "General Voice Index." Together, the measures in this index indicate if there is a voice disorder. Included are measures of functional impairment, measures of phonatory effort, and auditory-perceptual measures of voice.

Measures of functional impairment. Measures of functional impairment discussed as part of "Case History" in this chapter reflect the patient's self-perception of the degree of impairment in relation to voice.

The functional measures are appealing because they provide a direct means to estimate the severity of a voice problem from the patient's perspective. However, as yet, little is known about the reliability or validity of these measures.

Measures of phonatory effort. Phonatory effort measures were also discussed under "Case History." These measures reflect the patient's perception of how effortful it is to produce voice. These measures are included in the "General Voice Index" because disturbances in phonatory effort occur across a wide range of voice disorders. In fact, patients in almost every diagnostic category of voice disorders tend to complain about phonatory effort. (A primary exception may be patients with Parkinson's disease.)

The appeal of these measures is that, at least when obtained using a direct magnitude estimation scale as described previously, they seem to be reliable, that is, repeatable. They seem also to be valid; that is, they covary with acoustic and physiological variables such as fundamental frequency, intensity, and subglottal pressure (Colton & Brown, 1972; Wright & Colton, 1972a, 1972b). Thus, we think that these measures can tell us something about the overall severity of a voice problem at a general level.

Auditory-perceptual measures of voice. Auditory-perceptual evaluations of voice involve listening to the voice and describing and/or rating it. Auditory-perceptual evaluations represent a critical aspect of any voice assessment procedure. It would be virtually unthinkable to conduct a voice assessment without these evaluations. In fact, in a large study on the use of

---

[4] Laryngeal diadochokinetic tasks involve the repeated and rapid production of glottal plosives, or quiet "coughs," over a trial period of a predetermined length (generally several seconds).

Table 11-1. Data Summary ("Profile") Sheet.

Patient's Name: _____John Doe_____ Date: ✗ pre-tx
                                                              ✗ post-tx

Diagnosis: _____Unilateral paralysis_____ Clinician: _____

POORER THAN NORMAL	NORMAL	SUPERIOR

General Voice Index (raw data)

Functional Impairment

   Professional   5 ✗ 3 ✗   1

   Social   5 ✗ 3 ✗   1

   Communicative   5 ✗ 3 ✗   1

   Physical   5   4 ✗ ✗   1

   Psychological   5 ✗ 3 ✗   1

Phonatory Effort

   Speech   200 ✗ 150 ✗   100   75   50

   Singing   2✗ 175 150 ✗   100   75   50

Auditory-Perceptual Status *   **   ***   ****

   Speech   * ✗ *** **✗*   *****   ******

   Singing ✗   ** *** **✗*   *****   ******

Acoustic Index

$\overline{X}$ fo speech (z-score)   ±1.0   ✗✗

$\overline{X}$ I speech (raw data)   50 ✗ 55   60 ✗ 65   70

Physiological Index

Membranous VF closure

   MPT (z-score) ✗ -2.5 -2.0 -1.✗ -1.0   0   +1.0   +1.5   +2.0   +2.5

   S:Z (z-score) ✗ +2.5 +2.✗ +1.5 +1.0   0

   High-quiet (raw data) ✗ 2 3 4 ✗ 6 7   8   9   10

Neural Control

   L-DDK rate (z-score) -2.5 -2.0 -1.5 -✗0 ✗   0   +1.0   +1.5   +2.0   +2.5

   L-DDK strength   * ✗ *** ****   *****

   L-DDK consistency   *   ** *** ****   ✗✗ ✗

Respiratory Status
(z-score)   -2.5 -2.0 -1.5 -1.0   ✗ ✗   +1.0   +1.5   +2.0   +2.5

* severe
** moderately severe
*** moderate
**** mild
***** normal
****** superior

different measures in voice evaluation, clinicians from various parts of the world described auditory–perceptual measures as among the most useful clinically (Hirano, 1989). It is paradoxical that there is hardly a measure of voice that is surrounded by greater controversy than this family of measures. Among other things, this is because of shifting criteria within and across rating procedures.

Setting aside the problems for a moment, there are generally two aspects to the auditory–perceptual measure. One is the categorical description of voice, or labeling (common terms partly familiar to the layperson include "hoarse," "breathy," "pressed," "harsh," "rough," "diplophonic" or two-toned voice, etc.[5]). The second aspect is the actual ordinal severity rating (for example, mild, moderate, moderately severe, and severe). To make these assessments, the typical clinical procedure is simply to listen to the patient's voice, usually in conversational speech. If the patient is a singer or actor or otherwise uses the voice in unusual ways, you should listen to the voice during other relevant activities as well.

Returning to the controversies about auditory–perceptual measures, there has been concern about the consistency of auditory–perceptual measures within and across clinicians. According to some studies, consistency tends to be poor (see, for example, Bassich & Ludlow, 1986). According to other studies, agreement can be quite good (Sederholm, McAllister, Sundberg, & Dalqvist, in preparation). It turns out that some procedures tend to favor consistency and others tend to undermine it.

Specifically, it appears that consistent (or reliable) estimates of severity can be obtained by observing a series of constraints. The problem is that the constraints are not easily met in the clinical situation: a group of judges should be used to minimize the bias on the part of any one; the speech samples presented for evaluation should all be similar in *format*; the samples should be presented in back-to-back fashion; and judges should receive "anchors" (or examples of different severity levels) and training immediately prior to the task. Also, the fewer the points on the ordinal scale, the more reliable the rating is likely to be, both over time (same judge, time one versus time two) and between listeners (judge one versus judge two). So agreement is usually better with a 3-point scale (normal, some disorder, severe disorder) than with a 5-point scale (normal, mild, moderate, moderately severe, and severe disorder), or a 7-point scale (even more gradations). Of course, the flip side is that scales with fewer points allow for less sensitive differentiations.

Some adaptations can be made for the clinical situation. To minimize bias, use a standard task for all patients (modified for age groups). Taperecord the task to be judged later by you (again) and by a colleague unfamiliar with the patient and her complaint/history. Before initiating scaling procedures, use a brief training tape that includes some examples of normal, mild, and severe disorders to define the standards to be used. Choose a rating scale and stay with it. We advise using an Equal Appearing Interval (EAI) scale in which severity is assigned ordinally. As indicated earlier, a 3-point

Sharpen your judgment skills by listening to the voices of people around you and in the public arena.

---

[5] A written, verbal description of these terms is somewhat challenging because they refer to auditory concepts that are most easily demonstrated, not explained. For clarification, you can consult with an experienced clinician.

scale is probably more reliable than a 5- or 7-point scale, but obviously tells us less about gradations. Other psychological scaling methods such as direct magnitude estimation (DME: "Using 100 as a baseline for 'normal,' assign a number for this speech sample to indicate severity in relationship to that 100") or paired comparisons (PC: "Is this sample more severe than that one?") are also possible.

Acoustic Index

Acoustic measures may indicate something about the severity of the problem. They may also reflect structural and/or physiological abnormalities. However, the relations between structure/function and acoustic measures are not entirely straightforward. The reason is that similar underlying conditions can produce diverse acoustic outputs, and different underlying conditions can produce similar acoustic outputs.

With this caveat in mind, here is a description of the simplest acoustic measures that you should include in the voice assessment. A host of other measures also exist and are indicated later in this chapter. You should be familiar with those as well.

Average fundamental frequency (f_0) during speech.   You should obtain information about the patient's fundamental frequency (f_0, the acoustic equivalent of pitch) during speech. In rare cases, an abnormal f_0 may be a distinctive characteristic of a voice disorder. If it is, it may reflect either a cause or an effect of an underlying condition. For example, with laryngeal granuloma, a low f_0 might be a *causative* factor. Or, a low f_0 might reflect the *effect* of Reinke's edema. Conversely, a high f_0 might be the *effect* of vocal fold bowing.

Although we can speculate in this way, in fact, there are few data about the f_0 characteristics for different types of voice disorders. In our experience, f_0 abnormalities are less commonly encountered in persons with voice disorders than is sometimes anecdotally assumed.

Various types of equipment are available to establish f_0 during speech. Much of the equipment is expensive, ranging from about $500 for freestanding instruments to $1,000 or much more for a computer and software. We have found that, with some experience, most clinicians can use a portable electronic keyboard or even a simple pitch pipe to adequately extract information about patients' approximate average f_0 during speech.

Procedures that you can use to obtain f_0 information, and normative data, are given in Appendix 11-A. A pitch-to-frequency conversion chart, which you will need for this procedure, is in Appendix 11-B.

Average intensity during speech.   You should also obtain information about the patient's approximate average intensity during speech. As for the f_0, this measure may reflect causes or effects of a voice disorder. For example, a high intensity during speech might imply relatively strong vocal fold adduction and, possibly, high-impact forces, contributing to edema-based injury (nodules or polyps). (In fact, high intensities are rarely observed in the clinical situation probably because people tend to talk quietly in such settings.) Low intensities might reflect poor laryngeal valving because of

Information from the history about vocal use in the workplace will be useful in making these estimates.

space-occupying lesions of the membranous folds, vocal fold bowing, or paralysis.

Although these predictions are intuitive, there are actually few data about the intensity characteristics for patients with various voice disorders. An exception is a study by Hillman, Holmberg, Perkell, Walsh, and Vaughn (1989), who found that most of the subjects with voice disorders they examined (including subjects with nodules, polyps, contact ulcers, and nonorganic voice disorders) had speech intensities within the normal range, at least for a consonant–vowel task (repeated /pae/).

A procedure for establishing the average intensity during conversational speech and approximate normative information are in Appendix 11-A.

Physiological Index

In addition to the measures already described, an important part of your assessment will involve measures that more or less directly reflect critical aspects of laryngeal (and respiratory) functioning. These are "physiological measures," which can be subdivided in two: (a) those that may reflect membranous vocal fold closure patterns during phonation (including Maximum Phonation Time or MPT, the S:Z ratio, and high-quiet singing), and (b) those that may reflect neural control of the larynx (including laryngeal diadochokinetic or L-DDK rate, strength, and consistency). Together, these measures are vital in formulating a "4-dimensional picture" of the larynx.

In these measures, we attempt to describe physical aspects of the patient's voicing patterns.

Measures from the first set may reflect impairment in membranous vocal fold closure from discrete mass lesions of the vocal folds, bowing, vocal fold paralysis, or other conditions. Measures from the second set may be variously impaired with conditions that alter neural laryngeal control.

Note that some of these physiological measures (MPT and the S:Z ratio) are derived from tasks that require the maximum prolongation of phonemes. Such tasks may fatigue the patient. Thus, you should not repeat them back-to-back. You should intersperse them with other, nonsustained measures, or you should allow for adequate recovery time between repetitions by simply waiting.

Maximum phonation time. Maximum Phonation Time (MPT) involves the prolongation of a vowel, typically /a/, for as long as possible, on several trials. This measure is assumed to reflect the relative degree of closure of the membranous folds during phonation. Performance on this task might be poor whenever the membranous vocal folds do not close completely during phonation, for whatever reason (discrete mass lesions of the membranous folds, vocal fold bowing, peripheral paralyses, etc.) The rationale is that with healthy vocal fold functioning pulmonary airflow is restrained during the closed portion of the vocal fold vibratory cycle. In conditions that interfere with membranous vocal fold closure, considerably more airflow than usual may escape through the vocal folds during phonation. Thus, the pulmonary supply may be depleted more rapidly than normal and MPT shortened.[6]

---

[6] As it is typically obtained clinically, MPT is an inaccurate indicator of actual maximum phonation time (see Stone, 1983). However, clinicians do *not* use this measure as a reflection of actual maximum phonation time. Instead, they use it as a reflection of membranous vocal fold closure during phonation.

Having said as much, there are numerous problems with the MPT measure as a reflection of vocal fold closure. Empirically, the limited data that exist on its validity do not suggest a strong link to membranous vocal fold status, as might be predicted. As such, MPT results may frequently be misleading.

In fact, there is a large conceptual problem with MPT as a reflection of membranous vocal fold closure: it grossly confounds laryngeal and respiratory functions. If your patient has a poor MPT, it might be because her vocal folds are closing incompletely during phonation, or it might be because of limited pulmonary air supply. Conversely, if your patient's MPT is normal, good respiratory capabilities could be compensating for poor vocal fold closure.

Finally, there are also technical problems with MPT. For example, the measure is very sensitive to the number of trials. Improvements in performance are typically observed with increasing trial numbers without a plateau, even with numerous repetitions. MPT also heavily depends on the pitch of the vowel production (see Stone, 1983).

In view of these considerations, it might seem odd that we are discussing this measure at all. We are discussing it because a recent survey indicates that it is one of the most widely used clinical measures in voice assessment, worldwide (Hirano, 1989). Thus, you should be familiar with it and, if you use it, you should be aware of its limitations. In particular, if you use this measure, you should interpret it within the context of other measures, particularly respiratory ones (for example, prolonged /s/, described below).

To obtain MPT, you can use the procedures and norms in Appendix 11-C. Note that the procedures differ slightly for children and for adults. Across all age groups you should have the patient perform three trials. Then compute the z-score as follows:

> For both these measures, two or three trials may not be enough to yield a stable measure.

$$z = \frac{\text{patient's best performance} - \text{normative value}}{\text{standard deviation for the norm}}$$

The S:Z ratio.   The S:Z ratio is defined as the ratio of the maximum prolongation of /s/ in seconds, divided by the maximum prolongation of /z/ in seconds, over two trials (for adults) or over three trials (for children; see Appendix 11-C). As for MPT, this ratio is believed to reflect the completeness of vocal fold closure during phonation.

The S:Z ratio has distinct advantages over MPT as a reflection of membranous vocal fold closure. Conceptually, the advantage is that this ratio indicates the degree of vocal fold closure, *controlling for* respiratory functions. The reasoning is as follows: the primary difference between /s/ and /z/ production is vocal fold oscillation during /z/, but not during /s/. Thus, airflow should be relatively more inhibited during /z/, resulting in prolonged phonation compared to /s/. The result should be an S:Z ratio that is less than 1, assuming a normally functioning larynx. With incomplete vocal fold closure, airflow should be less inhibited during /z/ than otherwise. In this way, the /z/ prolongation value should be decreased relative to normal conditions and the value of the S:Z ratio should increase.

Empirical studies on the S:Z ratio seem to indicate quite good ability to reflect membranous vocal fold status, especially as compared to MPT. The primary empirical report is provided by Eckel and Boone (1981). In their study, S:Z ratios were obtained for control subjects (subjects with healthy larynges and no voice complaints), for subjects with nonorganic voice problems, and for subjects with vocal fold nodules. The results show that the average ratio was less than 1 (0.99) for the control subjects, as anticipated. It was 1.65 for subjects with nodules and it was intermediate (1.03) for subjects with nonorganic voice problems. Verdolini and Palmer (in preparation) further reported a reasonably good sensitivity of the S:Z ratio to correctly reflect known membranous vocal fold closure characteristics across a range of diagnostic conditions, including nodules, peripheral paralysis (poor closure), and granuloma, Parkinson's disease, nonorganic voice problems, and a control condition (relatively better closure, at least during the performance of the S:Z task).[7]

What are the limitations of the S:Z ratio? That is, what do you need to be careful about when interpreting the measure? First, questions have been raised in the literature about the validity of this ratio for children. Second, in our clinical experience, the ratio may not accurately reflect membranous vocal fold closure when the /s/ value is very long (e.g. more than one standard deviation above the norm). Although we can speculate on the reason, the bottom line is that we do not actually know.

To obtain the S:Z ratio, you should follow the instructions in Appendix 11-D (which provides also the norms). As for MPT, the procedures vary slightly, depending on your patient's age. The primary procedural difference across age groups is that for children, three trials of both /s/ and /z/ are needed; whereas for adults only two trials of each are needed. For both younger and older patients, you should vary the order of the phonemes across trials. Also for both age groups, take the longest /s/ and the longest /z/ to calculate the S:Z ratio (divide /s/ by /z/). Then compare this ratio to the norms by computing a z-score:

$$z = \frac{\text{patient's ratio } - \text{ normative ratio}}{\text{standard deviation for the norm}}$$

In addition to indicating the S:Z ratio on your Data Summary Sheet, you may find it useful to indicate the z-score for the /s/ prolongation value (norms in Appendix 11-D) as a gross reflection of respiratory capabilities. This information may be particularly important in interpreting the MPT measure, if you use it and its z-score. To calculate the z-score for the /s/, use the following formula:

$$z = \frac{\text{patient's longest /s/ } - \text{ norm}}{\text{standard deviation for the norm}}$$

---

[7] An interesting aspect of a high S:Z ratio with poor vocal fold closure is that the /z/ prolongation value is not only *not longer* than the /s/; the /z/ is actually *shorter*. This is, of course, the basis for a ratio that is greater than 1. Apparently, poorly closing vocal folds not only fail to inhibit glottal airflow; they actually *speed* the flow, compared to the glottis open situation. The aerodynamic reasons for this are unclear.

High frequency low intensity (high-quiet) singing.   In many conditions affecting the membranous vocal folds, patients' ability to produce high frequency, low amplitude vocal fold vibrations is impaired. With mass lesions, the reasons are intuitive. The increased mass in the vocal folds prevents very high frequency vibrations. Relatively greater subglottal pressures are also required to set the folds in motion and, as a consequence, once in motion the vibrational amplitudes will likely be relatively large. When patients with such lesions attempt high frequency, low amplitude ("high-quiet") phonation, the typical result is a delay in phonatory onset, discontinuous voicing once phonation is initiated, and failure to phonate quietly.

Preliminary data about the validity of the high-quiet singing task as a reflection of laryngeal status was reported in a study by Bastian, Keidar, and Verdolini-Marston (1990). In that study, clinical and normal subjects produced a few phrases from the song "Happy Birthday to You," starting at an (unspecified) high frequency and singing as quietly as possible. Falsetto registration was encouraged for males. Subjects' productions were rated on an ordinal scale (1 = extremely delayed phonatory onset, discontinuous phonation, and failure to phonate quietly, and 10 = immediate phonatory onset, continuous phonation, and quiet phonation). All subjects with a score from 1–4 had some impairment of the membranous vocal folds. Conversely, all subjects scoring from 8–10 were laryngeally normal. Some subjects with intermediate scores (5–7) had laryngeal findings and some did not.

One question about the high-quiet test regards judges' agreements on ratings. In the validation study mentioned above, agreement between judges was good. However, the judges in that study worked together on a daily basis and had developed consistent rating criteria. Agreement between judges may not be so good in all cases. In fact, in a study by Verdolini and Palmer (in preparation), it was found that the high-quiet test may not be sensitive to membranous vocal fold abnormalities in the hands of some clinicians. Another limitation is that the validity of this testing procedure has not been assessed for children.

If you want to obtain this measure, the appropriate methodology and norms are in Appendix 11-E. You should use the same rating scale as was used in the original validation study. Because this scale is an ordinal one, standard deviations are not available. Thus, to compare your patient's results to the norms, you should consider that lower scores (for example, 1–4) may reflect impaired membranous vocal folds and that higher scores (for example, 8–10) may imply healthy membranous folds.

Laryngeal diadochokinesis.   Laryngeal diadochokinesis (L-DDK) refers to the rapid, repeated production of glottal plosives over several seconds. For our purposes, there are three important parameters of L-DDK performance: (a) the rate of the productions (the number of glottal plosives per second), (b) the strength of the plosives, and (c) consistency or steadiness of productions across time.

Theoretically, performance on this test should grossly reflect neurological laryngeal functioning. In patients with paralyses, the glottal plosives should be weak and/or slow. However, there should be consistency across time. In patients with Parkinson's disease (an extrapyramidal disor-

> Some patients claim at first that they can't do this, but find that they can with some encouragement.

der), the results are somewhat more difficult to predict. However, either rate and/or strength and/or consistency might be poor. In contrast, patients with nonneurologically based voice disorders and vocally normal individuals should exhibit normal rate, strength, and consistency on the L-DDK task. A study by Verdolini and Palmer (in preparation) provided support for these predictions.

The methodology for eliciting L-DDK measures and the norms are in Appendix 11-F. For rate, compare the results for your patient to the norm by dividing the total number of glottal stops produced by the number of seconds for the task (typically 7), and then computing the z-score:

$$z = \frac{\text{patient's performance} - \text{normative performance}}{\text{standard deviation for the norm}}$$

For strength and consistency, simply indicate "good" (normal) or "poor" (mild, moderate, moderately severe, or severe).

Other Measures

In this chapter, we have focused on the simplest voice measures that you can make without expensive equipment. A large number of other measures are available. You should be familiar with them to evaluate their appropriateness for your own work setting and to interpret the findings that other clinicians may send you. You can consult other sources for a description of other measures (for example, Colton & Casper, 1990). The most important include acoustic measures (phonetograms, jitter, shimmer, signal-to-noise ratio), aerodynamic measures (subglottal pressures, maximum airflow, minimum airflow, and maximum flow declination rate), electroglottographic measures (closed quotient, open quotient), and videostroboscopic measures (particularly, vocal fold vibratory patterns).

Impressions

After you have completed the case history and the voice measures, you should form cohesive impressions about the results. You should discuss your impressions with the patient and/or family, and you should indicate the impressions in a specific section of the written report. In this section, include a description of the nature and severity of the disorder at a general level ("The patient has a moderately weak speaking voice . . ."), the immediate underlying causes (". . . consistent with the otolaryngological diagnosis of a unilateral laryngeal paralysis . . ."), and factors that may have contributed to the onset and maintenance of the problem (". . . that may have originated from a viral infection about two years ago.").

Eventually, we must put it all "together"!

Recommendations and Prognosis

Finally, you should make treatment recommendations and indicate your prognosis for improvement. Is voice therapy recommended? If so, how often and how long for each session? Over what period of time? What will be the focus of therapy? What is the likelihood of a partial or complete resolution of the problem with the treatment program recommended? Base your recommendations and prognostic statements on clinical experience and on reports available in the literature.

Section Summary

In this section on assessment, we have discussed the important concepts of voice assessment, in general, and specific assessment approaches. The important concepts, as we see them, are an understanding of voice and voice disorders and voice measures, how voice measures are properly elicited, and what measure limitations are. Using this information and by applying careful analytic thinking to the results, it is helpful to look for converging evidence across measures in answering critical clinical questions. In the next section we give examples of the findings from several different patients to illustrate some of these principles.

CASE EXAMPLES

Typical findings from five classes of voice disorders are discussed: (a) disorders caused by discrete mass lesions of the membranous vocal folds (Case 1), (b) those due to discrete mass lesions of the posterior larynx (Case 2), (c) those due to distributed vocal fold conditions (Case 3), (d) those due to a movement disorder (Case 4), and (e) those due to nonorganic conditions (Case 5). The findings are typical for the diagnostic categories discussed. However, you should not take any as absolute. Other outcomes are possible and, in fact, occur quite regularly.

Case 1: Vocal Fold Nodules

Relevant Case History

This patient is a 9-year-old boy who has moderate-sized, bilateral vocal fold nodules. According to his parents, he has been hoarse for about 2 years. Neither the parents nor the child recall any illnesses in conjunction with the onset of hoarseness. With the exception of common childhood illnesses (chicken pox, measles, and mumps) and vocal fold nodules, the general medical history is unremarkable by the parents' report. The child concedes that he often screams on the playground at school. He describes a moderate level of voice-related impairment in social and physical domains and a mild psychological impairment. He describes a moderate effort level during speech. He also reports a moderate motivation level to improve his dysphonia.

Measures

The findings for this child are shown in Table 11–2. The General Voice Index shows evidence of a voice disorder. As noted in the case history, the

Table 11-2. Data Summary ("Profile") Sheet.

Patient's Name: _____ Case 1 _____ Date: _____

Diagnosis: _____ Nodules _____ Clinician: _____

	POORER THAN NORMAL				NORMAL		SUPERIOR		
General Voice Index (raw data)									
Functional Impairment									
Professional	5	4	3	2					
Social	5	4		2	1				
Communicative	5	4	3	2					
Physical	5	4		2	1				
Psychological	5	4	3		1				
Phonatory Effort									
Speech	200	175	150	125	100		75	50	
Singing	200	175	150	125	100		75	50	
Auditory-Perceptual Status	*	**	***	****					
Speech	*	**	***	****	*****		******		
Singing	*	**	***	****	*****		******		
Acoustic Index									
X̄ fo speech (z-score)				±1.0	0				
X̄ I speech (raw data)			50	55	60 65	70			
Physiological Index									
Membranous VF closure									
MPT (z-score)	-2.5	-2.0	-1.5	-1.0	0	+1.0	+1.5	+2.0	+2.5
S:Z (z-score)	+2.5	+2.0	+1.5	+1.0	0				
High-quiet (raw data)	1	2	3	4 5 6 7	8 9	10			
Neural Control									
L-DDK rate (z-score)	-2.5	-2.0	-1.5	-1.0	0	+1.0	+1.5	+2.0	+2.5
L-DDK strength	*	**	***	****	*****				
L-DDK consistency	*	**	***	****	*****				
Respiratory Status (z-score)	-2.5	-2.0	-1.5	-1.0	0	+1.0	+1.5	+2.0	+2.5

* severe
** moderately severe
*** moderate
**** mild
***** normal
****** superior

child reports some functional impairments. He also describes a high phonatory effort level during speech and he is moderately hoarse. The Acoustic Index indicates a normal f_0 and intensity in speech. The Physiological Index indicates poor status on two of three measures assumed to reflect membranous vocal fold closure (the S:Z ratio and high-quiet singing). The third measure, MPT, is normal. Measures reflecting neural control (L-DDK measures) are also normal. Respiratory status, shown by prolonged /s/, appears superior.

Tying It Together

This voice profile is quite typical for patients with discrete mass lesions of the membranous vocal folds. In addition to phonatory effort and hoarseness, which are generic findings, the distinctive pattern is an overall impairment in measures reflecting membranous vocal fold closure, but normal neural control measures. The only finding that does not fit with the overall impression of poor membranous vocal fold closure is the normal MPT. As discussed in an earlier section, MPT is often misleading. In fact, note the superior respiratory measure. Good respiratory functions likely compensated for poor vocal fold closure for the MPT task. For this child, the treatment recommendation was to initiate voice therapy as an attempt to reduce the nodules and to improve the hoarseness.

Case 2: Discrete Mass Lesions of the Posterior Glottis (Contact Ulcers)

Relevant Case History

The patient is a 39-year-old car salesman who complains of a "catch in the throat" and a sensation of presence of a foreign body. He also describes his voicing as effortful and sometimes raspy. The otolaryngological report indicates contact ulcers on the medial surfaces of the arytenoids. The medical history obtained by both the physician and the speech-language pathologist points to the possible presence of gastric reflux. The patient describes a mild impairment in professional and social functioning related to voice and a moderate physical impairment (discomfort). He reports high phonatory effort during speech. Finally, he indicates a moderate motivational level to improve his voice.

Measures

The measures are shown in Table 11–3. The General Voice Index shows some functional impairments, high phonatory effort for speech, and normal voice quality or slight "raspiness." The Acoustic Index shows a low f_0 during speech, but normal intensity. Physiological measures are normal, including those that reflect membranous vocal fold closure (MPT, S:Z ratio, and high-quiet singing), and those that reflect neural control (L-DDK measures).

Table 11-3. Data Summary ("Profile") Sheet.

Patient's Name: _____ Case 2 _____ Date: _____

Diagnosis: _____ Granuloma _____ Clinician: _____

	POORER THAN NORMAL				NORMAL	SUPERIOR		
General Voice Index (raw data)								
Functional Impairment								
Professional	5	4	3	X	1			
Social	5	4	3	X	1			
Communicative	5	4	3	2	X			
Physical	5	4	X	2	1			
Psychological	5	4	3	2	X			
Phonatory Effort								
Speech	200	175	X	125	100	75	50	
Singing	200	175	150	125	100	75	50	
Auditory-Perceptual Status *	**	***	****					
Speech	*	**	***	****	*****	******		
Singing	*	**	***	****	X	*****	******	
Acoustic Index		(low)						
X fo speech (z-score)		X	-1.0		0			
X I speech (raw data)		50	55		60 X 65	70		
Physiological Index								
Membranous VF closure								
MPT (z score)	-2.5	-2.0	-1.5	-1.0	0 X	+1.0	+1.5	+2.0 +2.5
S:Z (z-score)	+2.5	+2.0	+1.5	+1.0	0 X			
High-quiet (raw data)	1 2 3 4 5 6 7				8 X 9	10		
Neural Control								
L-DDK rate (z-score)	-2.5	-2.0	-1.5	-1.0	0 X	+1.0	+1.5	+2.0 +2.5
L-DDK strength	*	**	***	****	***X**			
L-DDK consistency	*	**	***	****	***X**			
Respiratory Status (z-score)	-2.5	-2.0	-1.5	-1.0	X	+1.0	+1.5	+2.0 +2.5

* severe
** moderately severe
*** moderate
**** mild
***** normal
****** superior

Tying It Together

This profile is quite typical for discrete mass lesions that do not encroach on the membranous folds, such as contact ulcers (granuloma). Although the patient complains of some phonatory discomfort and the voice is perceived as marginally raspy, most other voice functions are largely unimpaired. In particular, physiological measures are normal. The reason is that the sound-producing elements of the larynx (the membranous folds) are not affected. The primary exception to normal acoustic and physiological functions is the somewhat low f_0 during speech. The low f_0 could have contributed to the onset and maintenance of the pathology. Because of this, and because of the possible presence of gastric reflux as an etiologic contributor, the combined treatment recommendation included medical (pharmaceutical) management of the gastric reflux and voice therapy. Surgical excision of the granuloma was withheld until a possible, later date.

Case 3: Distributed Mass Lesions of the Membranous Folds: Reinke's Edema

Relevant Case History

This patient is a 54-year-old telephone receptionist, a woman, with a 35-year smoking history (one pack per day). The otolaryngological diagnosis is Reinke's edema. The patient's primary complaint is that she is routinely mistaken for a man on the telephone. The functional impact is a moderately severe professional impairment and moderate psychological discomfort. Phonatory effort during speech is borderline high. The motivational level to improve the situation appears good.

Measures

The measures are shown in Table 11–4. The General Voice Index confirms the presence of a voice disorder. There are functional impairments, phonatory effort is high, and the speaking voice is considered moderately raspy. Acoustic measures confirm a low f_0 but a normal intensity during speech. Physiological measures fail to reveal distinctive impairments. In particular, two measures that screen for membranous vocal fold closure (MPT and S:Z) are normal. A third measure (high-quiet singing) is ambiguous. L-DDK measures are normal.

Tying It Together

This profile is quite typical for many patients with Reinke's edema. The cardinal findings are a low fundamental frequency during speech (probably from the added mass to the folds), together with normal membranous vocal fold closure measures and normal neural control measures. One might ask why the membranous vocal fold screening measures are normal with the added mass (edema) to the folds. The reason is probably that the added mass may be relatively evenly distributed up and down the folds. Thus,

Table 11-4. Data Summary ("Profile") Sheet.

Patient's Name: _____ Case 3 _____ Date: _____

Diagnosis: _____ Reinke's Edema _____ Clinician: _____

	POORER THAN NORMAL	NORMAL	SUPERIOR
General Voice Index (raw data)			
Functional Impairment			
Professional	5 ✗ 3 2	1	
Social	5 4 3 2	✗	
Communicative	5 4 3 2	✗	
Physical	5 4 3 2	✗	
Psychological	5 4 ✗ 2	1	
Phonatory Effort			
Speech	200 175 150 125 ✗	100	75 50
Singing	200 175 150 125	100	75 50
Auditory-Perceptual Status * ** *** ****			
Speech	* ** ✗ ****	*****	******
Singing	* ** *** ****	*****	******
Acoustic Index (low)			
$\overline{X}$ fo speech (z-score)	±1.0	0	
X I speech (raw data) 50 55		60 ✗ 70	
Physiological Index			
Membranous VF closure			
MFT (z score) -2.5 -2.0 -1.5 -1.0	✗ 0	+1.0 +1.5 +2.0 +2.5	
S:Z (z-score) +2.5 +2.0 +1.5 +1.0	✗ 0		
High-quiet (raw data) 1 2 3 4 5 ✗ 7	8 9 10		
Neural Control			
L-DDK rate (z-score) -2.5 -2.0 -1.5 -1.0	0 ✗	+1.0 +1.5 +2.0 +2.5	
L-DDK strength * ** *** ****	***✗*		
L-DDK consistency * ** *** ****	**✗*		
Respiratory Status (z-score) -2.5 -2.0 -1.5 -1.0	✗ 0	+1.0 +1.5 +2.0 +2.5	

* severe
** moderately severe
*** moderate
**** mild
***** normal
****** superior

the patient achieves good vocal fold closure during phonation. The primary treatment recommendation was to discontinue smoking. Supportive voice therapy was used.

Case 4: Parkinson's Disease

Relevant Case History

This patient is a 73-year-old retired male with progressive onset of Parkinson's disease over the past few years. He is followed by a neurologist. Under her direction, he takes medication daily for treatment of Parkinson's symptoms. An otolaryngological evaluation revealed mild vocal fold bowing that did not persist during purposefully effortful phonation. The patient walks with characteristically Parkinsonian small movements. His wife, who has a hearing impairment, complains that she cannot understand her husband because he talks so quietly. The patient describes a comfortable level of effort during conversational speech, and he notes only marginal functional impairments related to voice. However, his wife reports a significant disruption in their communication because her husband talks quietly: she seems more anxious for improvement than he does!

Measures

Table 11–5 shows the findings for this patient. Again, the General Voice Index indicates a disorder. Although the patient's ratings of functional impairments and of phonatory effort do not reveal problems, the clinician's auditory–perceptual evaluation indicates weak voice and monotone prosody (limited pitch and loudness variations during speech). The Acoustic Index confirms a somewhat high f_0 during speech and a low intensity, both consistent with vocal fold bowing. Despite the vocal fold bowing noted, physiological measures indicate good vocal fold closure during simple phonatory tasks (MPT, S:Z ratio, and high-quiet singing), but impaired neural control of voice (normal L-DDK rate, but poor strength and poor consistency).

Tying It Together

The profiles for patients with Parkinson's disease are variable, depending among other things on the stage of the disease and medication status. However, the profile for this patient is quite typical of medicated patients with a moderate disease stage, without dementia. The most tell-tale findings are monotone speech prosody, weak voice, and impaired neural control measures. Monotone prosody and weak voice reflect the limited range of motion in vocal fold elongation and amplitude characteristic of Parkinson's disease. The impaired neural control measures indicate a neurological problem. The marginally high fundamental frequency may reflect the vocal fold bowing noted by the otolaryngologist. Note that despite the bowing, the membranous vocal fold closure measures are normal. The reason is probably that the bowing does not persist for purposefully effortful tasks. For this patient, the medical treatment recommendation was to continue with

Table 11-5. Data Summary ("Profile") Sheet.

Patient's Name: _____ Case 4 _____ Date: _____

Diagnosis: _____ Parkinson's Disease _____ Clinician: _____

POORER THAN NORMAL				NORMAL	SUPERIOR
General Voice Index (raw data)					
Functional Impairment					
Professional	5	4	3	2	✗ (Normal)
Social	5	4	3	✗	1
Communicative	5	4	3	✗	1
Physical	5	4	3	2	✗
Psychological	5	4	3	2	✗
Phonatory Effort					
Speech	200	175	150	125	1✗0　　75　50
Singing	200	175	150	125	100　　75　50
Auditory-Perceptual Status	*	**	***	****	
Speech	*	✗ *** ****			***** 　 ******
Singing	*	** *** ****			***** 　 ******
Acoustic Index			(high)		
X̄ fo speech (z-score)			11.0		0
X̄ I speech (raw data)	50	✗ 55		60 65 70	
Physiological Index					
Membranous VF closure					
MPT (z-score)	-2.5 -2.0 -1.5 -1.0			0 ✗	+1.0 +1.5 +2.0 +2.5
S:Z (z-score)	+2.5 +2.0 +1.5 +1.0			0 ✗	
High-quiet (raw data) 1 2 3 4 5 6 7				8 9 10	
Neural Control					
L-DDK rate (z-score)	-2.5 -2.0 -1.5 -1.0			0 ✗	+1.0 +1.5 +2.0 +2.5
L-DDK strength	*	**	*** ✗*	*****	
L-DDK consistency	*	**	✗* ****	*****	
Respiratory Status (z-score)	-2.5 -2.0 -1.5 -1.0			✗ 0	+1.0 +1.5 +2.0 +2.5

* severe
** moderately severe
*** moderate
**** mild
***** normal
****** superior

the current medication. The speech/language recommendation was to perform a more complete evaluation of communication status, including an evaluation of speech and language. On the basis of the combined results, speech/voice therapy was recommended.

Case 5: Nonorganically Based Voice Disorder

Relevant Case History

This patient is a 24-year-old elementary school music teacher, a female, who complains of quick fatigue with voice use and occasional hoarseness. The otolaryngological examination failed to reveal notable findings. The patient is a nonsmoker and nonconsumer of alcoholic beverages and caffeine. She reports moderate to moderately severe disruption in professional, social, physical, and psychological domains related to voice use and moderate to moderately severe phonatory effortfulness during speech and singing. She appears highly motivated to improve her condition.

Measures

Table 11–6 shows the results for this patient. The findings are largely within normal limits. Measures of functional impairment, phonatory effort, and auditory–perceptual status are the only abnormal ones. The remaining measures, including membranous vocal fold closure measures, neurological control measures, and acoustic measures, are all normal (or at worst, ambiguous, for high-quiet singing).

Tying It Together

This profile is quite typical for a patient with a nonorganically based voice complaint. The distinctive pattern is elevated phonatory effort, possibly some hoarseness, but otherwise normal (or nearly normal) functioning.

Section Summary

In this section several examples of measures from different patients with a voice disorder have been presented together with illustrative typical findings for each type of patient, and some of the thinking that goes into interpreting the results.

SOME SPECIAL CONSIDERATIONS

The discussions here have been general to provide principles and procedures that can be applied to any patient with a voice disorder as defined here. Obviously, these principles and procedures must be modified to fit any specific patient. Further comments about special patient populations follow.

Table 11-6. Data Summary ("Profile") Sheet.

Patient's Name: _____ Case 5 _____ Date: _____

Diagnosis: _____ Non-organic _____ Clinician: _____

	POORER THAN NORMAL	NORMAL	SUPERIOR
General Voice Index (raw data)			
Functional Impairment			
Professional	5 ✗ 3 2	1	
Social	5 4 ✗ 2	1	
Communicative	5 4 3 2	✗	
Physical	5 ✗ 3 2	1	
Psychological	5 ✗ 3 2	1	
Phonatory Effort			
Speech	200 175 ✗ 125	100	75 50
Singing	200 ✗ 150 125	100	75 50
Auditory-Perceptual Status *	** *** ****		
Speech	* ** ✗ ****	*****	******
Singing	* ✗ *** ****	*****	******
Acoustic Index			
$\overline{X}$ fo speech (z-score)	±1.0	✗	
$\overline{X}$ I speech (raw data)	50 55	60 ✗ 65 70	
Physiological Index			
Membranous VF closure			
MPT (z-score)	-2.5 -2.0 -1.5 -1.0	0 ✗	+1.0 +1.5 +2.0 +2.5
S:Z (z-score)	+2.5 +2.0 +1.5 +1.0	✗ 0	
High-quiet (raw data)	1 2 3 4 5 6 7	✗ 8 9 10	
Neural Control			
L-DDK rate (z-score)	-2.5 -2.0 -1.5 -1.0	0 ✗	+1.0 +1.5 +2.0 +2.5
L-DDK strength	* ** *** ****	**✗**	
L-DDK consistency	* ** *** ****	**✗**	
Respiratory Status (z-score)	-2.5 -2.0 -1.5 -1.0	✗	+1.0 +1.5 +2.0 +2.5

* severe
** moderately severe
*** moderate
**** mild
***** normal
****** superior

Hoarseness and Throat Cancer

One example is our extreme concern that patients who are at-risk for throat cancer be referred promptly for otolaryngologic examination. Adults, older than 50, primarily men, who are hoarse or who have any change in voice for a period of 2 weeks or more that cannot be reasonably explained (a bad cold, the flu, hay fever) are clearly at-risk and should be referred to an otolaryngologist immediately.[8] This is a rule of public health that should be familiar to every speech-language pathologist, regardless of the nature of a particular clinical practice.

When the Patient Is a Child

Another example that requires additional special consideration is the child with a voice disorder. We have defined a voice disorder as a condition in which voice functioning is unacceptable to the user. Young children, particularly those age 4 and younger, may not recognize that they are hoarse. Further, even children who do recognize that they are hoarse may not note any particular functional impairments because of it. These considerations pose some problems for a voice assessment and for voice therapy. When a child does not recognize that he is hoarse, and/or when he does not note any particular functional disruptions because of hoarseness, there is no "voice disorder" as we have defined it! Should you perform a voice assessment or consider voice therapy, at all? Regarding the assessment, this question is particularly relevant because voice norms are relatively less well-established for children than they are for adults, and, therefore, the results may be tenuous. Further, hoarseness rarely signals a life-threatening condition in children — thankfully. Thus, health considerations rarely motivate an assessment of voice or voice therapy for children.

There are different opinions about how to proceed. You should be familiar with options and make your own decision. Some clinicians consider that hoarseness in children is maturational, in the sense that a large number of hoarse children develop clearer, normal voices as adults. This conclusion is implied by the relatively greater incidence of hoarseness in children, as compared to adults (see Wilson, 1987). Further, there is concern that voice therapy may lead the child to be unusually self-critical. Adding these to the considerations already mentioned, you might decide against voice therapy, and therefore you will not conduct a voice assessment. Or, if you do proceed, you will proceed in a guarded fashion.

Another view is that voice therapy and thus voice assessment may be valuable for many children. The child may not explicitly identify functional disruptions related to voice. However, disruptions may nonetheless exist, and therapy might improve them. For example, the child might suffer from low-grade, physical discomfort during voicing, but might not be aware of it because he has no other memory of voicing. Or, hoarseness may reflect problems with socialization patterns. A child may scream to get attention. Voice therapy might address these problems.

---

[8] Note that I prefer referral to an otolaryngologist for every patient that we see. I just emphasize the especially critical importance of a referral and a prompt referral, for cases such as these.

A complete discussion of such factors is beyond the scope of the present chapter. The point is that you will need to decide for yourself about the appropriateness of a voice assessment and voice therapy for children in general, and on a case-by-case basis. If you do proceed with an assessment and with therapy, you will need to adapt the usual procedures — taking the child's age, overall cognitive abilities, and motivational status into account.

When the Patient Is an Older Adult

Complaints about the voice by the older adult have a double focus. One focus, quite naturally, is about the possibility that voice problems indicate serious disease or disorder. Obviously, such a concern is appropriate and leads to a very close working relationship with the otolaryngologist and, for this age group, the neurologist. As indicated earlier, sometimes our assessment findings are highly indicative of such problems that require careful medical follow-up.

The other major focus is on functional losses. Common complaints are that the patient is no longer able to sing, or to be heard in a noisy room, or to call across the street to a neighbor, or to be heard easily by a hearing-impaired spouse or friend. These are very real problems, to be taken seriously. In the SLP assessment, you need to describe the nature and severity of the problem. In treatment, you need to assist the patient to accommodate as well as possible. Overall, the need is to be sensitive to the dimensions of the problem as it affects daily life.

The Linkage Between a Voice Disorder and Laryngeal Function During Swallowing

Older patients, particularly those with apparent or diagnosed laryngeal disorders characterized by impaired motor or sensitivity function, often have voice and swallowing problems (dysphagia) in tandem. The patient with paralysis of a vocal fold (or the muscles regulating the arytenoid cartilage, to which the vocal fold is "attached") in the open position probably has a breathy voice and, perhaps, aspiration during swallowing (leaking of some part of the bolus into the windpipe). Other patients, particularly older ones, report that the bolus "sticks" in the mid-throat and "I can't get it down right." Issues about dysphagia are discussed elsewhere in this book, but it is appropriate to remind ourselves of the relationship between voice and swallowing in this discussion of voice disorders as well.

What If the Patient Is a "Professional" Voice User?

For obvious reasons, there are many special considerations to be made when the patient uses the voice in a livelihood. Sometimes the questions are about competence ("I can't make myself heard as needed to do my job in that noisy machine shop/factory/tavern/classroom/courtroom".). Sometimes, they are about durability ("I'm okay in the morning, when I begin my workday, but by noon, my voice gives out"). In the case of the singer or actor, the complaint may be about the "quality" of voice. If you work clinically with these latter groups (professional singers and actors), you may need special skills in assessment and treatment to be helpful. You should also work in close collaboration with the singing teacher or vocal coach also assisting the patient in any treatment plan. If your caseload involves a great number of such patients, you might consider some formal voice training, yourself.

What About the Multicultural Perspective in Dealing With a Voice Disorder?

The need to be sensitive to differences among cultures in diagnosis in speech-language pathology is discussed in several sections of this book, and specifically in Chapter 2. This issue is also crucial in matters of a voice disorder. It is directly relevant to our definition of a voice disorder that requires identification of the "disorder" by the individual in the context of her social group, and her social and work activities, that is to say, her culture. These are the criteria against which her voice is measured, that you must consider carefully in assessment and treatment.

SUMMARY

In this chapter, we have discussed disorders and assessment of voice. To summarize, the following points are considered the important ones. First, the methodology that you use to assess the voice should be dictated by the clinical questions you want to answer. Second, the most important tools for conducting a good voice assessment are a solid understanding of basic voice science and voice disorders and good analytic thinking skills. Sophisticated equipment may be helpful, but is not necessary. Third, none of the available voice measures are without interpretative problems. You should be familiar with the rationale for each measure and its limitations. Fourth, although no single measure is without problems, you can use a battery of measures together to generate an overall impression, or more formally, a "voice profile," to help answer your clinical questions. It should be emphasized that there is no "cookbook" approach to voice assessment, even with a "profile" approach. You need to interpret each profile based on the unique ensemble of information that each patient presents. Finally, for individual measures to be meaningful, you should obtain the measures using the same procedures that were used to develop the related norms and you should compare the results to the norms.

Hopefully, these guidelines will provide you with a good start in the assessment of voice. With experience, you will develop more and/or other guidelines of your own. The important point is that your assessment procedure serve your patients well, and that it contribute to the development of treatment recommendations that will enhance their quality of life as much as possible.

REFERENCES

Bassich, C. J., & Ludlow, C. L. (1986). The use of perceptual methods by new clinicians for assessing voice quality. *Journal of Speech and Hearing Disorders, 51*, 125-133.

Bastian, R. W., Keidar, A. K., & Verdolini-Marston, K. (1990). Simple vocal tasks for detecting vocal fold swelling. *Journal of Voice, 4*, 172-183.

Butcher, P., Elias, A., Raven, R. (1993). *Psychogenic voice disorders and cognitive-behaviour therapy.* San Diego: Singular Publishing Group.

Colton, R. H., & Brown, W. S. (1972, November). Some relationships between vocal effort and intra-oral air pressure. Presented at the 84th meeting of the Acoustical Society of America, Miami.

Colton, R. H., & Casper, J. K. (1990). *Understanding voice problems: A physiological perspective for diagnosis and treatment.* Baltimore: Williams & Wilkins.

Eckel, F., & Boone, D. R. (1981). The s/z ratio as an indicator of laryngeal pathology. *Journal of Speech and Hearing Disorders, 46*, 147-149.

Fairbanks, G., Wiley, J. H., & Lassman, F. M. (1949). An acoustical study of vocal pitch in seven- and eight-year-old boys. *Child Development, 20*, 63-69.

Finnegan, D. E. (1984). Maximum phonation time for children with normal voices. *Folia Phoniatrica, 37*, 209-215.

Fitch, J. L., & Holbrook, A. (1970). Modal vocal fundamental frequency of young adults. *Archives of Otolaryngology, 92*, 379-382.

Fletcher, S. (1972). Time-by-count measurement of diadochokinetic syllable rate. *Journal of Speech and Hearing Research, 15*, 763-770.

Hillman, R. E., Holmberg, E. B., Perkell, J. S., Walsh, M., & Vaughn, C. (1989). Objective assessment of vocal hyperfunction: An experimental framework and initial results. *Journal of Speech and Hearing Research, 32*, 373-392.

Hirano, M. (1989). Objective evaluation of the human voice: Clinical aspects. *Folia Phoniatrica, 41*, 89-144.

Hollien, H., & Shipp, T. (1972). Speaking fundamental frequency and chronologic age in males. *Journal of Speech and Hearing Research, 15*, 155-159.

Horii, Y. (1983). Some acoustic characteristics of oral reading by ten- to twelve-year-old children. *Journal of Communication Disorders, 16*, 257-267.

Kent, R. D., Kent, J. F., & Rosenbek. J. C. (1987). Maximum performance tests of speech production. *Journal of Speech and Hearing Disorders, 52*, 367-387.

McGlone, R. E., & Hollien, H. (1963). Vocal pitch characteristics of aged women. *Journal of Speech and Hearing Research, 6*, 164-170.

Ptacek, P. H., Sander, E. K., Maloney, W. H., & Jackson, C. C. R. (1966). Phonatory and related changes with advanced age. *Journal of Speech and Hearing Research, 9*, 353-360.

Saxman, J. H., & Burk, K. W. (1967). Speaking fundamental frequency characteristics of middle-aged females. *Folia Phoniatrica, 19*, 167-172.

Sederholm, E., McAllister, A., Sundberg, J., & Dalqvist, J. Perceptual analysis of child hoarseness using continuous scales. In preparation.

Smith, E., Nichols, S., Lemke, J., Verdolini, K., Gray, S. D., Barkmeier, J., Dove, H., & Hoffman, H. (1993). Effects of voice disorders on patient lifestyle: Preliminary results. *NCVS Status and Progress Report, 4*, 237-248.

Stoicheff, M. L. (1981). Speaking fundamental frequency characteristics of nonsmoking female adults. *Journal of Speech and Hearing Research, 24*, 437-441.

Stone, R. E. (1983). Issues in clinical assessment of laryngeal function: Contraindications for subscribing to maximum phonation time and optimum fundamental frequency. In D. M. Bless & J. H. Abbs (Eds.), *Vocal fold physiology: Contemporary research and clinical issues* (pp. 410-424). San Diego: College-Hill Press.

Tait, N. A., Michel, J. F., & Carpenter, M. A. (1980). Maximum duration of sustained /s/ and /z/ in children. *Journal of Speech and Hearing Disorders, 45,* 239-246.

Verdolini, K., & Palmer, P. (in preparation). A profiles approach to voice measurement: Assessment of selected diagnostic categories.

Verdolini-Marston, K., Sandage, M., & Titze, I. R. (1994). Effect of hydration treatments on laryngeal nodules and polyps and related voice measures. *Journal of Voice, 8*(1), 30-47.

Wilson, D. K. (1987). *Voice problems of children* (3rd ed.). Baltimore: Williams & Wilkins.

Wright, H. N., & Colton, R. H. (1972a, November). Some parameters of autophonic level. Paper presented at the American Speech and Hearing Association, San Francisco.

Wright, H. N., & Colton, R.H. (1972b). Some parameters of vocal effort. *Journal of the Acoustic Society of America, 51,* 141.

RECOMMENDED READINGS

Discrete and Distributed Mass Lesions of the Vocal Folds

Bastian, R. W. (1986). Benign mucosal disorders, saccular disorders and neoplasms. In C. Cummings, J. Fredrickson, L. Harker, C. Krause, & D. Schuller (Eds.), *Otolaryngology — Head and neck surgery* (Vol. 3) (pp. 1965-1987). St. Louis: C. V. Mosby.

Bishop, M. J., Weymuller, E. A., & Fink, R. (1984). Laryngeal effects of prolonged intubation. *Anesthesia & Analgesia, 63,* 335-342.

Cherry, J., & Margulies, S. I. (1968). Contact ulcer of the larynx. *Laryngoscope, 78,* 1937-1940.

Delahunty, J. E., & Cherry, J. (1968). Experimentally produced vocal cord granulomas. *Laryngoscopye, 78,* 1941-1947.

Hillman, R. E., Holmberg, E. B., Perkell, J. S., Walsh, M., & Vaughn, C. (1989). Objective assessment of vocal hyperfunction: An experimental framework and initial results. *Journal of Speech and Hearing Research, 32,* 373-392.

Hirano, M., Yoshida, T., Kurita, S., Kiyokawa, K., Sato, K., & Tateishi, O. (1987). Anatomy and behavior of the vocal process. In T. Baer, C. Sasaski, & C. Harris (Eds.), *Laryngeal function in phonation and respiration* (pp. 3-13). Boston: College-Hill Press.

Jiang, J. J., & Titze, I. R. (in press). Measurement of vocal fold intraglottal pressure and impact stress. *Journal of Voice.*

Luchsinger, R., & Arnold, G. E. (1965). *Voice-speech-language. Clinical communicology: Its physiology and pathology.* Belmont, CA: Wadsworth.

McIlwain, J. (1991). Clinical aspects of the posterior glottis. *Journal of Otolaryngology, 20,* 74-87.

Monday, L. A., Cornut, G., Bouchayer, M., & Rich, J. B. (1983). Epidermoid cysts of the vocal cords. *Annals of Otology, Rhinology, and Laryngology, 92,* 124-127.

Peterson, K. L., Verdolini-Marston, K., Barkmeier, J. M., & Hoffman, H. T. (in preparation). Comparison of aerodynamic and electroglottographic parameters in evaluating clinically relevant voicing patterns.

Titze, I. R. (1981). Heat generation in the vocal folds and its possible effect on vocal endurance. In V. L. Lawrence (Ed.), *Transcripts of the Tenth Symposium: Care of the Professional Voice. Part I: Instrumentation in Voice Research* (pp. 52-59). New York: The Voice Foundation.

Verdolini, K., Druker, D., & Palmer, P. (submitted). Electroglottographic characteristics of pressed, normal, resonant, and breathy phonation. *Journal of Speech
and Hearing Research.*

von Leden, H., & Moore, P. (1958). *The larynx and voice: Laryngeal physiology under daily stress* (sound film). Chicago: The William & Harriet Gould Foundation.

von Leden, H., & Moore, P. (1960). Contact ulcer of the larynx: Experimental observations. *Archives of Otolaryngology, 72,* 746-752.

Ward, P. H., Zwitmen, D., Hanson, D., & Berci, G. (1980). Contact ulcers and granulomas of the larynx: New insights into their etiology as a basis for more ration-
al treatment. *Otolaryngology — Head and Neck Surgery, 88,* 262-269.

Movement Disorders of the Vocal Cords

Brodnitz, F. (1976). Spastic dysphonia. *Annals of Otology, Rhinology, & Laryngology, 85,* 210-214.

Darley, F. L., Aronson, A., & Brown, J. (1969a). Clusters of deviant speech dimensions in the dysarthrias. *Journal of Speech and Hearing Research, 12,* 462-496.

Darley, F. L., Aronson, A., & Brown, J. (1969b). Differential diagnostic patterns of
dysarthria. *Journal of Speech and Hearing Research, 12,* 246-249.

Dedo, H. H., Townsend, J. J., & Izdebski, K. (1983). Current evidence for the organic etiology of spastic dysphonia. *Otolaryngology, 86,* 875-880.

Kandel, E. R., & Schwartz, J. H. (1985). *Principles of neural science* (2nd ed.). New
York: Elsevier Publishers.

Kinzl, J., Biebl, W., & Rauchegger, H. (1988). Functional aphonia. A conversion
symptom as defensive mechanism against anxiety. *Psychotherapy and Psycho-
somatics, 49,* 31-36.

Ludlow, C. L., Naunton, R. F., Sedory, S. E., Schulz, G. M., & Hallett, M. (1988). Effects of botulinum toxin injections on speech in adductor spasmodic dysphonia. *Neurology, 38*(1), 1220-1225.

Moses, P. J. (1954). *Voice of neurosis.* New York: Grune and Stratton.

Ramig, L. O., Horii, Y., & Bonitati, C. M. (1993). The efficacy of voice therapy for patients with Parkinson's disease. *Journal of Medical Speech Pathology, 1,* 61-86.

Ramig, L. O., & Scherer, R. (1992). Speech therapy for neurological disorders of the
larynx. In A. Blitzer, C. Sasaki, S. Fahn, M. Brin, & K. Harris (Eds.), *Neurological
disorders of the larynx* (pp. 163-181). New York: Thieme Medical Publishers.

Robe, E., Brumlik, J., & Moore, G. P. (1960). A study of spastic dysphonia. *Laryngoscope, 70,* 219-245.

Rosenfield, D. B., Donovan, D. T., Sulek, M., Viswanath, N. S., Inbody, G. P., & Nudel-
man, H. B. (1990). Neurologic aspects of spasmodic dysphonia. *Journal of
Otolaryngology, 19,* 231-236.

Schaefer, S. D. (1983). Neuropathology of spasmodic dysphonia. *Laryngoscope, 93,*
1183-1204.

Nonorganic Disorders

Morrison, M. D., Rammage, L. A., Belisle, G. M., Pullan, C. B., & Nichol, H. (1983).
Muscular tension dysphonia. *Journal of Otolaryngology, 12,* 302-306.

Sodersten, M., & Lindestad, P. A. (1987). Vocal fold closure in young adult normal-
speaking females. *Phoniatric and Logopedic Progress Report* (pp. 5, 12-19).
Sweden: Karolinska Institute.

Sodersten, M., Lindestad, P. A., & Hammarberg, B. (1989). Vocal fold closure, perceived breathiness, and acoustic characteristics in young normal-speaking adults. In *Proceedings of the Vocal fold Physiology Conference 1989*. Stockholm.

Sodersten, M., & Lindestad, P. A. (1990). Glottal closure and perceived breathiness during phonation in normally speaking subjects. *Journal of Speech and Hearing Research, 33*, 601–611.

Auditory–Perception Evaluations of Voice

Bassich, C. J., & Ludlow, C. L. (1986). The use of perceptual methods by new clinicians for assessing voice quality. *Journal of Speech and Hearing Disorders, 51*, 125–133.

Kreiman, J., Gerratt, B. R., Kempster, G. B., Erman, A., & Berke, G. S. (1993). Perceptual evaluation of voice quality: Review, tutorial, and a framework for future research. *Journal of Speech and Hearing Research, 36*, 21–40.

Sederholm, E., McAllister, A., Sundberg, J., & Dalqvist, J. (in preparation). Perceptual analysis of child hoarseness using continuous scales.

Maximum Phonation Time

Hirano, M., Koike, Y., & von Leden, H. (1968). Maximum phonation time and air usage during phonation. *Folia phoniatrica, 20*, 185–201.

Ptacek, P. H., Sander, E. K., Maloney, W. H., & Jackson, C. C. R. (1966). Phonatory and related changes with advanced age. *Journal of Speech and Hearing Research, 9*, 353–360.

Stone, R. E. (1983). Issues in clinical assessment of laryngeal function: Contraindications for subscribing to maximum phonation time and optimum fundamental frequency. In D. M. Bless & J. H. Abbs (Eds.), *Vocal fold physiology: Contemporary research and clinical issues* (pp. 410–424). San Diego: College-Hill Press.

S-Z Ratio

Colton, R. H., & Casper, J. K., (1990). *Understanding voice problems: A physiological perspective for diagnosis and treatment*. Baltimore: Williams & Wilkins.

Eckel, F., & Boone, D. R. (1981). The s/z ratio as an indicator of laryngeal pathology. *Journal of Speech and Hearing Disorders, 46*, 147–149.

Tait, N. A., Michel, J. F., & Carpenter, M. A. (1980). Maximum duration of sustained /s/ and /z/ in children. *Journal of Speech and Hearing Disorders, 45*, 239–246.

Verdolini, K., & Palmer, P. (in preparation). A profiles approach to voice measurement: Assessment of selected diagnostic categories.

Young, M. A., Bless, D. M., McNeil, M. R., & Braun, S. R. (1983). Relation of physical condition to age-related voice changes. *Folia Phoniatrica, 35*, 185.

Laryngeal Cancer

Morris, H. L., VanDemark, D. R., Smith, A. E., & Maves, M. D. (1992). Communication status following laryngectomy: The Iowa Experience 1984–1987. *Annals of Otology, Rhinology, and Laryngology, 101*, 503.

High-Quiet Singing

Bastian, R. W., Keidar, A. K., & Verdolini-Marston, K. (1990). Simple vocal tasks for detecting vocal fold swelling. *Journal of Voice, 4*, 172–183.

Verdolini, K., & Palmer, P. (in preparation). A profiles approach to voice measurement: Assessment of selected diagnostic categories.

Laryngeal Diadochokinesis

Verdolini, K., & Palmer, P. (in preparation). A profiles approach to voice measurement: Assessment of selected diagnostic categories.

Other Voice Measures

Colton, R. H., & Casper, J. K., (1990). *Understanding voice problems: A physiological perspective for diagnosis and treatment.* Baltimore: Williams & Wilkins.

APPENDIX 11-A

Average Fundamental Frequency During Speech

Age/Sex	Norm	SD/Range	Authors[1]
7/F	294 Hz	—	Fairbanks, Wiley &
7/M	281 Hz	—	Lassman (1949)
8/F	297 Hz	—	
8/M	288 Hz	—	
10 to 12/F	237.5 Hz	198 to 271 Hz	Horii (1983)
10 to 12M	226.5 Hz	192 to 269 Hz	
17 to 25/F	217 Hz	1.7 semitones	Fitch & Holbrook (1970)
17 to 25/M	116.7 Hz	2.1 semitones	
20 to 29/F (nonsmoking)	224.3 Hz	192 to 275 Hz	Stoicheff (1981)
20 to 29/M	120 Hz	—	Hollien & Shipp (1972)
30 to 39/F (nonsmoking)	213.3 Hz	181 to 241 Hz	Stoicheff (1981)
30 to 40/F	196.3 Hz	171 to 222 Hz	Saxman & Burk (1967)
30 to 39/M	112 Hz	—	Hollien & Shipp (1972)
40 to 49/F (nonsmoking)	220.8 Hz	190 to 273 Hz	Stoicheff (1981)
40 to 50/F	188.6 Hz	168 to 206 Hz	Saxman & Burk (1967)
40 to 49/M	107 Hz	—	Hollien & Shipp (1972)
50 to 59/F (nonsmoking)	199.3 Hz	176 to 241 Hz	Stoicheff (1981)
50 to 59/M	118 Hz	—	Hollien & Shipp (1972)
60 to 69/F (nonsmoking)	199.7 Hz	143 to 235 Hz	Stoicheff (1981)
65 to 75/F	196.6 Hz	—	McGlone & Hollien (1963)
60 to 69/M	112 Hz	—	Hollien & Shipp (1972)
70+/F (nonsmoking)	202.2 Hz	170 to 249 Hz	Stoicheff (1981)
80 to 94/F	199.8 Hz	—	McGlone & Hollien (1963)
80 to 89/M	146 Hz	—	Hollien & Shipp (1972)

[1] For all these normative studies, subjects read a passage and the average fundamental frequency was extracted using relatively expensive equipment. For clinical purposes, we have found that similar values are obtained using a simpler counting task and a portable keyboard or a pitch pipe. The procedure is as follows. Ask the patient to count out loud slowly from 1 to 5. Match the patient's pitch contour with your own voice. Sustain the vowel on the word "three" as the patient continues counting. (You may want to warn the patient that you will be counting along, but to ignore you.) Then match this pitch to a keyboard or a pitch pipe. (The reason for selecting a vowel in mid-utterance is that pitch tends to fall below average values at the ends of utterances and may be higher than the average at the beginning.) Convert the pitch to frequency (Appendix 11-B). Use this as the average fundamental frequency in speech for that patient.

The comparison of this value to norms is straightforward when the *range* (in Hz) is given. If the value for your patient falls within this range, simply indicate "within normal limits." If the value falls above or below this range, indicate "higher" or "lower" than normal. If instead the standard deviation is given in semitones, the procedure is somewhat trickier. This is because the norm is given in Hz, corresponding to a logarithmic mapping onto the musical scale, whereas semitones are linear mappings onto the musical scale. In any event, adopt the following procedure. Using Appendix 11-B, identify the pitch that corresponds to the normative fundamental frequency for your patient. Count up from that pitch the number of notes (semitones) indicated as the standard deviation, and also down from that pitch the same number of semitones. If your patient's pitch falls within the range from the lowest to the highest of these pitches that you have identified, indicate the patient's pitch as "within normal limits," or "equal to or less than one standard deviation from the normative mean." If your patient's pitch falls outside this range, indicate that the pitch is greater than one standard deviation above or below the normative value, as appropriate.

Average Intensity in Speech

NORM = 65 dB at 3 feet

This norm may be an overestimation of the values that we tend to encounter clinically. Nonetheless, the procedure is to position a dB meter with a microphone-to-mouth distance of about 3 feet. Use the A-weighting, and slow response mode. Ask the patient to converse about some appropriate topic ("Tell me about your favorite vacation"). Note the approximate dB value around which the meter indicator fluctuates.

APPENDIX 11-B
PITCH TO FREQUENCY

Pitch	Frequency (Hz)	Pitch	Frequency (Hz)
B1	61.7	C#4	277.2
C2	65.4	D4	293.7
C#2	69.3	D#4	311.1
D2	73.4	E4	329.6
D#2	77.8	F4	349.2
E2	82.4	F#4	370.0
F2	87.3	G4	392.0
F#2	92.5	G#4	415.3
G2	98.0	A4	440.0
G#2	103.8	A#4	466.2
A2	110.0	B4	493.2
A#2	116.5	C5	523.2
B2	123.5	C#5	544.4
C3	130.8	D5	587.3
C#3	138.6	D#5	622.3
D3	146.8	E5	659.3
D#3	155.6	F5	698.4
E3	164.8	F#5	740.0
F3	174.6	G5	784.0
F#3	186.0	G#5	830.6
G3	196.0	A5	880.0
G#3	207.7	A#5	932.3
A3	220.0	B5	987.8
A#3	233.1	C6	1046.5
B3	246.9	C#6	1108.7
C4	261.6	D6	1174.7

APPENDIX 11-C
NORMATIVE DATA AND PROCEDURES

Maximum Phonation Time on /a/ in Seconds

Age/Sex	Norm	SD	Authors
3-6 to 3-11/F	6.28	1.76	Finnegan[1]
3-6 to 3-11/M	7.92	1.81	
4-0 to 4-11/F	8.86	1.84	
4-0 to 4-11/M	9.99	2.51	
5-0 to 5-11/F	10.47	2.57	
5-0 to 5-11/M	10.12	3.05	
6-0 to 6-11/F	13.81	3.65	
6-0 to 6-11/M	13.90	2.98	
7-0 to 7-11/F	13.68	2.45	
7-0 to 7-11/M	14.63	2.82	
8-0 to 8-11/F	17.12	4.62	
8-0 to 8-11/M	16.81	4.51	
9-0 to 9-11/F	14.47	3.78	
9-0 to 9-11/M	16.83	6.07	
10-0 to 10-11/F	15.88	5.99	
10-0 to 10-11/M	22.20	4.74	
11-0 to 11-11/F	14.76	2.06	
11-0 to 11-11/M	19.85	3.79	
12-0 to 12-11/F	15.16	3.87	
12-0 to 12-11/M	20.23	5.72	
13-0 to 13-11/F	19.24	4.58	
13-0 to 13-11/M	22.34	8.19	
14-0 to 14-11/F	18.85	5.15	
14-0 to 14-11/M	22.34	6.89	
15-0 to 15-11/F	19.53	4.66	
15-0 to 15-11/M	20.74	5.32	
16-0 to 16-11/F	21.85	4.47	
16-0 to 16-11/M	21.04	4.40	
17-0 to 17-11/F	21.99	4.47	
17-0 to 17-11/M	21.04	4.40	
18 to 38/F	20.90	5.70	Pracek, Sander,
18 to 39/M	24.60	6.70	Maloney, & Jackson[2]
66 to 93/F	14.20	5.60	(1966)
68 to 89/M	18.10	6.60	

[1] Finnegan's data collection procedure would not be tractible in most clinical situations, due to the number of trials (14) and due to fairly sophisticated equipment requirements. However, we have found it reasonable to use a modification of this procedure as follows: Instruct the child to take a deep breath and hold out /a/ for as long as possible. (Do not provide an explicit model so that the child won't copy your pitch and loudness.) Time the trial with a stopwatch. Repeat for 3 trials. Select the longest trial for comparison to norms.

[2] For these norms, the correct data collection procedure is: Instruct the patient to take a deep breath and sustain /a/ for as long as possible, with a constant pitch and loudness. For males, the pitch should correspond to 130 Hz (C_3), and for females, it should correspond to 210 Hz (G#3). The loudness should correspond to an approximately constant level on a VU meter of a tape recorder (or other apparatus), equivalent to about 82 dB at 2 inches. Repeat for 3 trials. Time each trial with a stopwatch. Take the average of the 3 trials for comparison to norms. (Note that Ptacek et al. do not explicitly say that their normative data for MPT are based on the average performance across 3 trials. We assume so.)

APPENDIX 11-D

S:Z Ratio (unitless)

Age/Sex	Norm	SD	Authors
5/F	0.83	0.50–1.14	Tait, Michel, & Carpenter[1]
5/M	0.92	0.82–1.08	(1980)
7/F	0.78	0.51–1.10	
7/M	0.70	0.52–0.97	
9/F	0.91	0.75–1.26	
9/M	0.92	0.66–1.50	
8 to 88/F, M	0.99	0.36	Eckel & Boone[2] (1981)

[1] To compare your patient's values with those reported by Tait et al., use the following procedures. Tell the child, "Take a deep breath and say /s/ (or /z/) for as long as you can … Ready? … Begin." Repeat for each phoneme three times, with a rest between trials. Time each trial with a stopwatch. Vary the order of the phonemes within each child, and vary order across different children. Select the longest /s/ and the longest /z/ to compute the s:z ratio (dividing /s/ by /z/). Compare to the norm.

[2] To compare the results for your patient to those reported here, use the following procedure. Tell your patients to take a deep breath and to hold out /s/ (or /z/) as long as possible at a comfortable pitch and loudness. (Give the patient an example without sustaining it maximally.) Time the patient's performance with a stopwatch. Repeat for two trials each of /s/ and /z/. Vary the order of /s/ and /z/ randomly within and across patients. Use the longest /s/ and the longest /z/ to compare the s:z ratio (divide /s/ by /z/), and compare it to the norm.

Note: For both children and adults, it is valuable to separately indicate the best /s/ prolongation value as a gross reflection of respiratory sufficiency. The norms are based on the same studies as for the s:z ratio, and are as follows:

Maximum Duration of /s/ in Seconds

Age/Sex	Norm	SD	Authors
5/F	8.3	4.0	Tait et al. (1980)
5/M	7.9	1.4	
7/F	10.2	2.6	
7/M	9.3	1.7	
9/F	14.4	3.1	
9/M	16.7	8.5	
8 to 88/F, M	17.73	7.65	Eckel & Boone[2] (1981)

APPENDIX 11-E

High-Quiet Singing (ordinal rating)

Age/Sex	Norm	SD	Authors
/F, M	8–10 (1–4 consistent with membranous vocal fold closure)	—	Bastian, Keidar, & Verdolini-Marston[1] (1990)

[1] The procedure is as follows. Tell the patient you will ask him to sing the first two phrases of "Happy Birthday" at a high pitch, as quietly as he can. Reassure that you are not interested in how pretty it sounds. Demonstrate (start at 329.6 Hz, or E_4, for men, and at 440 Hz, or A_4, for women and prepubescent males). Then ask the patient to perform the tasks. (We now prefer to place a dB meter at 3 feet from the patient's mouth to record intensity.) Rate the patient's performance on a scale on which 1 = extremely delayed phonatory onset and discontinuous phonation, and relatively louder phonation, and 10 = immediate onset and continuous phonation, and relatively quiet phonation (for example, 50–55 dB). Compare the score to the norm.

APPENDIX 11-F

Laryngeal Diadochokinesis (productions per second)

Age/Sex	Norm	SD	Authors
6/F, M	3.6	—	Based on Fletcher[1] (1972)
7/F, M	3.8	—	for /kʌ/
8/F, M	4.2	—	
9/F, M	4.4	—	
10/F, M	4.6	—	
11/F, M	5.0	—	
12/F, M	5.1	—	
14/F, M	5.4	—	
18 to 38/F	5.3	0.8	Pracek et al.[2] (1966)
18 to 39/M	5.1	1.0	
66 to 93/F	3.9	1.3	
68 to 89/M	4.1	0.9	

[1] We have not found norms for children for laryngeal diadochokinesis. Rather than eliminating this test for children or not interpreting it, we use the norms from Fletcher (1972) for repeated /kʌ/. These values seem to most closely approximate those for /ʌ/. We use the same procedure as for adults, below.

[2] The procedure for these norms is as follows. Show your patient the sound "uh" graphically and tell her you will ask her to produce it as rapidly as possible. Demonstrate. (In the demonstration, we include an initial glottal stop. It is unclear whether Pracek et al. did or not.) Then ask the patient to take a deep breath and make the sound as fast as possible until you say to stop (7 seconds). If the patient runs out of breath earlier, accept the trial if you think it is the best that can be done. In the absence of sophisticated counting devices, dot a pencil on paper for each production of "uh" for the duration of the trial (timed with a stopwatch). (Pracek et al. used a more sophisticated system, but we find this approach an adequate approximation.)

In addition to counting the *number* of tokens produced over the trial period, you should also note the strength and consistency of the tokens. Strong glottal plosives produced with a highly consistent rate would be considered "normal" on both strength and consistency parameters. With some clinical experience, you will be able to confidently scale poorer performance as "mild, moderate, moderately severe, or severe" impairment for both strength and consistency.

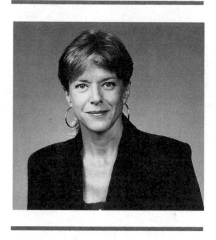

KATHERINE VERDOLINI, Ph.D.

M.A. 1982, Indiana University
Ph.D. 1991, Washington University

Dr. Verdolini is an Assistant Professor in the Department of Speech
Pathology and Audiology at the University of Iowa. Her primary
interest in speech pathology is voice, with research in voice
measurement, physiology, and efficacy of voice therapy; effects of
hydration on voice; and skill acquisition applied to voice. Her
previous positions and employment include Senior Speech Pathologist
at Barnes Hospital in St. Louis, teacher of singing at the University of
Missouri-St. Louis, and freelance vocal soloist based in Bologna, Italy.

CHAPTER

12

Head and Neck Cancer

Shirley J. Salmon, Ph.D.

Head and neck cancer is diagnosed in a laboratory by analysis of a tissue biopsy. Most often, the findings are interpreted to the patient and significant others by a physician. As you can imagine, receiving a diagnosis of cancer is devastating. Most individuals react with shock and, often, denial. When they do acknowledge the diagnosis, patients usually will agree to the recommended treatment and rehabilitation procedures. Because more men than women have cancer of the oral tract and/or larynx, hereafter, I will use male pronouns to refer to patients and female pronouns to refer to speech pathologists or significant others.

The cancer may be dealt with medically by surgery, irradiation therapy, chemotherapy, or a combination. These treatments may cause speech, voice, resonance, and/or swallowing problems. When such problems are anticipated, a speech pathologist will be asked by the surgeon to see the patient and significant others for pretreatment counseling.

Following treatment, a speech pathologist will be involved with appraisal and diagnosis of the communication and/or swallowing disorders, counseling, and follow-up therapy. Because oral communication is such an integral part of an individual's personality, you must consider your patient's lifestyle, occupation, availability of family support, and other pertinent factors when carrying out these responsibilities. Also, you must thoroughly

The speech pathologist is an important member of the treatment team for these patients.

understand the related anatomy and physiology, the ramifications of various cancer treatment procedures, and the psychosocial implications of head and neck cancer. This chapter will (a) acquaint you with some of the issues involved in the appraisal of speech and/or voice that is impaired or lost because of cancer, and (b) sensitize you to the emotional reactions of those involved with such losses or impairments.

These emotional reactions are never to be minimized!

MULTIDISCIPLINARY INTERACTIONS

After head and neck cancer is diagnosed, the physician will recommend that it be treated by surgery, radiation, chemotherapy, or any combination of these. The treatment may differ from one person or place to another, depending on such factors such as site and size of lesion, general health and age of the patient, physician preference, equipment availability, expertise of support personnel, and patient input. Regardless of the treatment selected, a number of changes may result that could be temporary, fluctuating, or permanent. Many of the changes are predictable, but some are not. Consequently, you must be knowledgeable about the most common types of aftereffects and be flexible enough to deal with those that are unexpected.

In larger facilities, a team of professionals will meet in pretreatment planning conferences to discuss the selection of treatment, a rehabilitation strategy, and the emotional state of the patient (Logemann, 1989). Generally, the team is headed by a surgeon and includes representatives from dentistry, dietetics, nursing, oncology, pharmacy, physical medicine, psychology, radiology, social work, and speech pathology. In smaller facilities, formal pretreatment planning conferences may not be held. Nevertheless, depending on the complexity and severity of the case, the surgeon will consult with those professionals expected to be involved in the rehabilitative process. It is essential that each professional understand and respect the unique contributions made by the others.

Treatment of the WHOLE person can only be accomplished with a team effort.

Factors associated with the voice and speech problems that generally require speech pathologists' involvement are considered in the remaining pages of this chapter. Factors associated with swallowing disorders (dysphagia) will be presented in Chapter 15.

ORAL CANCERS

The American Cancer Society (1992) estimated that there were 30,000 new cases of oral cancer in 1992. This number represents approximately 3% of all cancers in that year.

Conventional methods of treatment for oral cancers are surgery, radiation therapy, or both. With selected cases, chemotherapy is used in combination with radiotherapy and/or surgery. Depending on the location, size, and treatment of the cancer, the patient will be faced with cosmetic alterations, dental modifications, swelling or hardening of tissue, drooling or pooling of saliva, dysphagia, resonance changes, and impaired speech production. If swallowing, speech, or voice is impaired, the patient will be referred to the speech pathologist.

Pretreatment Counseling

Surgical reconstruction and/or prosthetic management of the oral structures or oral and nasal cavities usually will affect resonance, swallowing, and speech production. Of particular concern is the possibility of partial (under 75%) or total (75% or more) glossectomy (surgical excision of the tongue). The tongue is vital for speech and swallowing, and it cannot be replaced by a prosthesis. When these problems are anticipated, the surgeon will request the speech pathologist to provide pretreatment counseling. It is essential that you review the medical chart and determine the treatment plans before you meet with the patient and significant others.

> Demonstrating familiarity with the patient's history will increase your credibility with him and his family.

Your goals will be to help the patient understand the treatment plan, be cognizant of the major ramifications of treatment, be aware of the services that will be provided by speech pathology, and be prepared for posttreatment rehabilitation.

After a few social exchanges with the patient, I try to determine how well he understands the planned treatment procedure. Depending on the patient's response, I reiterate, clarify, or expand on his knowledge base and correct any misunderstandings. Concurrently, I include family members in the conversation and correct any of their misconceptions. I make a real effort to use lay terms, imagining that I am talking to my father or the neighbor down the street. If I use diagrams, I draw simple lines to illustrate basic structures and function. Often, we laugh about my ineptness and lack of artistic talent; momentarily, it lightens the somberness of the situation. I avoid predicting specific problems to anticipate. I acknowledge that the patient will experience difficulties with speech and swallowing, but point out that individual differences and variations of treatment determine the extent of deficits and, also, whether they will be transitory or permanent. In other words, I encourage a "wait and see" attitude.

> A friendly, gentle, clinical manner is important in this situation.

At this point, I usually mention that, because speech will be affected, we need to consider a temporary alternative means of communication. Writing is the most commonly used method unless either the patient or caregiver is illiterate. In such cases, a picture board should be provided. If writing is to be used, I always obtain a sample of the patient's writing or printing to determine legibility.

> **Warning:** Some of these patients are reluctant to admit that they have limited literacy skills.

I do not rush these sessions and, typically, plan for them to last 60–90 minutes. Always, I listen for comments that may reveal attitudes about the patient's willingness to comply and to participate in the rehabilitation process, as well as the various family members' perception of their own involvement. When a spouse uses the pronoun "we" in place of a singular pronoun "he," I am always encouraged.

Posttreatment Counseling

The posttreatment counseling and assessment sessions blend together in terms of professional goals and interactions with the patient. In the case of those who have undergone glossectomy (partial or total removal of the tongue), the goal is to determine if intelligible speech likely can be developed. When soft palate or pharynx is involved, the goal is to determine if velopharyngeal closure can be attained, with or without a palatal prosthesis.

Because the tongue is the primary structure used for vowel and consonant articulation, it is amazing that any intelligible speech can be produced following glossectomy. However, some patients demonstrate that it can be accomplished — presumably by compensatory strategies using any remaining tongue structure and other pharyngeal and oral structures. It remains a mystery as to how some individuals are able to compensate and overcome severe deficits in ways that might never have been predicted. In your rehabilitation planning, you should never discount the potential resources or resiliency of some human beings.

When the wound is sufficiently healed and pain has subsided, I conduct a careful evaluation of function. The results will help me formulate plans for speech and swallowing therapy. I begin from the outside and work inward. First, I observe facial structures, noting symmetry, muscle tone, ability to maintain closure of the mouth, flaring of the nares, or drooling. Asymmetry, or drooping of one side of the face, might signal poor coordination and precision during articulation. Drooling or inability to maintain closure of the mouth might indicate swallowing problems, and flaring of the nares may be an indication of inadequate velopharyngeal closure.

Next, I perform an oral mechanism examination that begins with an assessment of lip mobility, range of motion, and strength. I then check the presence of teeth and note the extent of mouth opening. I do this because I know that compensatory lip movements against teeth, the alveolar ridge, or a dental plate are used frequently by some patients to produce consonants formerly made with the tongue tip. Obviously, teeth and jaw movements also contribute to precise articulation. Providing a mirror and demonstration when necessary, I next instruct the patient to puff out his cheeks so I can assess the contribution of the buccal musculature, the strength and completeness of the lip seal, and the ability to attain intraoral pressure, all of which contribute to intelligible articulation.

Simultaneously, I watch to see whether intraoral pressure can be maintained and listen for nasal emission. Air leakage through the nose may indicate velopharyngeal incompetence. Because resection of some portion of the velopharynx is relatively common with oral cancer patients, velopharyngeal competency always must be evaluated. Such competency is vital for swallowing, intelligible speech production, and normal vocal resonance. Specific techniques related to diagnosis and appraisal of velopharyngeal insufficiency are discussed in the "Cleft Palate" chapter.

When I examine the residual tongue, I first observe how it rests on the floor of the mouth and note asymmetries in structure. Then, I assess movement — focusing more on mobility and strength than on mass (Imai & Michi, 1992). I instruct the patient to look at my modeling and then into the mirror to observe his attempts to imitate. First, I appraise the vertical and anteroposterior range of motion. Then, using a tongue blade to provide resistance, I note the strength of the tongue remnant during lateralization and elevation. I want to determine which areas the tongue cannot reach or contact. Recent findings indicate that patients with anterior tongue involvement tend to have more difficulty producing intelligible consonants, and that those with posterior tongue involvement experience more difficulty producing intelligible vowels. These findings also indicate that patients who undergo mandibulectomy (excision of the mandible) that crosses the

We must be careful in predicting, before surgery, his range of ability, after surgery.

During these examinations, we're trying our best to determine *what* the patient is capable of doing.

midline or who are edentulous (without teeth) exhibit a high risk of speech impairment (Leonard, Goodrich, McMenamin, & Donald, 1992).

At this point, I may instruct the patient to produce a few selected vowels and consonants in isolation. However, because speed and coordination of the articulators are better taxed during the act of speaking, I continue my appraisal by administering an articulation test. I believe that the pictures used in articulation tests to elicit single word responses are too juvenile for use with adults. Consequently, I ask the patient to read sentences from the *Fisher-Logemann Test of Articulation Competence* (Fisher & Logemann, 1971), or the *Sentences For Phonetic Inventory* (Fairbanks, 1960). In addition, I make an audiotape recording of the patient reading a standard passage, "The Rainbow Passage," from the *Voice and Articulation Drillbook* (Fairbanks, 1960). If the patient cannot read, I ask him to repeat sentences from one of the tests mentioned and audiorecord his responses during a conversational interview. We all must remember that these tests are not easy for the patient to endure, physically or emotionally. Consequently, we must frequently reward the patient's efforts and provide reassurance that we need the information to determine speech rehabilitative treatment plans.

When scoring these assessment tools I am, of course, interested in the sounds produced correctly, but, for treatment plans, I focus more on those that are omitted or distorted. Depending on the structures involved, possible compensatory articulation mechanisms include pharyngeal widening or narrowing and exaggerated tongue, lip, jaw, epiglottis, or larynx movements (Weber, Ohlms, Bowman, Jacob, & Goepfert, 1991). The distortions may help me decide what exercises to recommend so that compensatory movements may become more accurate. The omissions may indicate compensatory movements toward the articulatory target that are imperceptible and need to be strengthened or articulatory positions that the patient cannot achieve. For example, if tongue mobility is significantly reduced vertically or laterally, the contact between the tongue and palate may be incomplete. In such cases, I may want to recommend that a palate-lowering or augmentation prosthesis be constructed soon after surgery. If you are interested in a detailed description of how such a device is constructed and utilized, see Logemann (1989).

This information will be helpful when we begin to plan treatment.

Finally, in my assessment, I evaluate the patient's ability to modify rate, pitch, and loudness. Patients who have undergone glossectomy sometimes speak too rapidly; use a low, monotonous pitch; and an inappropriate loudness level for conversation (Skelly, Donaldson, Fust, & Townsend, 1972). The adverse impact glossectomy often has on swallowing is profound. The consequences must not be neglected and are discussed in Chapter 15. You should address all of the parameters mentioned in this section when developing your treatment plan.

Section Summary

In this section, issues involved in the appraisal of speech and/or voice impairment due to oral cancer have been covered. I have suggested ways to approach the patient and to evaluate his deficiencies as well as his remaining abilities. Always, the goal is to determine the potential for compensatory articulation movements and to recommend treatment procedures that will facilitate viable communication.

CANCER OF THE LARYNX

If you are interested in meeting laryngectomized individuals and observing their compensatory skills, I recommend a visit to a New Voice or Lost Cord Club meeting. There are more than 300 such clubs throughout the world. All are affiliated with the International Association of Laryngectomees (IAL), which is sponsored by the American Cancer Society (ACS). Their primary purpose is to serve as support groups for laryngectomized individuals and their significant others. The individual clubs, the IAL, and the ACS are valuable resources for both professionals and patients. I use the literature and videotapes they provide extensively in my practice.

The address: American Cancer Society, 1599 Clifton Rd. NE, Atlanta, GA 30329.

The American Cancer Society (ACS) (1992) estimates that 12,500 new cases of laryngeal cancer were diagnosed in the United States in 1992. This represented less than 2% of all cancers diagnosed in that year. Even considering the 50,000 laryngectomized individuals in the current United States population, this is not a large number of people. Yet, their rehabilitation needs are so conspicuous that they are given primary consideration by most speech pathologists. The average age of these individuals is 62.5 years, so usually they are employed. The ratio of men to women is 4.5:1.

Surgical Procedures

Small, less invasive cancers of the larynx commonly are treated by irradiation therapy; patients with such cancers usually are not referred for speech appraisal. Generally, more advanced cancers of the larynx are treated with surgery preceded or followed by radiotherapy. In these instances, the surgery is considered a lifesaving procedure.

Surgeons are acutely aware of the traumatic consequences associated with loss of voice due to total removal of the larynx. Consequently, they are diligent about developing better or newer surgical techniques to permit salvage of whatever part of the larynx is free from cancer, so that some type of laryngeal voice can be achieved and oral feeding can be maintained without chronic aspiration. Depending on site and extent of the lesion, a surgeon may perform a total laryngectomy or a partial laryngectomy. Total laryngectomy is excision of the entire larynx. Partial laryngectomies include (a) hemilaryngectomy, (b) supraglottic laryngectomy, (c) subtotal laryngectomy, and (d) near total laryngectomy. Therefore, it is important for you to know which surgical procedure is planned, as your counseling, assessments, and rehabilitation plans will vary accordingly.

Preoperative Counseling

Let's begin this discussion with a general precaution. It is that the patient and family are likely coming to grips with the reality of cancer, the prospect of surgery, and the changes it will bring, as well as fears of pain and death. They may or may not show much interest in what you need to discuss with them. Nevertheless, there is information they should have and so we proceed, in as much or as little detail as we judge they can follow. For example, my explanation of the various methods of speech following laryngeal surgery are fairly brief, unless they ask for more detailed information.

Before meeting with the patient and significant others, I review the medical chart to determine the specific surgical procedure planned. If a partial laryngectomy is proposed, you must be sure that the patient and family members understand that his voice will be different; swallowing may be more difficult; and he may breathe, permanently or temporarily, through a hole in his neck. If a total laryngectomy is anticipated, you should determine if radical neck surgery will be included and whether a tracheoesophageal fistula (TEF) is planned as a primary procedure in conjunction with the laryngectomy or as a secondary procedure after total laryngectomy is performed. Unilateral or bilateral radical neck surgery will cause the patient more discomfort with arm raising and neck turning immediately following surgery; a referral to physical therapy is appropriate. Neck surgery also may influence the choice of an artificial larynx. If a TEF is planned as a primary procedure, you should provide much more information about this method of alaryngeal speech preoperatively (refer to final paragraphs of this section).

Obviously, a close working relationship with the surgeon is required if this preoperative counseling is to be maximally helpful to the patient and family.

The patient's general health also should be considered. Previous cancer or irradiation treatments, hiatal hernia, ulcer, or respiratory difficulties may have adverse effects on some types of speech after laryngeal surgery.

When you meet with the patient and family members, try to gain some insight about the patient such as personality, motivation, coping strategies, and inquisitiveness. Does he express an interest in voice and speech rehabilitation? Is he attentive? Do his questions or responses reflect an orientation to reality? Does he appear shy or outgoing? Do the spouse and he share in their communication or does she seem to do all the talking for him? Laryngectomized individuals who receive emotional support from peers and family tend to move more rapidly through the rehabilitative process, so try to glean some information about family relationships. Do family members show or express concern for each other and talk about their plans to help the patient after surgery?

Other areas to probe are the patient's vocation and avocations. To what extent does he rely on speech for his job, homelife, and social activities? Does he plan to return to his current job, request a transfer to a different position that is less demanding of oral communication skills, or to retire? Would he be interested in discussing these issues with an appropriate counselor?

Finally, you will want to assess his speech and language behaviors. Typically, this is carried out in a fairly informal way. After all, you have been conversing with him throughout the interview and so already should have reached some conclusions. The patient's voice quality may be impaired because of the cancer, but what about resonance? Does velopharyngeal closure seem adequate? Is his speech rate within normal limits? Is he missing teeth or does he wear dentures? Are his articulation skills proficient? What percent of his conversational speech would you judge to be intelligible? Does he use gestures and facial expressions? Does he exhibit manual dexterity and coordination? Also, ask about his and his spouse's hearing. Consider a referral of one or both for an audiological evaluation.

Before discussing anything about the surgery or its ramifications, determine the patient's perception of what he already has been told. He may not understand that, when he wakes up in the recovery room, he will be breathing through an opening in his neck (tracheostoma) and mouthing words without a voice. At the very least, it is imperative that he understand these two basic consequences of laryngectomy. Ask the patient, "What have you been told about the surgery that is planned?" Or say, "Well, it sounds as if you are scheduled for some pretty serious surgery. Tell me about it." Listen carefully to his response. Reinforce or elaborate upon his accurate information; correct any misconceptions.

Typically, I explain that, when all or a portion of the larynx is removed, a tracheostomy must be performed to protect the lungs from being filled with food or liquid. I estimate that the tracheostoma will range in size from a dime to a quarter. Finally, I mention that in the future, if the tracheostoma will be permanent, the patient will wear homemade or commercially available stoma covers for both aesthetic and hygienic reasons.

My explanation of the various methods of speech following partial laryngectomies is fairly brief and includes mention of possible swallowing problems. If total laryngectomy is planned, I first explain why an alternative source for voice is required following removal of the larynx. I do this by drawing a simple line sketch of the involved structures (nose, mouth, tongue, pharynx, area from where larynx was excised, trachea, lungs, esophagus, and stomach). To lighten the moment, I personalize the drawing with curly hair, a pug nose, or a long, thin neck (Figure 12–1). At this point, I am ready to provide a simple explanation of the relevant anatomy and physiology. My goal is to increase the patient's understanding, so I use layman's terminology in both my discussion and on the diagram. I explain that food or liquid moves from the mouth, into the back of the throat (pharynx), through a ring of muscles at the top of the esophagus (pharyngoesophageal [PE] segment), into the food tube (esophagus), and down into the stomach. I explain that these structures comprise one set of plumbing that is primarily designed for food intake. Also, I mention that the important biologic function of the larynx and vocal cords is to prevent food and water from entering the lungs. When the larynx is no longer available to serve as a trap door, the windpipe (trachea) must be diverted and an opening into the trachea (stoma) must be created. The trachea and lungs function as a second set of plumbing designed for breathing in and out to stay alive. Finally, I show that when the windpipe was connected to the larynx, air from the lungs could pass through the vocal cords and cause them to vibrate for the production of vocal sound. Without the larynx, a substitute sound source is necessary to produce voice. The sound source may be a speech aid (an artificial larynx) or the ring of muscles (PE segment) at the top of the esophagus. At this point, I am ready to discuss the three methods of alaryngeal speech.

The emphasis here is on what he understands, not on what we assume he has been told!

Using lay terminology is very important here!

Artificial Larynx Speech

I explain that most speech aids are battery operated and, when activated, they produce a sound. If an intraoral device is used, the sound is transmit-

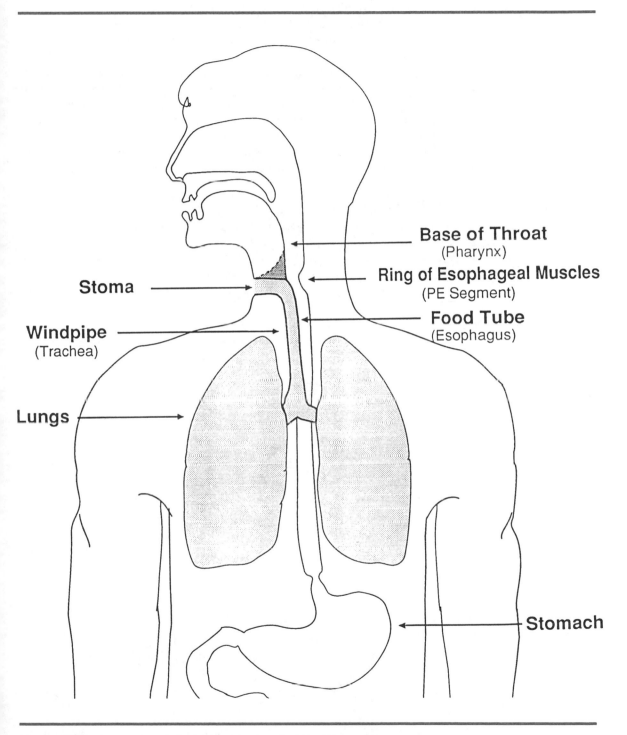

Figure 12-1. Anatomy and physiology associated with total laryngectomy.

ted through a mouthtube into the oral cavity. If a neck-type device is used, the sound is transmitted through the neck tissue into the pharynx and oral cavity (see Figure 12–2). In either case, the artificial larynx sound is modified by the resonators and is shaped into artificial larynx speech by the articulators.

These instruments are not as easy to learn to use as some people might think. However, unless demented or retarded, most patients can acquire intelligible artificial larynx speech, if they receive appropriate speech therapy. You should assure the patient that you will help him select a device from the variety that is available and begin teaching him how to use it as soon as his feeding tube is removed. The goal is for him to be able to express intelligibly a few short, functional phrases by the time he leaves the hospital.

Esophageal Speech

Next, I explain how standard esophageal speech is attained. On the line drawing, I point out the area of the PE segment and talk about the importance of it for the production of esophageal voice. By opening and closing my fist, I illustrate how the PE segment instantaneously opens to allow air from above it to enter the esophagus for insufflation. Then, with a rapid

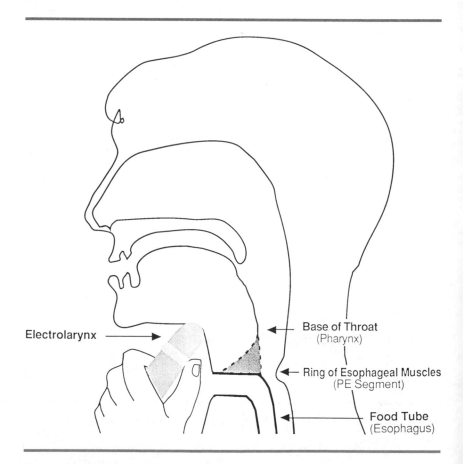

Figure 12-2. Artificial larynx speech.

opening and closing of my fist, I illustrate how this ring of muscles can be activated to vibrate and produce sound when air is expelled from the esophagus and passed upward through the segment (see Figure 12–3). The esophageal sound (voice) is transmitted into the pharynx where it is altered by the resonating cavities and formed into esophageal speech by the articulators.

Esophageal speech cannot be attained by everyone. In fact, it is estimated that about 60% of all laryngectomees do not or cannot use esophageal speech as their sole means of oral communication. Some people are highly motivated to learn it because they want to speak without having to depend on any type of prosthetic device.

Tracheoesophageal Fistula Speech

Finally, I explain how esophageal voice is attained when a tracheoesophageal fistula (TEF) procedure has been performed. The TEF can be performed either as a primary procedure at the time of laryngectomy or at a

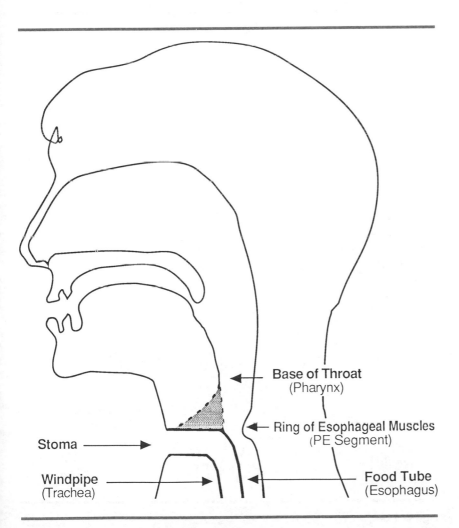

Base of Throat
(Pharynx)

Ring of Esophageal Muscles
(PE Segment)

Stoma

Windpipe
(Trachea)

Food Tube
(Esophagus)

Figure 12–3. Esophageal speech.

later date as a secondary procedure. I indicate that after the larynx is removed and a tracheostoma has been created, the surgeon will make a small tunnel (fistula) through the tracheal wall into the esophagus. Allowing several days for healing, the surgeon or speech pathologist will insert a small voice prosthesis into this opening (see Figure 12–4). When the patient uses his thumb or finger to occlude his tracheostoma, air from the lungs will be shunted through the voice prosthesis and into his esophagus. This air will cause vibration of the PE segment that results in sound. The esophageal sound that travels into his oral and nasal cavities can be used to articulate speech.

While I am explaining these steps, I try to underscore the patient's eventual responsibilities for removing, cleaning, and reinserting the prosthesis. Then, I present a list of the criteria for TEF candidacy and, together, we appraise his abilities to meet them. The criteria may differ slightly from

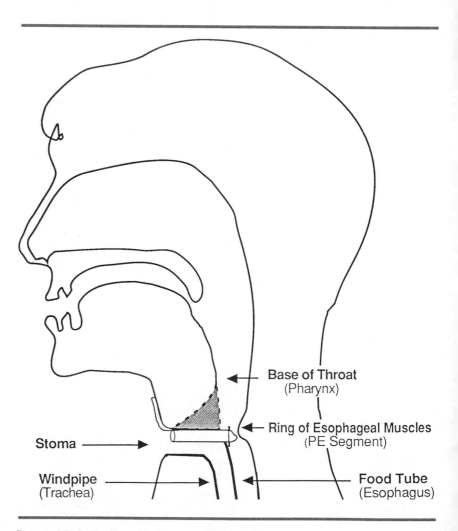

Figure 12-4. Tracheoesophageal fistula speech.

those originally established by Singer and Blom (1980). Requirements where I work include (a) patient motivation with the ability to comprehend the method of voice production and a willingness to accept responsibility for care of the voice prosthesis, (b) sufficient manual dexterity and visual acuity to insert the prosthesis and occlude the stoma, (c) ability to generate adequate pulmonary pressure to activate the voice prosthesis, (d) sufficient hearing acuity to detect and monitor phonations, and (e) no evidence of alcohol abuse. Patients who elect TEF as a secondary procedure after a laryngectomy must meet four additional requirements. These are (a) adequate size and shape of the stoma so the fistula can be surgically performed and the stoma can be totally occluded by the patient's thumb or finger during sound production, (b) stoma occlusion will not elicit sustained coughing, (c) patient is 3-6 months postirradiation, and (d) patient performs satisfactorily on an esophageal air insufflation test described by Blom, Singer, and Hamaker (1985).

Before terminating the preoperative session for those who will undergo total laryngectomy, I make an effort to relieve some immediate concerns that are discussed at length in the literature (Salmon, 1986). I tell the patient and spouse that it is not at all likely that he will die on the operating table and that he will be well cared for by a competent nursing staff. Pain medication will be available; however, most patients report that the pain is no worse than a sore throat and a stiff neck — when radical neck dissection is required. I mention that trained, well-rehabilitated individuals with laryngectomies and their spouses from the New Voice Club are available to make pre- and postoperative visits. Because there is controversy about whether such a visit should be scheduled before or after surgery, I let the patient and spouse decide.

I advise all patients that staples or insoluble stitches will be used to close the incisions. Because the sutures need time to heal, the patient will not be allowed postoperatively to swallow food or liquids. Instead, a feeding tube will be in place for 7-10 days. Dressings and other tubes also may be present, but their use is routine and should not be considered extraordinary.

If the spouse expects to visit the patient in his room immediately before surgery, I suggest she be there at least an hour before the operation is scheduled. Otherwise, he may already have been sedated and/or taken to the operative area before she arrives. Also, I indicate how long the surgery might take. I suggest she may want someone to wait with her during a relatively long day. I note the day of surgery and plan a short visit with her in the surgical waiting room.

Lastly, you will want to determine which means of communication might be most appropriate immediately following surgery. When the patient wakes in the recovery room, he will not be able to make sound for talking. Is the patient literate? If not, after surgery, he may have to mouth words, use a picture communication board, or be taught to use an artificial larynx. If he is literate, obtain a sample of his writing to determine legibility. He will require a pad and pencil or magic slate on which to write. Unless the patient or spouse requests additional information, I usually terminate the session at this point. I do so by saying I will see the patient bedside 5-7 days postoperatively.

Postoperative Counseling

I plan my visit with the patient and significant others several days after surgery. The first few sessions are purely educational. I provide them with written descriptions about his type of surgery; many are published by the American Cancer Society. Also, when appropriate, I explain resuscitation procedures for neckbreathers. If available, I show videotapes or play audiotapes that demonstrate the methods of speech he might use. If the patient who has undergone total laryngectomy is interested, I schedule an appointment with trained visitors from the New Voice Club.

Movements of the articulators are impaired by pain and swelling. Velopharyngeal closure and some tongue movements are affected by a nasogastric feeding tube. Therefore, I delay formal assessment until the patient's condition improves.

Partial Laryngectomy Appraisal

You must always appraise voice and swallowing problems of patients who have undergone a partial laryngectomy. Sometimes, the swallowing problems are transitory. When they persist, there is a risk of aspiration and pneumonia. Decisions must be made about continuing dysphagia therapy, subjecting the patient to long-term feedings through a stomach tube, or performing a total laryngectomy. A tracheostomy also may be permanent or transitory, so you may need to teach the patient to occlude his stoma to produce voice. Initially, with or without a tracheostomy, the patient may be voiceless or exhibit a breathy voice quality. Determine if the patient achieves improved voice quality when you instruct him to vary pitch and loudness. You should encourage the positive changes in follow-up voice therapy. Simultaneously, you should assess the patient's speech rate and articulation. Usually, a reduced rate of speaking tends to provide more pulmonary support for increased volume and more deliberate articulation will improve intelligibility.

Total Laryngectomy Appraisal

Artificial Larynx Speech

I encourage all laryngectomized patients to learn to use an artificial larynx speech aid (see Figure 12–5). I display several devices on a table and discuss the distinctive features of each. I assist patients in holding and operating them. I give each patient a list of supply sources and current prices for later reference. There is no set formula for helping a person select a device; suitability must be determined on an individual basis. Following are some factors to consider when helping patients select an instrument.

An intraoral device may be used if the patient undergoes postoperative radiotherapy and the neck becomes too sore to tolerate the pressure of a neck-type device. Also, if radical neck surgery has been performed that substantially changes the neck structure, a neck-type device may not work well. In both instances, an oral adaptor for a neck-type device, or an intra-oral artificial larynx like the Cooper-Rand or Tokyo, pictured in Figure 12–5, would be appropriate.

Various types of the neck-type electrolarynx differ in terms of weight, shape, size, and diameter of the vibrating head. Obviously, there are differences among patients in neck size and density. A thick, fleshy or swollen neck will absorb rather than transmit sound delivered by the device, so an instrument that produces a more powerful sound should be selected. A person with a small, thin neck may be able to use a less powerful device. Soft, supple tissue is required to embed the vibrating head; when no such tissue can be located around the neck or chin area, cheek placement may be necessary.

In addition to these considerations, one should take into account differences in cost, ease of manipulation, cradling comfort, and subjective preferences of patient and spouse. In many clinics, when the final selection is made, a loaner device of that type is made available. Then, therapy should be initiated before hospital discharge.

Tracheoesophageal Fistula (TEF) Speech

Criteria to be met by those interested in a TEF have been discussed previously. Recovery time differs for these patients, depending on whether the TEF was performed as a primary or secondary procedure and if other related surgery was also performed. While patients are recovering, they can meet individuals who use TEF speech or view them on videotape. Even if the patient viewed it preoperatively, I like to show him a videotape of a person demonstrating the removal, cleaning, inserting, and taping of his voice prosthesis. At that time, we use a mirror to examine the shape of the pa-

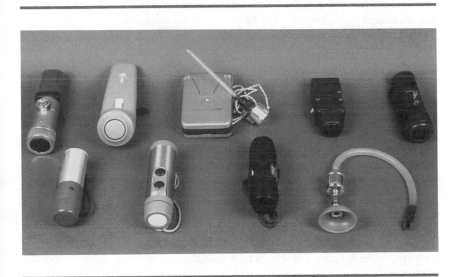

Figure 12–5. Artificial larynx devices. Aurex, AT&T, Cooper-Rand, Denrick, Jedcom or Bruce, Romet, Servox Intron, SPKR, and Tokyo. (Left to right from top and bottom)

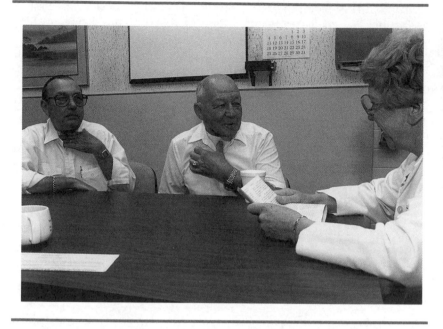

Figure 12-6. Therapy with two laryngectomized individuals using TEF speech.

Successful use of the TEF procedure requires considerable cooperation by the patient and the family.

tient's stoma and consider if a finger or thumb occlusion will be used. Also, we look at the surface surrounding his stoma and discuss the likelihood of his being able to wear a tracheostoma valve (eliminating the need for finger or thumb occlusion). I want to appraise these factors and stimulate the patient's thinking about his responsibility in the speech rehabilitation process. Whenever he is scheduled for voice prosthesis placement, the feeding tube is removed from the puncture site, the functioning of the pharyngoesophageal (PE) segment is tested, and an appropriately sized voice prosthesis is inserted. At this point, treatment begins, during which the patient must be instructed how to maintain and use the prosthesis.

Esophageal Speech

The surgeon determines when patients can begin esophageal speech therapy. Some prefer the instruction be delayed for 30 days postoperatively; others believe it can begin after the patient is able to swallow solid foods. While still recovering in the hospital, the patient should be taught the basic skills of using an artificial larynx and be encouraged to use one during his initial esophageal speech training. He can meet esophageal speakers or view them on videotape.

I explain that adequacy of the patient's "plumbing" to produce esophageal voice will need to be determined later in trial therapy or with an esophageal air insufflation test. When he is able to swallow, I assess tongue, lip, and jaw movements, as these are typically used to insufflate the esophagus. I also talk with the patient to assess his willingness to persist and his understanding that acquisition of proficient esophageal speech generally takes at least 6 months.

Motivation is an important factor in the ability to acquire esophageal speech (Shanks, 1986). Other psychological or physiological characteristics that have a positive effect are extroversion, independence, younger age, adequate hearing, and sufficient tongue mobility. All of these factors must be considered in your appraisal. However, you must consider also the plea by Shanks (1986, p. 346) "it has not been said that if someone fails to meet the different criteria, that person should be denied the chance to try to speak [with esophageal speech] after laryngectomy. It is a person's right to talk."

Section Summary

In this section, I have discussed surgical procedures and ramifications associated with laryngeal cancer. I have suggested ways to counsel patients and their significant others so their acquired knowledge might lessen the emotional impact of their losses. Finally, I have offered suggestions you may incorporate when observing and assessing behaviors to enhance your appraisal process.

SUMMARY

The speech-language pathologist is an important member of the team providing services to the patient with head and neck surgery, as well as to the patient's family. Our major goals with these patients is to assess the impact of the disease and its treatment on the communication skills of the patient and to provide means for rehabilitation of those skills.

There is considerable diversity among these patients in range of disease, residual capabilities, and personal characteristics. As a consequence, diagnostic and treatment methods frequently must be planned on an individual basis.

REFERENCES

American Cancer Society. (1992). *Cancer Facts & Figures — 1992.* Atlanta, GA: Author.

Blom, E. D., Singer, M. I., & Hamaker, R. C. (1985). An improved esophageal insufflation test. *Archives of Otolaryngology, 111,* 211–212.

Fairbanks, G. (1960). *Voice and articulation drillbook* (2nd ed.). New York: Harper & Row.

Fisher, H., & Logemann, J. (1971). *Fisher-Logemann Test of Articulation Competence.* Boston: Houghton Mifflin.

Imai, S., & Michi, K. (1992). Articulatory function after resection of the tongue and floor of the mouth: Palatometric and perceptual evaluation. *Journal of Speech and Hearing Research, 35,* 68–78.

Leonard, R., Goodrich, S., McMenamin, P., & Donald, P. (1992). Differentiation of speakers with glossectomies by acoustic and perceptual measures. *American Journal of Speech-Language Pathology, 1,* 55–63.

Logemann, J. A. (1989). Speech and swallowing rehabilitation for head and neck tumor patients. In E. N. Myers & J. Y. Suen (Eds.), *Cancer of the head and neck* (2nd ed.) (pp. 1021–1043). New York: Churchill Livingstone.

Salmon, S. J. (1986). Adjusting to laryngectomy. In W. H. Perkins & J. L. Northern (Eds.), *Seminars in speech and language: Current strategies of rehabilitation of the laryngectomized patient, 7,* 67–94. New York: Thieme.

Shanks, J. C. (1986). Essentials for laryngeal speech: Psychology and physiology. In R. L. Keith & F. L. Darley (Eds.), *Laryngectomee rehabilitation* (2nd ed.) (pp. 337–349). Austin, TX: Pro-Ed.

Singer, M. I., & Blom, E. D. (1980). An endoscopic technique for restoration of voice after laryngectomy. *Annals of Otology, Rhinology and Laryngology, 89,* 529–533.

Skelly, M., Donaldson, R. C., Fust, R., & Townsend, D. (1972). Changes in phonatory aspects of glossectomy intelligibility through vocal parameter manipulation. *Journal of Speech and Hearing Disorders, 37,* 379–389.

Weber, R. S., Ohlms, L., Bowman, J., Jacob, R., & Goepfert, H. (1991). Functional results after total or near total glossectomy with laryngeal preservation. *Archives of Otolaryngology Head and Neck Surgery, 117,* 512–515.

RECOMMENDED READINGS

Gargan, W. (1969). *Why me? An autobiography.* New York: Doubleday & Company.

Lanpher, A. (1965). Hello, Tallulah. In W. Ross (Ed.), *The climate is hope* (pp. 35–50). Englewood Cliffs, NJ: Prentice-Hall.

Moss, D. G. (1988). *Why didn't they tell me?* Seattle: Laryngectomee Supply Company.

Nicholson, E. (1975). Personal notes of a laryngectomy. *American Journal of Nursing, 75,* 2157–2158.

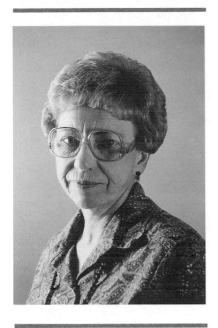

SHIRLEY J. SALMON, Ph.D.

M.A. 1961, The University of Iowa
Ph.D. 1965, The University of Iowa

Dr. Salmon is presently Speech Pathologist at the VA Medical Center
in Kansas City, MO and Professor in the Hearing and Speech
Department at the University of Kansas Medical Center. She reports
special interest in treating patients with laryngectomy and teaching
about their total rehabilitation.

CHAPTER

13

Traumatic Brain Injury

Ann A. VanDemark, Ph.D.

As a speech-language pathologist, you will find individuals with traumatic brain injury (also identified by some writers as head injury or closed head injury) to be among the most complex and challenging clients you will encounter in your professional career. The communication disorders that may result from traumatic brain injury are as diverse, as complicated, and as fascinating as the human brain itself.

Traumatic brain injury (TBI) may occur at any time in an individual's life. It is not a disorder of childhood, nor is it the result of aging or disease, genetic defect or faulty learning. It occurs in an instant, most often the instant of a motor vehicle accident or a fall, or some other event resulting in a blow to the head. The damage to the brain from trauma was described as follows in a recent issue of the *Asha* magazine (American Speech-Language-Hearing Association, 1989):

> Here's what happens to the brain in a collision: the head whips forward and hits the windshield. The brain, like gelatin, continues to move after the skull stops. It bounces off the inside of the skull and rubs against the bony prominences within. Blood vessels break and form a pool. The pool has no place to go because the skull cannot expand. Pressure inside the skull increases. This pressure pushes the brain toward the hole at the base of the skull. Simultaneously, there is tearing and shearing of the nerve fibers as the brain moves. (p. 83)

It's not a pretty picture! The resulting brain damage is usually widespread and presents a combination of localized and diffuse injury. It involves multiple systems and many areas of the brain, and produces a wide range of symptoms, including physical, cognitive, psychological, and behavioral impairments. The degree of severity extends from extreme impairment and total disability through barely visible, though still troublesome, residuals of the injury. A communication disorder is usually only one of the problems that the individual with TBI will have to face.

COMMUNICATION DISORDERS IN TBI

If we were to look at a group of individuals, all with TBI, we would probably find as many different combinations and patterns of communication disorder as there are individuals in the group. Most common are the impairments caused by diffuse, generalized injury — impairments in areas I think of as the "cognitive infrastructure" that supports human communication. These include perception, attention, concentration, memory, sequencing, information processing, reasoning, problem solving, and executive functioning. Impairments in these areas have led one writer to observe that, although most persons with certain classic types of aphasia communicate better than they talk, individuals who have sustained a head injury often appear to talk better than they communicate (Sohlberg & Mateer, 1989). Our profession has chosen the label "cognitive/communicative" disorders for the group of impairments that follow traumatic brain injury (American Speech-Language-Hearing Association, 1987).

Izaak Walton wrote about *The Compleat Angler*. Working with traumatic brain injury requires "the compleat speech-language pathologist."

Some individuals also experience impairments that are more likely to be related to localized brain damage on the cortical surface and subsurface and in the brain stem. These include impairments of speech intelligibility, fluency, motor planning, voice, language, hearing, and/or swallowing. These may be so severe that the individual is unable to communicate at all, or may be so mild that only the injured individuals and their most perceptive clinicians are aware that something is "different."

This chapter details assessment rationales and procedures that address cognitive/communicative impairment and will refer you to other chapters for the areas of voice, fluency, intelligibility, and so on.

DIAGNOSTIC SETTINGS

It is important to be aware of the wide variety of settings in which evaluation of the client with TBI may take place. The services of the speech-language pathologist may be called for in several different hospital settings, including the acute care trauma center, intensive care, neurology, neurosurgery, and inpatient or outpatient rehabilitation units. TBI rehabilitation also takes place extensively in community-based residential, outpatient and day rehabilitation programs, vocational rehabilitation settings, and in schools. There is a very strong relationship between the length of time since the injury and the type of rehabilitation program or facility where the speech-language pathologist will be assessing and treating the client.

THE INTERDISCIPLINARY MODEL

We have learned from experience that the most effective way of managing the multiple problems of the individual with traumatic brain injury is the *interdisciplinary* treatment model. The concept of interdisciplinary practice is growing, as the rehabilitation professions become more aware of the benefits of a truly integrated and coordinated approach to treatment. The multiple problems of the client with TBI require a tremendous amount of coordination and team decision making, beyond what the traditional multidisciplinary model provides. For a good discussion of the differences between multidisciplinary and interdisciplinary treatment, read Michael Howard's (1989) chapter in *Innovations in Head Injury Rehabilitation* (Deutsch & Fralish).

Team players are essential to effective TBI rehabilitation. Close harmony is more effective than solos!

The *interdisciplinary team* includes all of the professional and support staff who work with a client, as well as the client or client's representative. Depending on the client's needs, the professional staff may include speech-language pathology, physical medicine, neuropsychology, occupational therapy, physical therapy, rehabilitation nursing, social work, vocational services, therapeutic recreation, and dietetics. If the client is of school age, a teacher or special education specialist may also be included. The support staff may include nursing assistants, rehabilitation aides, direct-care staff from residential settings, and family members. One of the hallmarks of the interdisciplinary model is the inclusion of the client on the team and the consideration of the client's goals and desires when formulating the treatment plan. When the client is not able to participate, a spouse or other family member or a designated representative, such as a guardian, joins the team. The interdisciplinary team creates and then works together toward a common set of functional goals, none of which are easily identified with or exclusive to a single discipline. An example of a functional goal is "Independent mobility in the community." To achieve this goal, a client might need to improve in the areas of walking (physical therapy), driving (occupational therapy), reading street signs and transportation schedules (speech-language pathology), behaving appropriately (psychology), and so on. The client might practice these skills with support staff or family as well as with the professional staff.

"Empowerment" is an important concept in rehabilitation; here's a good example.

The purpose of this discussion, in addition to acquainting you with the concept of interdisciplinary treatment, is to point out that the evaluation process that the speech-language pathologist designs for each client with TBI must provide information that can be utilized by the interdisciplinary team to engage in functional, outcome-based treatment planning.

CHARACTERISTICS OF THE EVALUATION PROCESS

Let's consider first the *purpose* of the evaluation. These are some of the reasons why a speech-language pathologist might do a cognitive/communicative evaluation:

1. Establish the presence or absence of deficits and collect baseline information on them.

2. Make a prognosis or a prediction about the amount of recovery an individual might expect.

3. Determine readiness for transfer to a rehabilitation program.

4. Conduct an in-depth, comprehensive evaluation to be used in planning and implementing a rehabilitation program.

5. Assess a client's progress in a rehabilitation program.

6. Determine if a client's cognitive/communicative abilities will support returning to work or living safely alone in the community.

7. Do a follow-up evaluation to ascertain if a client has maintained progress made in the rehabilitation program.

The nature of the evaluation process will vary with the setting in which the client is being seen, which is likely, in turn, to vary with the severity of the injury and the length of time since the injury took place. The client's awareness, stamina, and ability to participate in the evaluation will also affect the nature of the process.

In the trauma center or acute care setting, clients' behaviors will often be changing rapidly, and they may have limited ability to focus on and attend to formal testing. You will also have limited time in which to conduct the evaluation; in most hospitals there is a good deal of competition for opportunities to work with a client. You will be establishing the presence of deficits and gathering baseline data, but you will probably not be thinking in terms of long-term intervention. You will most often choose evaluation components that can be administered rather quickly, and you may have to rely on those that can be completed using observational data rather than formal test data.

By contrast, in a rehabilitation setting, you are more likely to have the luxuries of time and easy access to the client, and the client will probably have reached a level of recovery that permits improved ability to attend and participate. You will be focusing on the information you need to plan a longer rehabilitation program, and you will turn to more formal testing procedures that take longer to administer and yield more norm-referenced and criterion-referenced data. You will also be likely to incorporate more naturalistic and community-based assessment tasks. When you need to answer specific questions about return-to-work or safety in independent living, you will also be more likely to rely on standardized assessment data and community observation.

In designing any evaluation, the first step will be to gather as much background information as possible about the client. Obviously, the more you know, the more efficiently you will be able to target your evaluation toward the important areas. In our program, it is not uncommon for the interdisciplinary team to meet before anyone sees the client, to share information and to focus on the most important areas to assess. You will by now have read Chapter 3, about the clinical history, which will provide you with starting points. My goal here is to indicate some of the sources of information that should be available to you and some of the special questions that need to be asked about the client with TBI.

Planning is an important cognitive ability; many clients with TBI find it difficult.

The client will almost certainly either be or have been hospitalized, so the reports of the physicians, nurses, and other hospital services will be valuable resources. If the client has been receiving rehabilitative services before you are asked to do your evaluation, you will gain valuable information from the reports of those other disciplines/services. The client's family is always a valuable resource, particularly about the client's preinjury communication skills in home, school, and work settings. Depending on the amount of cognitive/communicative impairment, the client may also be able to give you useful information.

You will need to know what kind of injuries the individual sustained, how much time has elapsed since the trauma, and what the course of treatment has been. You will want to learn as much as you can about the location and extent of the brain damage, also looking for information about the length of time the individual was unconscious, if there was a coma, and for how long. The client's responsiveness on a day-to-day basis early in the recovery period is useful to know; how soon after the injury was the client talking again, how much and how well, and how have the client's communicative abilities changed over time since the injury? All of this will prove useful as you plan your evaluation, formulate a prognosis, and develop a direction for intervention.

THE ASSESSMENT BATTERY

When you have completed your gathering of background information, you will have a good idea of the questions you need to answer about the client. Now let's consider some of the ways to get the information to answer those questions: the actual assessment tools.

Assessment tools for cognitive/communicative disorders typically fall into four categories:

1. **Rating scales** that are used in many settings to make broad, general statements about a client's level of function.

2. **Assessments of cognitive/communicative competence**, which are most often administered in a clinic or hospital setting.

3. **Assessments of other communicative impairments** such as voice, hearing, motor speech, or swallowing, also done most often in a clinic or hospital setting.

4. **Assessment of functional performance**, which is usually carried out in a more natural, environmental setting such as the home or the community.

Rating Scales

Most everyone who works professionally with TBI is aware of and usually quite familiar with the *Rancho Los Amigos Scale of Cognitive Levels and Expected Behavior* (Hagen & Malkmus, 1979). You will find this scale in Figure 13-1. It gives us a kind of "shorthand" description of a head-injured

Level I	No Response	Unresponsive to all stimuli
Level II	Generalized Response	Inconsistent, nonpurposeful, non-specific reactions to stimuli. Responds to pain, but response may be delayed.
Level III	Localized Response	Inconsistent reaction directly related to type of stimulus presented. Responds to some commands. May respond to discomfort.
Level IV	Confused Agitated Response	Disoriented and unaware of present events. Agitated with frequent bizarre and inappropriate behavior. Attention span is short and ability to process information is impaired.
Level V	Confused Inappropriate Nonagitated Response	Nonpurposeful random or fragmented responses when task complexity exceeds abilities. Patient appears alert and responds to simple commands. Performs previously learned tasks but is unable to learn new ones.
Level VI	Confused Appropriate Response	Behavior is goal-directed. Responses are appropriate to the situation with incorrect responses due to memory difficulties.
Level VII	Automatic Appropriate Response	Correct routine responses which are robot-like. Appears oriented to setting, but insight, judgment and problem solving are poor.
Level VIII	Purposeful Appropriate Response	Correct responding, carryover of new learning. No required supervision, poor tolerance for stress and some abstract reasoning difficulties.

Figure 13-1. Rancho Los Amigos Scale of Cognitive Levels and Expected Behavior. From *Rancho Los Amigos Scale of Cognitive Function* by C. Hagen and D. Malkmus, 1979, Downey, CA: Adult Brain Injury Service, Rancho Los Amigos Medical Center. Copyright by Professional Staff Association, Rancho Los Amigos. Reprinted by permission.

person from observations of particular behaviors such as orientation, attention span, level of agitation, ability to learn new information, and so on. The scale is hierarchial, with the lowest numbers indicating the greatest impairment. You will hear professionals say things like "He's a Rancho IV," or "She's a Rancho II moving toward III," or "clients admitted to this program must be at Rancho V or above." Of course, the scale is only as good as our observations and our agreement as to what constitutes a "Rancho _____." The scale focuses more on the similarities between clients than the individual differences; nevertheless, it is a useful place to start.

Clients who are in acute care settings are often rated on the *Glasgow Coma Scale* (Jennett, Shook, Bond, & Brooks, 1981), which uses the observations of degree of eye opening, the best verbal response, and the best motor response to describe the level of disability the client is experiencing. Here, too, a small sample of behavior is used to make a broad categorization of an individual and the observations are relatively subjective.

A third scale that has been used extensively since its introduction is the *Functional Independence Measure* (Diller & Ben-Yishay, 1987). This scale looks at a client's performance in selected key activities of daily living and measures the level of dependence/independence the individual displays.

Rating scales provide a relatively efficient means of describing and categorizing a client's behavior and for tracking the rate and direction of improvement. Scales present a more global picture of the client and do not represent a detailed description of the individual's impairments.

Cognitive/Communicative Assessment Batteries

Until rather recently, speech-language pathologists typically evaluated clients with TBI using items selected from a variety of sources, a kind of "personal test battery" because there were no standardized batteries for the evaluation of cognitive/communicative impairment. Adamovich, Henderson, and Auerbach (1985) provided a hierarchy of cognitive processes to be tested and suggested informal, nonstandardized ways of assessing them. Although this type of evaluation gave the individual clinician a good deal of information about a particular client, there was no good basis for comparison with other clients and it was difficult, if not impossible, to make statements about the severity of impairment or the prognosis for recovery.

Recently, we have seen the development of test batteries that are standardized and take into consideration a larger sample of measured behavior. With these batteries we can assign a level of severity to a client's impairments in several different areas as well as deriving an overall cognitive/communicative impairment score. The description of assessment instruments that follows is not intended to be complete; rather, it provides examples of some of the most current and better-standardized examples of cognitive/communicative assessment batteries.

The *Western Neuro Sensory Stimulation Profile* (WNSSP), which was developed by Ansell, Keenan, and de la Rocha at the Western Neuro Care Center and published in 1989, is designed specially for evaluating the severely impaired, slow-to-recover head-injured individual, particularly those at Rancho levels II–V. It assesses arousal and attention, expressive communication, and response to auditory, visual, tactile, and olfactory stimuli. The test uses a multipoint scoring system that takes into account not only the accuracy of the client's response, but also the amount of cuing (prompts, "hints") required to obtain the response, plus the response latency (the length of time it takes for the client to respond). The WNSSP is particularly effective for gathering baseline data and tracking a client's recovery pattern; it is not intended to compare a client with TBI's performance to that of a "normal" individual.

The Brief Test of Head Injury (BTHI) was developed by Helm-Estabrooks and Hotz and published in 1991. It is intended to be administered in 20–30 minutes, hence the title "Brief." The test assesses orientation/attention, following commands, linguistic organization, reading comprehension, naming, memory, and visual spatial skills, and it, too, is intended for use with individuals who have sustained severe head injuries. The total score on the test can be reported as a percentile rank, a standard score, or a severity score (severe, moderate, mild, or borderline-normal).

The *Scales of Cognitive Ability for Traumatic Brain Injury* (SCATBI), published by Adamovich and Henderson in 1992, consist of five subtests that measure orientation, perception and discrimination, organization, recall, and reasoning. The range of difficulty within the test items is sufficient to test a range of clients from very low functioning to very high functioning. The test was standardized on both normal and TBI clients, so comparisons can be made between a client's performance and normal expectations. The results can be shown as percentile ranks or standard scores, and direct comparison among the performance levels on the different subtests is also possible.

The *Ross Information Processing Assessment* (RIPA) was developed by Deborah Ross in 1986 to assess cognitive and linguistic deficits following closed head injuries to adolescents and adults. The test samples several areas basic to cognitive/communicative functioning: immediate memory, recent memory, temporal orientation for recent and remote memory, spatial orientation, orientation to the environment, recall of general information, problem solving and abstract thinking, organization, and auditory processing and retention.

No test battery will answer all of your questions about a client's cognitive/communicative abilities; however, completion of a battery such as those listed above accomplishes several things. It provides a baseline against which you will be able to measure future changes in the client's performance. It yields an overall level of severity, and depending on the test battery given, it may also identify specific deficit areas you will want to investigate more thoroughly. Sohlberg and Mateer (1989, p. 33) provide an excellent list of tests and tasks that can be used for a more in-depth investigation of specific cognitive/communicative deficit areas, if your chosen test battery does not yield enough detail.

Assessment of Other Aspects of Communication

In addition to the cognitive/communicative assessment, you will, of course, need to explore any other aspects of communication that may be impaired. Because TBI frequently produces damage to the brain stem, it is not uncommon to find impairments of motor speech, swallowing, and respiration. If the client presents some of the symptoms of aphasia (see Chapter 7), you may wish to do further assessment of specific language abilities. Keep in mind, though, that the diffuse brain injury typical of TBI does not usually produce the classic types of aphasia that are associated with localized, focal injuries. You will, of course, screen the individual's hearing and make a referral to an audiologist if indicated. If the individual is unable to speak, you will want to assess the potential to use an augmentative communication device. Other chapters in this book provide information that will be useful in the assessment of these areas with TBI clients and I will not repeat that information here. One observation, however; I do feel it is best to do the cognitive/communicative assessment first, because those deficits are likely to have an impact on the client's performance in all areas. Without an understanding of the client's level of cognitive/communicative abilities, the speech-language pathologist could make an incorrect interpretation of the data from other assessments. For example, a client might fail to perform well on a hearing screening because of hearing impairment, or because of difficulty with attention and concentration — reflecting cognitive/communicative impairment. Sometimes it is hard to decide "which is the chicken and which is the egg," but knowing the client's cognitive/communicative limitations first should make it easier to interpret the data from other assessments.

Observations of Functional Performance

The traditional "testing" approach to assessment of the client with TBI tends to yield information about "processes" and "components" of cognitive/communicative deficits. This is valuable information; however, evaluation and rehabilitation of clients with TBI has also come to focus very strongly on the broader concept of *function*, that is, the client's ability to carry out the communicative activities needed in the everyday environment. Beukelman, Yorkston, and Lossing (1984) have pointed out that assessment of function requires two components, identifying the client's communicative *needs* and then observing how well the client is able to meet those needs. Observation of the client in a variety of real-world situations provides valuable information about the client's ability to function outside the clinic setting. Many TBI rehabilitation programs use a combination of "real" tasks in the clinic, in the living setting, and in the community, with the community-based assessment consisting of direct observation of the client in normal community activities such as shopping, dining out, managing money, using community transportation, and so on. Key factors in functional assessment are explained clearly by Sohlberg and Mateer (1989, pp. 19–23). Most important is the development of measurement parameters; that is, we must be able to describe the client's performance in quantifiable terms. Examples might be: recording the length of time needed to complete a task, recording the number of cues or prompts the client requires, counting the number of errors made, noting the effect of environmental variables such as noise, interruptions, and so on.

What works in the "real world" is what counts!

In our program, we have developed a Behavioral Rating Scale that takes into account three parameters: the amount of physical assistance needed to perform a task, the amount of cuing or prompting needed, and the quality of performance. Each of these parameters is rated on a scale from 0–7, with 0 representing "cannot perform the task under any circumstances" and 7 representing performance "within normal limits." This scale is useful in quantifying observations of the client's communication skills in community and functional tasks.

COMPLEMENTARY EVALUATIONS

Impaired communication is only one of a complex of problems that may face the client with TBI. We need to remind ourselves often that communication disorders not only coexist with other disorders, but also interact with them and may influence the client's performance in areas not directly involving communication.

Concurrently with your evaluation, a client will probably be undergoing assessment by the other members of the interdisciplinary team. There is much complementary information that can and should be shared during and after all of these evaluations. Each discipline will be approaching the client's impairments from its own vantage point and sharing of information is one of the hallmarks of interdisciplinary practice.

A SPECIAL WORD ABOUT CHILDREN WITH TBI

Most of the information in this chapter has addressed the assessment of adults with traumatic brain injury, because by far the highest incidence of TBI is found in the young adult population who are involved in automobile accidents and sports injuries. Children are not immune to TBI, of course, and although this chapter does not specifically address the assessment of children, there are some important points to keep in mind.

When the client is an adult, we assume that the effects of the injury are imposed on an *already developed* neuromotor system. When a child incurs a traumatic brain injury, the effects of the injury interact with and may dramatically affect the child's *still developing* neuromotor system. This is a complex issue; some of the progress a child makes may be the result of recovery and intervention and some the result of maturation; further, normal development will almost certainly be affected by the extent and nature of the brain injury. In addition to all of the cognitive and physical variables we consider when assessing an adult with TBI, we also need to keep developmental milestones in mind when assessing a child.

As always when dealing with children, it is crucial to use age-appropriate materials. Most of the standardized cognitive/communicative assessment tools are normed for adults; some can be used appropriately with older adolescents. There are at this time no *standardized* cognitive/communicative assessment batteries specifically for children with TBI. Many of the tools and techniques appropriate for children with language disorders will yield useful information and functional observation is particularly valuable in the assessment of a child with TBI.

SUMMARY

The points to remember from this chapter are: (1) the individual who suffers a TBI is likely to have impairment of the cognitive infrastructure that supports communication; our profession labels this cognitive/communicative impairment; (2) cognitive/communicative impairment coexists with and interacts with the other impairments that typically result from TBI; (3) clients with TBI are evaluated in many settings, for numerous purposes, and at many points along the way to recovery; and (4) the interdisciplinary model of rehabilitation is the most effective model for the client with a TBI.

REFERENCES

Adamovich, B., Henderson, J., & Auerbach, S. (1985). *Cognitive rehabilitation of closed head injured patients: A dynamic approach.* San Diego: College-Hill Press.

Adamovich, B. B., & Henderson, J. (1992). *Scales of Cognitive Ability for Traumatic Brain Injury (SCATBI).* Chicago: The Riverside Publishing Company.

American Speech-Language-Hearing Association. (1987). Role of speech-language pathologists in the habilitation and rehabilitation of cognitively impaired individuals: A report of the subcommittee on language and cognition. *Asha, 29,* 55.

American Speech-Language-Hearing Association. (1989). Traumatic brain injury: Rebuilding shattered lives. *Asha, 31,* 83–106.

Ansell, B. J., Keenan, J. E., & de la Rocha, O. (1989). *The Western Neuro Sensory Stimulation Profile.* Tustin, CA: Western Neuro Care Center.

Beukelman, D., Yorkston, K., & Lossing, C. (1984). Functional communication assessment of adults with neurogenic disorders. In A. Halpern & M. Fuhrer (Eds.), *Functional assessment in rehabilitation* (pp. 101–114) Baltimore: Brookes.

Deutsch, P. M., & Fralish, K. B. (Eds.). (updated annually). *Innovations in head injury rehabilitation.* New York: Matthew Bender.

Diller, L., & Ben-Yishay, Y. (1987). Analyzing rehabilitation outcomes of persons with head injury. In M. Fuhrer (Ed.), *Rehabilitation outcomes: Analysis and measurement* (pp. 209–220). Baltimore: Brookes.

Hagen, C., & Malkmus, D. (1979). *Rancho Los Amigos Scale of Cognitive Function.* Downey, CA: Adult Brain Injury Service, Rancho Los Amigos Medical Center.

Helm-Estabrooks, N., & Hotz, G. (1991). *Brief Test of Head Injury (BTHI).* Chicago: The Riverside Publishing Company.

Howard, M. (1989 update). Interdisciplinary team treatment in acute care. In P. M. Deutsch & K. B. Fralish (Eds.), *Innovations in head injury* (pp. 3.1–3.26). (updated annually). New York: Matthew Bender.

Jennett, B., Shook, J., Bond, M., & Brooks, N. (1981). Disability after severe head injury: Observations on the use of the Glasgow Outcome Scale. *Journal of Neurology, Neurosurgery, and Psychiatry, 44,* 285–293.

Ross, D. (1986). *Ross Information Processing Assessment (RIPA).* Chicago: The Riverside Press.

Sohlberg, M., & Mateer, C. (1989). The assessment of cognitive-communicative functions in head injury. In K. Butler (Ed.), *Topics in Language Disorders, 9*(2). Frederick, MD: Aspen Publishers.

RECOMMENDED READINGS

American Congress of Rehabilitation Medicine. (1993). *Guide to interdisciplinary practice in rehabilitation settings.* Skokie, IL: ACRM Publication Orders, 5700 Old Orchard Road, Skokie IL 60077-1057.

DePompei, R., & Blosser, J. L. (1991). Functional cognitive-communicative impairments in children and adolescents: Assessment and intervention. In J. Kreutzer & P. Wehman (Eds.), *Cognitive rehabilitation for persons with traumatic brain injury* (pp. 215–235). Baltimore: Paul H. Brookes.

Sohlberg, M. M., & Mateer, C. A. (1990). Evaluation and Treatment of Communicative Skills. In J. S. Kreutzer & P. Wehman (Eds.), *Community integration following traumatic brain injury* (pp. 67–84). Baltimore: Paul H. Brookes.

Twelfth Institute on Rehabilitation Issues. (1985). Report of the Study Group on Rehabilitation of Traumatic Brain Injury (pp. 9–85). Menomonie: University of Wisconsin-Stout.

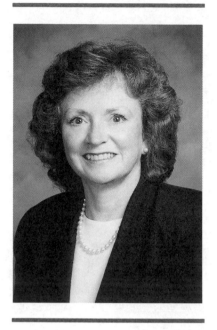

ANN A. VANDEMARK, Ph.D.

M.A. 1962, The University of Iowa
Ph.D. 1964, Indiana University

Dr. VanDemark is Director of Clinical Rehabilitation Services for Special Tree, Ltd., a comprehensive rehabilitation program based in Romulus, Michigan specializing in the treatment of traumatic brain injury. Her previous employment settings have been Indiana University, the University of Iowa, VA Medical Center in Iowa City, the University of Michigan, and Wayne State University. Her special interests are neurogenic speech, language, and cognitive-communicative disorders.

C H A P T E R

14

Cleft Palate

Sally J. Peterson-Falzone, Ph.D.

This chapter deals with the diagnostic questions, methodology, and decisions for patients with clefts at all developmental and treatment stages. The special diagnostic procedures generally available only in medical settings are discussed briefly. The majority of the information is about the assessment tasks faced by the speech-language pathologist in nonmedical settings such as public schools and private practice. The discussion is based on a wide variety of research studies, some of which are listed among the References and Recommended Readings, and on *Parameters for the Evaluation and Treatment of Patients with Cleft Lip/Palate or Other Craniofacial Anomalies* (1993).

AN OVERVIEW

It's highly probable that you know someone with cleft lip and palate but you may not know much about the disorder. Briefly, it is a birth defect that occurs once in about 750 live births. It is a highly variable defect that may include cleft lip, cleft palate, or both, and may be a complete cleft (extending through all affected structures) or incomplete (only a partial extension). In any case, the cleft is the result of incomplete development during early pregnancy. In many families, clefts follow a fairly clean line of inheritance. In others, there is no previous history.

    If there is a cleft lip, there will be facial disfigurement. If the cleft extends through the gum ridge (the alveolus), there will be dental problems ranging from missing teeth to a marked misfit (malocclusion) between the upper jaw (the maxilla) and the lower jaw (the mandible). If the cleft extends through the palate (the roof of the mouth), the baby will initially have problems sucking and later will not be able to direct the airstream through the mouth during speech. Instead, there will be nasal emission of air during consonants and hypernasal voice quality during vowels (an oversimplified description of speech, but one that is helpful). See Figures 14-1 to 14-3 for examples of cleft lip and palate before and after surgical repair.

With this brief background, we proceed to discuss diagnosis of communication status.

THE FIRST FEW MONTHS OF LIFE

The speech-language pathologist on a cleft palate/craniofacial team typically meets the child and family during the first critical weeks of life. At this stage, our diagnostic concerns include (1) the effects of the cleft on prelinguistic vocal output, (2) how the presence of the cleft may affect the family emotionally and thus influence their stimulation of the child, (3) the high probability of middle ear fluid and hearing loss, and (4) the possibility of associated malformations and/or syndromes (more than 50% of children with clefts have at least one associated minor or major malformation).

When you see the child and family at this early stage, you have an excellent opportunity to prevent or minimize later problems in communication development. This text contains chapters on assessment of various aspects of communication behavior in infants and young children. Depending

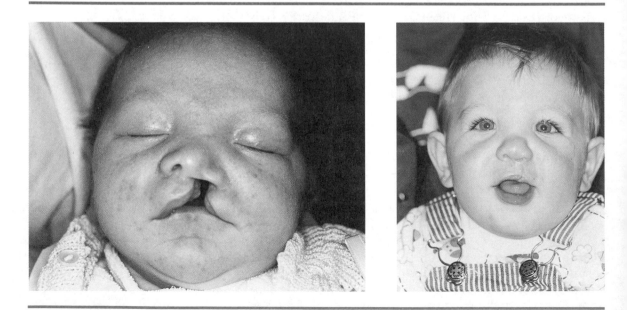

Figure 14-1. Infant with unilateral cleft lip and palate before and after lip repair. Center for Craniofacial Anomalies, University of California-San Francisco, William Y. Hoffman, surgeon.

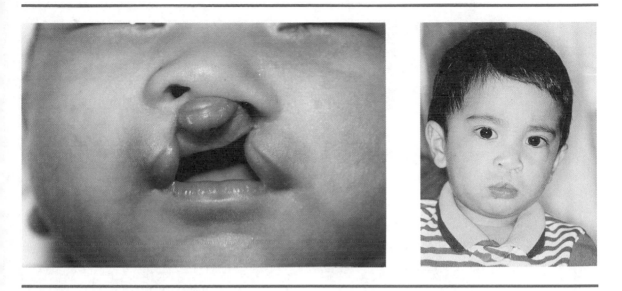

Figure 14-2. Child with incomplete bilateral cleft before and after lip repair. Center for Craniofacial Anomalies, Univerity of California-San Francisco, William Y. Hoffman, surgeon.

on both the time available and the particular setting in which you meet with the child and family, you may use a variety of tools to assess early development. As an example, the *MacArthur Communicative Development Inventories* (Fenson, Dale, Reznick, Thal, Bates, Hartung, Pethick, & Reilly, 1989) consist of two parent-inventory scales, one for infants up to the age of 15 months and one for toddlers aged 16 to 30 months. The information derived with these inventories can predict later problems in language development, and investigators have found them to be useful in identifying deficits in children with cleft palate.

In the last decade, there has been a welcome burst of studies of prelinguistic vocalizations and of early phonetic and phonologic development in children with clefts. Investigators have studied the differences between the early vocalizations of babies with clefts and those of babies without clefts, and offered theories about how these differences influence later speech development. Following is a list of the key findings from four such studies (Chapman, 1991; Grunwell & Russell, 1987; O'Gara & Logemann, 1988, 1990; Philips & Kent, 1984):

Most infants in the United States and Europe do not undergo surgical closure of the palatal cleft during the first 6 months of life. So most of these studies are of children with open cleft palates.

- In their reduplicated babbling (like "bababa"), babies with clefts show a relative lack of the normal acoustic cues for the differences between consonants and vowels. Parents of babies with clefts often report that their babies were late in babbling, perhaps because they simply cannot recognize the babbling behavior when the normal acoustic cues are absent.

- Babies with clefts produce many more sounds made at the boundaries of the vocal tract (the lips and the vocal cords) as opposed to sounds made within the mouth, and at 6 months of age they do not show the "take-over" of alveolar consonants heard in noncleft babies by this age.

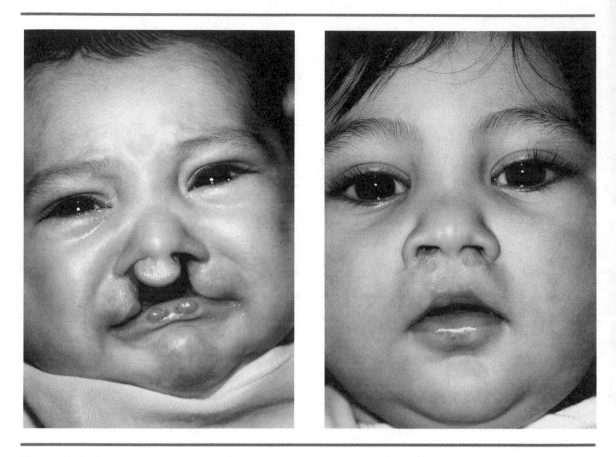

Figure 14-3. Pre- and post-operative pictures of an infant with an incomplete bilateral cleft (complete on the left side, incomplete on the right) and lower lip mounds. The mounds signal the presence of Van der Woude syndrome, a condition combining lower lip pits or mounds with various forms of clefting. This syndrome is autosomal dominant, meaning the risk for recurrence in the family, or in this child's own children, is 50%. Center for Craniofacial Anomalies, University of California-San Francisco, William Y. Hoffman, surgeon.

Some infants have been fitted with palatal plates prior to surgical closure of the palate to try to promote more normal articulation development. This is technically difficult to do, especially if the child advances to the toddler stage and removes the plate at will, usually feeding it to the dog!

- Babies with clefts use more nasals, glides and the glottal fricative /h/ than the stop-plosives preferred by noncleft babies.

- Babies with clefts also use fewer syllables in their early vocalizations than do noncleft babies.

Clinically, these findings tell us that there will be some early, unavoidable differences in speech sound development in infants with clefts. Our first diagnostic task is to assess the infant's general communicative development, to be certain that it is in line with the child's overall development. Second, we want to study early vocalizations carefully so that we can explain to parents (1) what they are hearing from their child, (2) how this may be different from early speech sound development in normal infants, and (3) ways in which they may help to promote normal speech and language development in their child.

AFTER PALATE CLOSURE

Surgeons, speech pathologists, orthodontists, and other members of cleft palate/craniofacial teams are still trying to determine an optimum age range for surgical closure of the palatal cleft. Currently, the most common ages for palatal surgery in the United States fall in the range of 9 to 18 months. Within the team context, postoperative evaluations typically begin 2 to 3 months after surgery and are carried out periodically as the child grows. Specifically, we want to determine if palatal surgery has been successful in providing the child with velopharyngeal closure. We also want to determine if language and speech development is within normal limits and, if not, in what way. One obvious possibility is that the child may have learned some abnormal speech production patterns in her attempt to compensate for the open cleft palate.

> We are still trying to determine the best time for palatal surgery to promote normal speech development without causing problems in later growth of the midface. A lot of data have been put forth, but the argument is far from over.

Determining Adequacy of Velopharyngeal Function in Toddlers

With the very young child, we are usually entirely dependent on perceptual evaluation of speech in determining if the palatal surgery has "worked." Most instrumental assessments of the function of the velopharyngeal mechanism *for speech* are not applicable, because the patient's cooperation is required and small children typically do not! Because standardized articulation tests (don't confuse with tests of language development) are unlikely to elicit sufficient output in children under the age of 3 years, clinicians have generally resorted to toys or other objects selected to elicit the particular speech sounds of concern (e.g., the stops, fricatives, and affricates, which require high intraoral pressure) and to observations of the child's verbal interactions with a parent.

> If you have the equipment, *videotape* your evaluations of infants and toddlers! The information you get will be even more valuable than from audiotaped samples.

As you carry out these examinations, you must be familiar first of all with the normal sequence of development of speech sounds to compare the output of the individual child with other children of his age. For example, it is important to remember that voiced consonants precede voiceless consonants in normal acquisition. Speakers with inadequate velopharyngeal function may have difficulty making the normal contrasts between voiced and voiceless consonants, but if more voiced than voiceless consonants are heard in a toddler with a repaired cleft, this may simply reflect his developmental stage, not residual velopharyngeal inadequacy. Of equal importance when you are assessing a child with a repaired cleft is your experience in distinguishing consonants produced with correct placement but nasal emission (nasal escape of air) from those produced with inappropriate articulatory placement. It is a troublesome but relatively common finding that young children may persist in nasal emission of the airstream on pressure consonants, even if the surgery has provided them with a functional or potentially functional velopharyngeal system — particularly if the surgery was performed well after the child started producing meaningful speech. In these cases, it is helpful to explore the child's ability to direct the airstream orally in play activities and "nonsense" speech play.

You need to be particularly concerned about the presumably "compensatory" articulations that appear in some children with clefts in the early stages of speech sound development and frequently persist after a functional velopharyngeal system has been provided through surgery or prosthetic care. These errors may be the most frequent examples of the effects of early articulatory/phonetic constraints on phonologic development, discussed in the following section. Textbooks on cleft palate have described glottal stops and pharyngeal fricatives for decades. Pharyngeal stops, pharyngeal affricates, velar fricatives, middorsum palatal stops, and the "posterior nasal fricative" have been described as additional types of errors that seem to be heard more often in speakers with cleft palates than in noncleft individuals, and more recently pharyngeal affricates have been added to the list. Clinicians have verified the occurrence of these misarticulations in children with either current velopharyngeal inadequacy or a history of such inadequacy. Glottal stops, pharyngeal fricatives, and posterior nasal fricatives may occur either as substitutions or as "coarticulations;" that is, as simultaneous articulatory maneuvers, with other places of production. Fortunately, Trost-Cardamone's instructional videotape (1987) provides practical experience in listening for and transcribing these errors.

Performance on stimulability tasks is revealing when you are trying to decide on the adequacy of velopharyngeal closure. For example, the response to auditory–visual stimulation may indicate that, even though a little boy typically nasalizes a plosive or fricative during speech, he can, with help, produce it in a normally oral fashion. That tells us that he may well have the physiologic potential for velopharyngeal closure in speech. By the way, sometimes we get better results from stimulability testing when we use nonsense syllables instead of words, because young children are less likely to be restricted by previous learning than when words are used.

A Word About the Examination of Oropharyngeal Structures

Optimally, any child with a cleft is already being followed by a cleft palate/craniofacial team and thus receives periodic assessments of the integrity of oropharyngeal structures. But, even in these cases, you will have to make your own evaluation of the child's status. Assessment of the oral structures, in general, has been discussed in Chapter 4. For children with repaired clefts, the following points should help you:

1. The repaired lip is rarely of consequence in the speech problems in individuals with clefts. However, if the lip is abnormally short, bilabial consonants may be produced as labiodentals. A more frequently observed problem is a discrepancy in position of the upper and lower lips due to retrusion of the maxilla. If the upper lip is significantly behind the lower lip, labiodental targets may be produced with the lower incisors against the upper lip or may be produced as bilabials. Tip-dental consonants may become "tip-labials," e.g., contact between the tongue-tip and the upper lip for /t/, /d/, and /n/.

2. In any child, forceful pressing down on the dorsum of the tongue with a tongue depressor can elicit a gag and/or a cessation of cooperation for

the rest of the exam. In the child with a repaired cleft the muscular link between the tongue and the velum — the palatoglossus muscle — may be tighter than normal and pushing down on the tongue dorsum may interfere with upward movement of the velum, thus giving false information about velar movement.

3. In virtually any speaker, "velopharyngeal closure" is not visible on the intraoral view, because the site of closure is hidden behind the velum itself. In the young child with or without a cleft, "velopharyngeal closure" is actually "velum-adenoid" closure; that is, the velum is closing against the adenoid pad and not directly against the posterior pharyngeal wall. The adenoid pad is not normally visible on the direct intraoral examination.

4. Precisely because the direct intraoral view limits what the examiner can see and understand about velopharyngeal closure, it is important to remember the "nonvisible" factors that can influence velopharyngeal closure; that is, factors that cannot be adequately assessed on this view. These include mechanical interference with velar movement (such as enlarged tonsils or pharyngeal webbing), a deficiency of muscle mass on the nasal surface of the velum, abnormal direction of pull of the velar musculature, and inadequate movement of pharyngeal musculature towards closure.

Effects of Early Phonetic Constraints on Postclosure Phonetic, Phonologic, and Language Development

Most of the studies listed above regarding early vocalizations and phonetic development in children with clefts were longitudinal studies, providing information on development in these children following palatal closure. These studies, together with research on postsurgery communicative development, provide us with critical information about what to expect in children with clefts during their toddler and preschool years. Following are some of the important findings:

- A higher percentage of glottal placements (glottal stops and the glottal fricative /h/) than heard in noncleft children.

- A delay in the appearance of "oral stop predominance" and also in the use of oral fricatives.

- A preference for mid vowels over high or low vowels.

- A sort of "chain reaction" from early phonetic constraints to phonologic problems to influences in early language development. For example, toddlers targeted and produced more words beginning with nasals, vowels, and approximants and infrequently targeted words beginning with stops, fricatives, or affricates (Estrem & Broen, 1989). In essence, they selected words that contained the sounds they were capable of producing.

- Limited phonetic inventories and differences in phonologic process usage that may become more apparent with increasing age or, more likely, with the increasing language output of the child.

- An apparent decrease or disappearance in the above differences as children mature.

The results of the studies providing us these generalizations serve as a warning on assessment of phonologic development and expressive language development in children with clefts. They are subject to structural influences that do not affect other children and that may exert an effect long after the structural problem has been eradicated. Be careful to examine phonetic and phonologic aspects of speech sound development separately, and also to place your observations of early language development within the context of these influences. There are, of course, other factors that can affect language development in children with clefts. These include adverse reactions of adults and peers to facial appearance, increased vulnerability to ear disease and hearing loss, interruptions in social and educational development from hospitalizations, and so on.

FOLLOW-UP EVALUATIONS IN THE TODDLER AND PRESCHOOL YEARS

Within the team context, regular follow-up evaluations of children in this age range are typically scheduled every 6 to 12 months, because this is a period of rapid development. Now the child can cooperate more fully for instrumental evaluation of velopharyngeal function. Nasopharyngoscopy is feasible in children as young as 4 years, and multiview videofluoroscopy may be used with even younger children as long as they are able to cooperate sufficiently and perform the tasks appropriately so that clear views may be obtained with a minimum of radiation exposure. Aerodynamic studies and acoustic studies using instrumentation such as the Nasometer™ are also feasible with fairly young children. An important warning here is that no instrumental technique can prove that a velopharyngeal system is capable of adequate closure if the child is "bypassing" the system, that is, if he is relying exclusively on glottal placements or other speech sounds that do not require velopharyngeal closure. The validity of the information is dependent not just on the phonemes modeled by the examiner, but on the child's own phonologic "matches" to those targets.

When you are examining a child with a cleft in the toddler and preschool years, accuracy of your assessment will depend, in large part, on a knowledge of the particular problems to which these children may be vulnerable: hypernasal resonance on vowels and vocalic segments, nasal air loss on pressure consonants, use of "compensatory" articulations and other atypical backed articulations, phonetic errors that may be related to structural problems in the developing dental and jaw relationships, and errors in placement that may be related to a palatal fistula. A palatal fistula is an opening between the oral and nasal cavities, often the result of surgical breakdown. Depending on size and location, a fistula results in nasalization of speech in somewhat the same way, though usually to a lesser extent, as dysfunction of the velopharyngeal mechanism.

With specific regard to nasal air loss on pressure consonants, a key diagnostic question is related to consistency. If the air loss is present on all pressure consonants, there is most likely a physical inadequacy in the function of the velopharyngeal mechanism. If the air loss is heard on pressure consonants produced at all oral placements but is not consistently audible on each token, the velopharyngeal system may be closing inconsistently, subject to such factors as phonetic context. If the air loss is limited to anterior pressure consonants, a palatal fistula may be present or, conversely, the lack of air loss on velar stops may simply reflect a lingual assist to the velum in closure. If the air loss is limited to a specific consonant or class of consonants, the speaker may be exhibiting phoneme-specific nasal air loss. Phoneme-specific nasal air loss, like the compensatory articulations that may persist after physical management of velopharyngeal inadequacy, reflects an error in learning and should not be taken as indicative of a velopharyngeal mechanism that is truly incapable of closure.

Because assessment will vary with the child's age and with linguistic and cognitive functioning, your testing should include a sample of connected speech (preferably spontaneous), a speech sound inventory such as that typically elicited through picture articulation tests, and stimulability testing. It is a good idea to audiotape the entire speech sample so you can replay it as often as necessary to facilitate accurate, reliable transcription and also to provide a baseline for later comparisons. Your analysis of the speech sample should include an estimate of overall intelligibility, comparison of productions to developmental norms, a phonetic inventory, and a phonological pattern analysis. "The main goal in all evaluations is to distinguish speech errors that may be due to faulty velopharyngeal or other structural deviations from speech errors that are compensatory or developmental in nature" (Trost-Cardamone & Bernthal, 1993, p. 317). These authors provide a chart of guidelines for deciding on appropriate management, depending on the results of the assessment of the child's sound system.

Some clinicians have reported that problems in velopharyngeal function can lead to secondary problems in laryngeal function, specifically overdrive or "hyperfunction" of the laryngeal system presumably caused by partial loss of the vocal airstream through an inadequate velopharyngeal port. Speech evaluations of children with clefts should include perceptual evaluation of laryngeal function and referral for medical assessment of the laryngeal system when indicated.

EVALUATION OF VELOPHARYNGEAL FUNCTION

By the time the child has reached the preschool years and often earlier, parents, surgeons, and treating speech-language pathologists are concerned about "objective" evaluation of the status of velopharyngeal closure. How can we be certain that the palatal surgery worked, or that further physical management (surgical or prosthetic) of the velopharyngeal mechanism will be needed? Even within the context of the cleft palate/craniofacial team functioning in a medical setting where elaborate instrumentation is available, evaluation of velopharyngeal function follows a hierarchical approach that begins with a perceptual evaluation.

In nonmedical settings, we can use some simple and safe techniques to obtain a gross index of the presence or absence of air leakage through the nose. A mirror held beneath the nose during production of speech samples containing pressure consonants or a sustained fricative will fog if there is nasal air loss; in the case of a child with a cleft, it is wise to "test" both sides of the nose because various degrees of nasal obstruction are common in these children. The same is true for the commercially available See-Scape™, which consists of a nasal olive connected through a section of flexible plastic tubing to an upright section of rigid, clear tubing containing a small piece of Styrofoam™. When the nasal olive is held in the naris as the subject produces the desired speech sample, airflow through the tube causes the Styrofoam™ to rise in the rigid tubing. With either this device or the mirror test, the examiner must be cautious to hold the olive or the mirror in place only during the production of oral pressure consonants, not during production of nasal consonants or during normal nasal respiration. An additional problem with the See-Scape™ is that small children are often delighted to see the Styrofoam™ rise in the tube and may begin to direct the airstream nasally even though their velopharyngeal mechanisms are functioning adequately. In the "modified tongue-anchor technique," you can use a small piece of sterile gauze to gently hold the tip of the child's tongue outside the mouth, and direct the child to close his lips around the rest of the tongue and inflate his cheeks. The theory behind this approach is (a) that inflation of the cheeks is impossible in the presence of inadequate velopharyngeal function, and (b) that anchoring the tongue forward keeps the dorsum of the tongue out of the area of the velopharyngeal port, preventing a lingual assist to the velum for closure. It is critical to bear in mind that each of these techniques is crude and subject to influences that may not be immediately apparent to you; *none is capable of actual measurement of the function of the velopharyngeal system.*

Imaging of the Velopharyngeal System

With rare exception, visualization of the velopharyngeal system cannot be accomplished outside a medical setting. However, this brief synopsis of imaging techniques is included to give you a feel for the more sophisticated procedures available. For a detailed discussion, please see Moon (1993).

Still Cephalometric X Rays

Orthodontists use lateral, frontal, and oblique films to assess craniofacial structure and growth in their patients. These films are taken with the head in a fixed position and a standardized X-ray tube-to-focal-plane distance. A lateral film focussed at the midsagittal plane may be used for assessing the size and relationship of velopharyngeal structures at rest and perhaps during sustained production of a pressure consonant. The advantages of this approach are the relatively low dose of radiation, about .01 rads for a single film (Moon, 1993); the common availability of the instrumentation; and the standardization. The disadvantages are that the velopharyngeal system cannot be studied during actual speech production and that the image is a two-dimensional representation of a multidimensional system.

Multiview Videofluorography

Fluorography is essentially "motion picture X ray." With the advent of videorecorders, it became possible to record these examinations on videotape, requiring far less radiation than was previously necessary for the exposure of movie film. Most cleft palate/craniofacial centers now use multiview videofluorography as one means of visualizing the velopharyngeal mechanism. The typical views are lateral, frontal, and base, which gives a cross-sectional, or horizontal, view of the velopharyngeal port. In the lateral view, the examiner can see the movement of the velum and any forward excursion of the posterior pharyngeal wall. The amount and level of medial movement of the lateral pharyngeal musculature can be studied in the frontal view. The base view shows the contribution of all of these structures — the velum, lateral walls, and posterior wall — towards closure, but the vertical level of movement of each structure is obscured. Oblique views are useful if asymmetric movement is suspected. (Please see Witzel & Stringer, 1990, for a description of additional useful views.) The major disadvantages of multiview videofluorography are the lack of a standardized head position (although some facilities have added head-holders to their units), and the radiation exposure. The amount of exposure varies, of course, with the specific equipment and the length of the study, but dosage estimates offered by Skolnick and Cohn (1989) indicated that a multiview workup could reach as much as 2.5 rads. This can be consequential for a small child.

Computerized Tomography

To date there has been relatively little application of CT scans, or cine-CT scans, to the study of the velopharyngeal mechanism, quite likely because of expense and also the limitations of the procedure. We may see more research using this instrumentation, but routine clinical use for study of the velopharyngeal mechanism even in large craniofacial centers does not seem imminent. The same is true for magnetic resonance imaging (MRI), which does not involve radiation; future advances in MRI technology could lead to wider application in the imaging of the velopharyngeal mechanism.

Ultrasonography

In the 1970s, there were a few investigations on the use of ultrasonography to study the movement of the lateral pharyngeal walls in speech. The interest in this technique was sparked by problems in imaging the lateral walls with other techniques and also because ultrasound does not involve radiation. Moon (1993) discusses the limitations of this instrumentation in the study of the speech mechanism, and points out that there are no published reports of its use with patients exhibiting problems in the function of the velopharyngeal mechanism.

Oral Endoscopy

A rigid endoscope, inserted orally, was used in the 1960s for evaluating velopharyngeal function, but has such severe limitations that the technique is now rarely used. One limitation is that when the velum elevates and closes against the posterior pharyngeal wall, the oral view can provide little information. Another is that, even in the rare instance in which the mechanism for closure is visible on this view, the presence of the rigid scope in the mouth obviously limits the speech sample.

Nasopharyngoscopy

Nasal endoscopy for study of the velopharyngeal mechanism was first reported by Pigott (1969), who used a rigid, side-viewing endoscope of small diameter. Nasal endoscopy allows study of the velopharyngeal system from above, without interfering with speech production. Flexible fiberoptic nasopharyngoscopy is more widely used than oral endoscopy and, together with multiview videofluorography, has become a fairly common technique of assessment in cleft palate/craniofacial centers. Technical advances have led to scopes of decreasing diameter, allowing for greater patient comfort and compliance. The quality of the information derived is at least as dependent on the expertise of the examiner as on the characteristics of the individual scope. The use of nasopharyngoscopy is not recommended in a nonmedical setting because of the invasive nature of the technique and because a topical anesthetic is usually needed for comfortable insertion of the scope.

Measuring the Function of the Velopharyngeal System

The major approaches to measuring the consequences of velopharyngeal closure or lack of closure during speech can generally be classified into acoustic and aerodynamic studies. The instrumentation is noninvasive, but can be very expensive.

Spectrography

Researchers first began to understand the effects of inadequate velopharyngeal function on the acoustic energy distribution of speech through the use of spectrographic analysis. These studies began to appear in the mid-1950s, and spectrography remained a popular research tool into the mid-1980s. However, spectrography is not a practical or commonly used tool in the evaluation of velopharyngeal function.

Accelerometry

Accelerometers are small, vibration-sensitive transducers. In the study of nasality in speech, one accelerometer is placed on the side of the nose and another on the thyroid lamina. The accelerometric "index" of oral–nasal coupling is the ratio of output of the two transducers. Nasal accelerometry has been advocated as a useful tool in the assessment of speakers with suspected problems in velopharyngeal closure, and the relatively small amount of published data seem to indicate a significant relationship between accelerometer ratios and the amount of nasality heard by listeners. The instrumentation can be used outside a medical setting, but the technical requirements (transducers, amplifiers, rectifiers, computer or oscilloscope screens, etc.) have limited its use.

Measurement of Sound Pressure Level

For several decades, researchers have tried to compare the pressure level of the sound signal emitted from the nose to that emitted from the oral cavity and to use this comparison as an index of velopharyngeal function. Currently, the most popular instrument for making these measurements is the Nasometer™, a commercially available, computer-based device, which is the outgrowth of the earlier TONAR I and TONAR II devices developed by Fletcher (1970, 1972). There has been a recent flourish of studies correlating Nasometer™ measurements to listener judgements of nasality, as well as to other indices of velopharyngeal adequacy. It may have promise for corroborating clinical impressions of hypernasality. The cost of the instrumentation may be prohibitive to many potential users.

Aerodynamic Studies

Historically, clinicians and researchers have used various approaches to detecting nasal airflow (the mirror test and See-Scape™, described previously), measuring nasal or oral airflow (pneumotachographs), and measuring oral air pressure (e.g., the oral manometer). Warren and Dubois (1964) developed a quantitative technique of using measurements of nasal air flow, nasal air pressure, and oral air pressure to calculate the cross-sectional area of the velopharyngeal (VP) orifice area during speech. This approach has been used to categorize patients into adequate closure, adequate/borderline closure, borderline/inadequate closure, and inadequate closure groups based on pressure-flow estimates of VP orifice size. Investigators have not been in complete agreement about the correlation of listener judgments to pressure-flow estimates of orifice size, but active research continues. There is a commercially available hardware and software package for pressure-flow studies, the PERCI-PC (Microtronics Corporation, Carrboro, NC). As stated by Warren (1989, p. 234), "This system is used to collect pressure-flow data and the software provides analysis modes for measuring the pressure, air flow, volume, sphincter area, resistance, conductance, and timing variables associated with palatal closure and breathing." Either the full laboratory instrumentation array or the PERCI-PC is in use in several cleft palate/craniofacial centers around the world. Both are noninvasive. The instrumentation and hardware for the PERCI-PC are less formidable than the laboratory array, but nevertheless require considerable financial investment and training for the examiner.

A Further Note on Instrumental Assessment

Other types of instrumentation have been used in investigations of velopharyngeal activity, but generally only in laboratory settings as opposed to clinical assessments. Please see Moon (1993) for a discussion of electromyography, phototransduction, and mechanical-electrical "movement transduction." Of these three, there does seem to be a potential for clinical applicability for the photodetector.

THE SCHOOL-AGE CHILD

Because of improvements in surgical care and also earlier diagnosis and intervention for communication problems in young children with clefts, it is now far more common for these children to reach school age exhibiting good velopharyngeal closure for speech and age-appropriate articulation skills. For example, two decades ago, Morris (1973) surveyed the published data and estimated that approximately 25% of the children who had repaired cleft palates had inadequate velopharyngeal closure for speech requiring further surgical or prosthetic treatment. In a retrospective analysis modeled after Morris's study but limited to personal experience with 240 children treated in three major cleft palate/craniofacial treatment centers, I found this percentage to have dropped to 16% (Peterson-Falzone, 1990). Chapman (1993) reported "catch-up" in phonologic development in children by the age of 5 years that would not have been expected based on results of earlier studies of articulation competency in school-age children with clefts and attributed the discrepancy to changes in management. Nevertheless, in dealing with children in this age group, you will be faced with at least four diagnostic questions: (1) What are the possible effects of adenoid involution and of natural craniofacial growth on velopharyngeal closure? (2) What are the effects of changing dental and occlusal factors on articulation and to what extent should these alter decisions about therapy? (3) What surgical procedures may be taking place in a child of this age and what may be the impact on plans for therapy? (4) What goals are appropriate in therapy?

Adenoid Growth and Involution

The adenoid pad is visible on radiographic views of the nasopharynx by 6 weeks of age and increases in size thereafter until it reaches a peak size and begins to involute (atrophy). Investigators disagree regarding the age at which the maximum size is reached, indicating two possible peak ages: around 5 years (Linder-Aronson & Leighton, 1983), and 9 to 10 or 11 years (Subtelny & Koepp-Baker, 1956). In any child under the age of 5 years, the adenoid pad is probably increasing in size. At any age over 5 years, the pad may be either still enlarging or undergoing natural resorption. After that age period, in most people, the adenoid pad gradually shrinks or atrophies until, in most adults, the pad is barely noticeable. Although there have been very few reported cases of the onset of velopharyngeal inadequacy secondary to natural involution of the adenoids in children without clefts (Peterson-Falzone, 1985), the gradual disappearance of the adenoids in children with clefts, combined with the natural downward-and-forward growth of the face, can lead to late onset of velopharyngeal inadequacy in a child whose original palatoplasty had provided him with good velopharyngeal closure. The number of such reported cases is small, but certainly enough to alert us to the possibility of changing velopharyngeal status in the school-age child.

Dental and Occlusal Factors

As in every other child in the early school-age years, the sequenced loss of deciduous dentition and eruption of the permanent dentition may temporarily interfere with articulatory accuracy in children with clefts. However, children with clefts may also have (1) absence of the lateral incisor and/or canine on the side of the cleft, (2) malalignment of the dentition in the area of the cleft, (3) lateral crossbite on the side of the cleft, and (4) anterior crossbite due to maxillary retrusion. In addition to the natural changes in dental status, there may be changes secondary to dental, orthodontic, or prosthetic intervention. It is impossible to predict how the individual child will respond to these fluctuating states. Some children adapt well to even multiple missing teeth and an accompanying malocclusion; others seem unable to improve articulatory placement in the presence of a relatively minor dental anomaly. Such problems are more likely to cause problems in speech if they are present in combination (e.g., missing teeth plus a crossbite) rather than as isolated entities and if they occur during the child's speech-learning years as opposed to adult years. You have to decide if the articulation problems you are trying to eradicate are due to a dental/occlusal anomaly for which the child cannot realistically compensate, at least for the present. Stimulation testing provides part of this answer; response to therapy over a specified time period should provide the rest. Depending on the maturational status and motivation of a child and also on the schedule of therapy (individual versus group, intensity, length of sessions), if production does not improve during a predetermined time frame, you should reconsider if therapy is a good idea. In any case, consultation with the craniofacial team and specifically with the child's dentist and/or orthodontist is critical before therapy is initiated. It is possible that time spent in therapy may be time lost, either because progress is temporarily impossible or because the "misarticulation" will spontaneously improve once the dental/occlusal situation improves.

A related problem may be the presence of a residual defect through the alveolus (gum ridge) on the cleft side. In most cleft palate treatment centers in the United States, bone grafting of this defect is not done until the ages of 9 to 12 years, depending on the dental development of the child. If the defect is large enough, there may be a patent opening from the oral cavity into the buccal sulcus or even up into the nasal cavity. In the former case, the child may exhibit a slight puffing out of the lip on production of /p/ and /b/. If the opening extends into the nose, there may be nasal air loss on all anterior pressure consonants. If this constitutes a significant speech problem for the child, you can consult with the cleft palate/craniofacial team or the child's dentist regarding the possibility of the use of a dental plate constructed to close the space. The same is true, of course, for fistulae through the palate into the nasal cavity.

Surgical Procedures

Surgical repair of a residual alveolar defect (discussed above) or a palatal fistula may take place during the child's school-age years. The effect of these defects on speech varies with size and location, and is not predictable from child to child. Successful repair of even a small palatal fistula can be much more difficult than one would expect.

If secondary management of the velopharyngeal system is needed, the options are (1) a dental prosthetic speech bulb, (2) a variety of surgical techniques for lengthening the soft palate, and (3) a variety of surgical procedures, generically termed pharyngoplasties, for altering the configuration of the velopharynx. The decision that such management is needed should be the result of collaboration between the cleft palate/craniofacial team and the treating speech-language pathologist, particularly because the child's history of progress in therapy will play a key role in that decision.

Selecting Appropriate Goals for Therapy

For the child with a repaired cleft palate, the critical questions regarding appropriateness of therapy center on the compensatory articulations and other atypical "backed" placements. Certainly therapy to teach correct oral placements is indicated if the repaired velopharyngeal mechanism is intact. However, therapy to teach correct placements may also be appropriate even in the presence of an inadequately functioning velopharyngeal mechanism. The modification of placements from glottal and pharyngeal to oral may actually result in a change in the behavior of the velopharyngeal mechanism in speech, in the optimum case completely eliminating the need for further surgical or prosthetic management. In any event, if a child is producing nothing but glottal and pharyngeal placements, secondary surgery on the mechanism should not be performed until an attempt has been made to modify these placements through therapy.

Elimination of compensatory articulations can be quite difficult. Again, a key question is the amount of time to be spent on these efforts. If production does not improve within a predetermined time frame, the efficacy of therapy should be reconsidered. That time frame should be specified in weeks or months, not years. "Burn-out" on the part of the child is always a possibility and becomes inevitable once he knows that therapy is not making it easier for him to make himself understood.

With regard to therapy to eliminate nasal emission, the decision for or against therapy is simplest when the problem is one of phoneme-specific nasal emission. This is a problem that will not be eradicated by anything other than speech therapy. If nasal emission and hypernasality are consistent but mild in degree, clinicians in medical settings may use nasopharyngoscopy to provide biofeedback to the speaker in the effort to modify velopharyngeal closure. However, this is not applicable in other professional settings. Finally, if nasal emission and hypernasality are consistent and severe in degree, consideration must be given to further physical management of the velopharyngeal mechanism.

THE TEENAGER AND YOUNG ADULT

Although most of the habilitative procedures that a youngster with a cleft palate will need are accomplished before her teenage years, there are some "end-stage" phases of management that can still affect her communication skills. Completion of orthodontic therapy usually takes place during this time. If congenitally missing teeth have not been replaced by implants before this age, replacement either by implants or a fixed bridge will probably be accomplished in the teenage years. If a surgical advancement of the midface is needed to bring the upper and lower jaws into good alignment, that surgery will most likely take place after completion of facial growth (age 15 to 16 in girls, a year or so later in boys). This surgery can have a beneficial effect on speech if there were preoperative misarticulations related to malalignment of the jaws. However, in some cases, the forward movement of the midface may result in inadequate velopharyngeal closure. If this postadvancement inadequacy does not disappear spontaneously over time, further physical management of the velopharyngeal system will be necessary.

Throughout this chapter, I have assumed that the child with a cleft palate is under appropriate multidisciplinary care from the early days of life. This assumption leads, in turn, to the assumption that the habilitative process is essentially complete by the late teenage or early adult years. In reality, there are still significant numbers of teenagers and young adults who come to cleft palate/craniofacial centers for the first time in their lives with incomplete, inadequate care. In the worst cases, the cleft has not been successfully repaired, and speech is characterized by severe hypernasality, pervasive nasal air loss, and often a heavy reliance upon compensatory articulations. These individuals become "salvage" cases for the team and for the treating speech-language pathologist, alike. Although the team surgeons may be able to repair the velopharyngeal mechanism successfully, it is more than likely that extensive and intensive therapy will be required to improve speech. Although successful habilitation is not impossible, the multiple difficulties in communication and social acceptance experienced by these late-presenting patients constitute the ultimate justification for early referral of infants with clefts to multidisciplinary teams for timely intervention and rigorous longitudinal monitoring.

Some important aspects of treatment will not be completed by this time, such as follow-up genetic counseling as the teenager prepares for his own family life.

SUMMARY

We have reviewed the principle points of diagnosing speech problems in children with clefts from the early months of life through the early adult years. The information should serve as an introduction that leads the clinician on to sources of more detailed, advanced material on diagnosis and treatment, such as that found in professional journals and graduate-level texts. Information prepared specifically for patients, families and the lay public may be obtained through the American Cleft Palate-Craniofacial Association, 1218 Grandview Drive, Pittsburgh, PA, 15211, telephone (800) 24-CLEFT.

REFERENCES

The First Few Months of Life

Chapman, K. L. (1991). Vocalizations of toddlers with cleft lip and palate. *Cleft Palate-Craniofacial Journal, 28*, 172-178.

Fenson, L., Dale, P. S., Reznick, S., Thal, D., Bates, E., Hartung, J. P., Pethick, J., & Reilly, J. S. (1989). *The MacArthur Communicative Development Inventories.* Developmental Psychology Lab, San Diego State University.

Grunwell, P., & Russell, J. (1987). Vocalizations before and after cleft palate surgery: A pilot study. *British Journal of Disorders of Communication, 22*, 1-17.

O'Gara, M. M., & Logemann, J. A. (1990). Early speech development in cleft palate babies. In J. Bardach & H. L. Morris (Eds.), *Multidisciplinary management of cleft lip and palate* (pp. 717-721). Philadelphia: W. B. Saunders.

Parameters for the Evaluation and Treatment of Patients with Cleft Lip/Palate or Other Craniofacial Anomalies. Maternal & Child Health Consensus Statement. *Cleft Palate-Craniofacial Journal, 30* (Suppl. 1).

Philips, B. J., & Kent, R. D. (1984). Acoustic-phonetic descriptions of speech production in speakers with cleft palate and other velopharyngeal disorders. In N. J. Lass (Ed.), *Speech and language: Advances in basic research and practice* (Vol. 11, pp. 113-168). New York: Academic Press.

Recommended Readings

Brookshire, B. L., Lynch, J. L., & Fox, D. R. (1980). *A parent-child cleft palate curriculum: Developing speech and language.* Tigard, OR: C. C. Publications.

Dorf, D. S., Reisberg, D. J., & Gold, H. O. (1985). Early prosthetic management of cleft palate. Articulation development prosthesis: A preliminary report. *Journal of Prosthetic Dentistry, 53*, 222-226.

O'Gara, M. M., & Logemann, J. A. (1988). Phonetic analyses of the speech development of babies with cleft palate. *Cleft Palate Journal, 25*, 122-134.

After Palate Closure

Estrem, T., & Broen, P. A. (1989). Early speech productions of children with cleft palate. *Journal of Speech and Hearing Research, 32* 12-23.

Trost-Cardamone, J. E. (1987). *Cleft palate misarticulations: A teaching tape.* Videotape produced by the Instructional Media Center, California State University, Northridge.

Recommended Readings

Chapman, K. L., & Hardin, M. A. (1992). Phonetic and phonologic skills of two-year olds with cleft palate. *Cleft Palate-Craniofacial Journal, 29*, 433-441.

Chapman, K. L. (1993). Phonologic processes in children with cleft palate. *Cleft Palate-Craniofacial Journal, 30*, 64-72.

Lynch, J. L., Fox, D. R., & Brookshire, B. L. (1983). Phonological proficiency of two cleft palate toddlers with school age follow-up. *Journal of Speech and Hearing Disorders, 48*, 274-285.

Powers, G. R., Dunn, C., & Erickson, C. B. (1990). Speech analyses of four children with repaired cleft palates. *Journal of Speech and Hearing Disorders, 55*, 542-549.

Trost, J. E. (1981). Articulatory additions to the classical description of the speech of persons with cleft palate. *Cleft Palate Journal, 18,* 193-203.

Follow-up Evaluations in the Toddler and Preschool Years

Trost-Cardamone, J. E., & Bernthal, J. E. (1993). Articulation assessment procedures and treatment decisions. In K. T. Moller & C. D. Starr (Eds.), *Cleft palate: Interdisciplinary issues and treatments* (pp. 307-336). Austin, TX: Pro-Ed.

Recommended Readings

McWilliams, B. J., Morris, H. L., & Shelton, R. L. (1990). *Cleft palate speech* (2nd ed.). Toronto: B. C. Decker.

Morris, H. L. (1990). Clinical assessment by the speech pathologist. In J. Bardach & H. L. Morris (Eds.), *Management of cleft lip and palate* (pp. 757-762). Philadelphia: W. B. Saunders.

Evaluation of Velopharyngeal Function

Fletcher, S. (1970). Theory and instrumentation for quantitative measurement of nasality. *Cleft Palate Journal, 7,* 601-609.

Fletcher, S. (1972). Contingencies for bioelectric modification of nasality. *Journal of Speech and Hearing Disorders, 37,* 329-346.

Moon, J. B. (1993). Evaluation of velopharyngeal function. In K. T. Moller & C. D. Starr (Eds.), *Cleft palate: Interdisciplinary issues and treatments* (pp. 251 306). Austin, TX: Pro-Ed.

Pigott, R. (1969). The nasoendoscopic appearance of the normal palato-pharyngeal valve. *Plastic and Reconstructive Surgery, 43,* 19-24.

Skolnick, M. L., & Cohn, E. R. (1989). *Videofluoroscopic studies of speech in patients with cleft palate.* New York: Springer-Verlag.

Warren, D. W. (1989). Aerodynamic assessment of velopharyngeal performance. In K. Bzoch (Ed.), *Communicative disorders related to cleft lip and palate* (3rd ed., pp. 230-245). Boston: College-Hill Press.

Warren, D. W., & Dubois, A. (1964). A pressure-flow technique for measuring velopharyngeal orifice area during continuous speech. *Cleft Palate Journal, 1,* 52-71.

Witzel, M. A., & Stringer, D. A. (1990). Methods of assessing velopharyngeal function. In J. Bardach & H. L. Morris (Eds.), *Management of cleft lip and palate* (pp. 763-776). Philadelphia: W. B. Saunders.

Recommended Readings

Dalston, R. M. (1982). Photodetector assessment of velopharyngeal activity. *Cleft Palate Journal, 19,* 1-8.

Dalston, R. M., Warren, D. W., & Dalston, E. T. (1991). Use of nasometry as a diagnostic tool for identifying patients with velopharyngeal impairment. *Cleft Palate-Craniofacial Journal, 28,* 184-189.

Fox, D. R., & Johns, D. (1970). Predicting velopharyngeal closure with a modified tongue-anchor technique. *Journal of Speech and Hearing Disorders, 35,* 248-251.

Horii, Y. (1983). An accelerometric measure as a physical correlate of perceived hypernasality in speech. *Journal of Speech and Hearing Research, 26,* 476-480.

Karnell, M. P., & Morris, H. L. (1985). Multiview endoscopic evaluations of velo-pharyngeal physiology in 15 normal speakers. *Annals of Otology, Rhinology and Laryngology, 94,* 361-365.

Karnell, M. P., Seaver, E. J., & Dalston, R. (1988). A comparison of photodetector and endoscopic evaluations of velopharyngeal function. *Journal of Speech and Hearing Research, 31,* 503-509.

Redenbaugh, M., & Reich, A., (1985). Correspondence between an accelerometric nasal/voice amplitude ratio and listeners' direct magnitude estimations of hy-pernasality. *Journal of Speech and Hearing Research, 18,* 273-281.

Shprintzen, R. J. (1989). Nasopharyngoscopy. In K. Bzoch (Ed.), *Communicative disorders related to cleft lip and palate* (3rd ed., pp. 211-229). Boston: College-Hill Press.

The School-Age Child

Linder-Aronson, S., & Leighton, B. C. (1983). A longitudinal study of the develop-ment of the posterior pharyngeal wall between 3 and 16 years of age. *European Journal of Orthodontics, 5,* 47-58.

Morris, H. L. (1973). Velopharyngeal competence and primary cleft palate surgery, 1960-1971: A critical review. *Cleft Palate Journal, 10,* 62-71.

Peterson-Falzone, S. J. (1985). Velopharyngeal inadequacy in the absence of overt cleft palate. *Journal of Craniofacial Genetics and Developmental Biology* (Suppl. 1), 97-124.

Peterson-Falzone, S. J. (1990). A cross-sectional analysis of speech results follow-ing palatal closure. In J. Bardach & H. L. Morris (Eds.), *Management of cleft lip and palate* (pp. 750-757). Philadelphia: W. B. Saunders.

Subtelny, J. D., & Koepp-Baker, H. (1956). The significance of adenoid tissue in ve-lopharyngeal function. *Plastic and Reconstructive Surgery, 17,* 235-250.

Recommended Readings

Hoch, L., Golding-Kushner, K. J., Siegel-Sadewitz, V. L., & Shprintzen, R. J. (1986). Speech therapy. In B. J. McWilliams (Ed.), Current methods of assessing and treating children with cleft palates. *Seminars in Speech and Language, 7,* 313-325.

Morris, H. L., Wroblewski, S. K. M., Brown, C. K., & VanDemark, D. R. (1990). Velar-pharyngeal status in cleft palate patients with expected adenoidal involution. *Annals of Otology, Rhinology, and Laryngology, 99,* 432-437.

Peterson-Falzone, S. J., & Graham, M. S. (1990). Phoneme-specific nasal emission in children with and without physical anomalies of the velopharngeal mecha-nism. *Journal of Speech and Hearing Disorders, 55,* 132-139.

The Teenager and Young Adult

Recommended Readings

Kummer, A. W., Strife, J. L., Grau, W. H., Creaghead, N. A., & Lee, L. (1989). The effects of Le Fort I osteotomy with maxillary movement on articulation, resonance, and velopharyngeal function. *Cleft Palate-Craniofacial Journal, 26,* 193-199.

Vallino, L. D. (1990). Speech, velopharyngeal function, and hearing before and after orthognathic surgery. *Journal of Oral and Maxillofacial Surgery, 48,* 1274-1281.

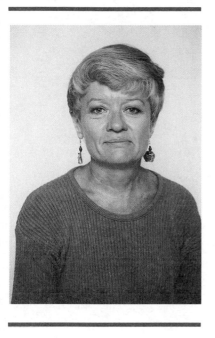

SALLY J. PETERSON-FALZONE, Ph.D.

M.A. 1965, The University of Illinois at Urbana
Ph.D. 1971, The University of Iowa

Dr. Peterson-Falzone is the speech-language pathologist for the Center
for Craniofacial Anomalies and a clinical professor in the Department
of Growth and Development at the University of California-San
Francisco. Previous employment was at the University of Illinois
Center for Craniofacial Anomalies. She is a past president of the
American Cleft Palate-Craniofacial Association, and editor of the
document *Parameters for the Evaluation and Treatment of Patients
with Cleft Lip/Palate or Other Craniofacial Anomalies* (Maternal and
Child Health Consensus Statement, 1993). Her special interests are in
cleft lip and palate, craniofacial anomalies, and related disorders.

C H A P T E R

15

Disordered Swallowing

Adrienne L. Perlman, Ph.D.

Many speech-language pathologists work with patients who have problems chewing or swallowing. This problem is called dysphagia, which comes from the Greek word phagein, meaning "to eat." Although dysphagia can occur anywhere along the path from the lips to the stomach, speech-language pathologists are primarily concerned about problems in the oral cavity, pharynx, or larynx. And so, to be precise, speech-language pathologists (SLPs) treat oropharyngeal dysphagia. Similarly, gastroenterologists (physicians who diagnose and treat disorders of the esophagus, stomach, and intestinal tract) also use the term dysphagia when referring to esophageal dysphagia.

dısfeɪʒə is the commonly accepted pronunciation; although some people insist on saying dısfɑʒə.

Because patients with dysphagia are frequently identified in association with other medical problems, the majority of speech-language pathologists who diagnose and treat dysphagia work in the hospital setting. Although physicians are the most likely to identify a patient with dysphagia, it is not uncommon for a parent, teacher, nurse, occupational therapist, or speech-language pathologist to observe or suspect problems with swallowing.

Once dysphagia is suspected, the adult or child should be referred to a physician. The physician can then refer the patient for special examinations. Because schools and nursing homes do not have the equipment necessary for complete dysphagia diagnosis, patients usually go to hospitals for diagnostic workups. After the hospital evaluation, school clinicians and clinicians who work in nursing homes can then become responsible for the therapy recommended for their patients.

Because initial identification of the problem can occur in any of the environments in which one finds a speech-language pathologist, a background in dysphagia is important for all clinicians. Much of the basic information you need to begin understanding normal and disordered swallowing is presented in your courses on anatomy, speech science, neuropathologies, and voice disorders. However, to be qualified to work with this population, you will need advanced courses specific to the physiology and pathophysiology of swallowing, as well as on diagnosis, treatment, and team management.

This chapter will provide you with introductory information about the normal swallow, identification of a swallowing problem, techniques currently used by SLPs for diagnosis of swallowing problems, and details on some of the other professions involved in management of dysphagic patients.

This chapter is intended to provide beginning students with no more information than they can safely swallow.

NORMAL SWALLOWING

In your anatomy course you were introduced to the sensorimotor function of the cranial nerves and the role of those nerves in innervating the muscles of speech and voice production. The cranial nerves that innervate the muscles of speech and voice production (V, VII, IX, X, and XII) also contribute to the sensory and motor function of the face, mouth, larynx, and pharynx during chewing and swallowing. A thorough discussion of the cranial nerves and the mucosa and muscles they innervate is presented elsewhere (Perlman, 1991). If you choose to read that paper, I suggest that you have a textbook by your side that shows the origins and insertions of the muscles of the face, mouth, pharynx, and larynx, as well as the paths of the cranial nerves.

It is important for you to learn this information. It will relate directly to your work, particularly with adults and children who have experienced acquired or congenital neuromuscular diseases or disorders, stroke, certain systemic diseases, or head and neck cancer.

There are, of course, certain structures that play a particularly significant role in the assessment of swallowing disorders. Those structures are identified in Figure 15-1. The following sections will try to describe the function of the mouth, pharynx, and larynx during the oral and pharyngeal stages of swallowing.

The Oral Stage of Swallowing

The oral stage of swallowing can be divided into the oral preparatory and the oral transport phases (Figure 15-2). During the preparatory phase, the lips, jaw, tongue, soft palate, muscles of mastication, and buccal muscles all work to move the bolus (food or liquid) around in the mouth. This phase can last for extended periods if the taste is particularly good, but be very short if the flavor of the bolus is unpleasant. Along with taste, other factors that may influence the duration of this phase among individuals with normal oral function are the temperature, viscosity, and size of the bolus. Factors such as degree of oral sensitivity, rate of secretion of saliva, the viscosity of saliva, and if the patient is edentulous (toothless), can also affect this phase of swallowing.

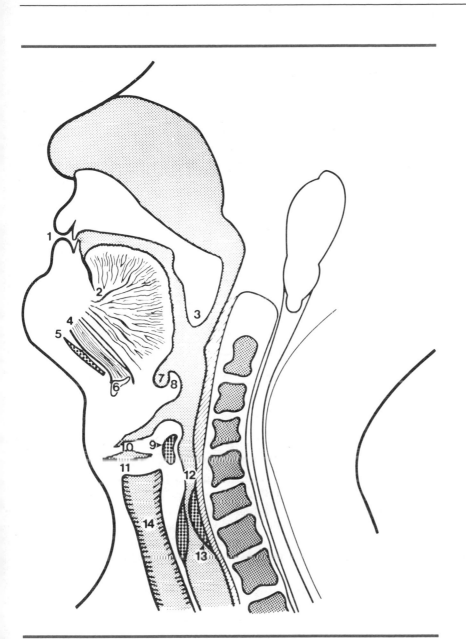

Figure 15-1. Structures that are important in the assessment and treatment of disordered swallowing:

1. lips
2. tongue
3. soft palate
4. geniohyoid m.
5. mylohyoid m.

6. hyoid bone
7. vallecula
8. epiglottis
9. arytenoid cartilage
10. false vocal fold

11. true vocal fold
12. pyriform sinus
13. cricopharyngeus m.
14. trachea

If the food bolus requires mastication, the oral preparatory phase includes a reduction phase, which is, simply, the phase during which the food is chewed. The bolus is placed between the molars, chewed until it is

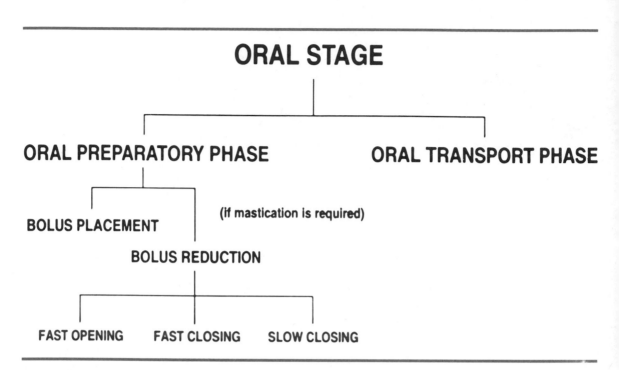

Figure 15-2. Phases of the oral stage of the swallow.

broken into small pieces, mixed with sufficient saliva, and then appropriately placed on the tongue for oral transport.

The reduction phase can be divided into fast opening, fast closing, and slow closing phases, each a reflection of mandibular movement. The fast opening stage occurs as the mandible descends, the fast closing stage as the mandible ascends, and the slow closing phase begins when the teeth make contact with the food in preparation for the grinding process. And so, the muscles of mastication must be strong and very well-coordinated and the jaws must be reasonably well-aligned for chewing to occur properly.

During the oral preparatory phase, the soft palate generally touches the posterior tongue. As the oral transport phase begins, the lips and buccal muscles contract, the posterior tongue depresses, and the remainder of the tongue performs a stripping action against the hard palate as it propels the bolus (mass of food or liquid) toward the oropharynx. The muscles of the floor of the mouth contract and the soft palate elevates.

The Pharyngeal Stage of Swallowing

After the bolus enters the oropharynx, the pharyngeal stage of the swallow begins. This stage consists of a series of rapid, coordinated motions that work to propel the bolus into the esophagus. The pharyngeal stage is very complex and it may be difficult for you to follow these actions with just one reading of the following paragraphs. I suggest that you suck on a piece of hard candy or sip a favorite beverage while reading (and rereading) the following two paragraphs. The purpose is not to keep you awake, but to make it easier for you to do repeated swallows. Keep swallowing and try to visualize the actions that are described. Refer to Figure 15-1 or a favorite anatomy book, if you need to.

During the oral transport phase, the muscles of the floor of the mouth begin to contract. As these muscles contract, the hyoid bone is pulled into a more anterior–superior position and the larynx also elevates and moves somewhat forward. The movement of these two structures helps to open the entrance to the esophagus at the level of the cricopharyngeus muscle. This is the muscle that must also relax when patients use esophageal or tracheoesophageal puncture speech.

Once the bolus enters the oropharynx, the false vocal folds and true vocal folds contract and the other adductory muscles of the larynx help to close the laryngeal aditus. That closure protects the airway from penetration of the food or liquid. Additionally, the epiglottis covers the entrance to the larynx, providing further protection for the airway, reshaping the anterior portion of the pharynx so that the pharynx becomes more cylindrical, and diverting the bolus toward the pyriform sinuses, which are just above the entrance to the esophagus. As the larynx closes, there is a period of apnea (absence of respiration) that is usually followed by an expiration.

It takes less than 1 second (about 800 milliseconds) from the time the bolus enters into the oropharynx until it passes into the esophagus. Considering the precise coordination needed during swallowing, it is easy to understand why so many individuals develop swallowing problems. On the other hand, given this complex organization, it is impressive that so many of us do so well.

CAUSES AND EFFECTS OF OROPHARYNGEAL DYSPHAGIA

Oropharyngeal dysphagia generally results from neuromuscular or structural changes in the oral cavity, pharynx, or larynx. Among infants and children, the more frequent causes of dysphagia include developmental or traumatic neuromotor disorders and congenital anatomical defects. Problems in feeding and swallowing in the pediatric population can be different than those of adult populations (Arvedson & Brodsky, 1993).

Among the adult population, dysphagia is most commonly associated with stroke, neurologic disease, systemic disease, head and neck cancer surgery, radiation therapy for head and neck cancer, traumatic brain injury, and cervical spine disease. Changes in the efficiency of the swallow have been found to result from certain medications. Also, healthy individuals of advanced age can demonstrate swallowing problems that are reflective of the general changes that occur in the sensorimotor system with aging. And, just like a speech or language disorder, dysphagia may be a symptom of a yet undiagnosed disease.

The astute student will recognize from the previous list that many of the causes of dysphagia in both children and adults are also causes of communication disorders. And so, some of the patients who are treated by speech-language pathologists for disordered swallowing may also be treated for communication problems. Two examples are patients with Parkinson's disease who may have dysarthria as well as dysphagia and patients who have had all or a portion of their tongue removed (total or partial glossectomy) for oral cancer.

Respiratory complications, malnutrition, and dehydration are critical health problems that can result from dysphagia. Along with these potential physical health problems, the inability to eat normally often limits the social interactions that so frequently center around food in our society. Not being to able to share a meal with family and friends can have serious emotional effects on individuals who are swallowing-impaired.

Imagine having to take all nourishment through a tube in your stomach and never again eating a pizza or Grandma's cookies or even drinking a glass of water.

THE SWALLOWING EVALUATION

As indicated earlier, the complexity of dysphagia and associated disorders and diseases requires study and treatment by a number of specialists. Consequently, a thorough examination and accurate diagnosis often requires the participation of several different healthcare professionals. Here we are most interested in the role of the speech-language pathologist, but we will consider also the role of other specialists.

Case History

The evaluation begins by reading the patient's hospital chart or whatever other records are available. The intent is to learn about the individual's past medical history as well as the current medical diagnosis, coexisting problems, medications taken by the patient, respiratory status, nutritional, dietary and hydration status, and the general physical condition of the patient. We are looking for indicators that suggest that the patient may be at-risk for malnutrition, dehydration, or aspiration (the penetration of food or liquid into the trachea), as well as for clues as to what may be the cause of the dysphagia.

Information about the respiratory status is important because we will want to know if the patient has a history of aspiration pneumonia or other respiratory complications. A patient with a history of such problems is generally treated more conservatively than one who has a healthy, robust set of lungs.

Of special interest is whether the patient has a tracheotomy and, if so, what type of tracheostomy tube has been placed. If a patient requires an inflatable tracheostomy tube to protect his lungs from the aspiration of oral secretions, then it is highly unlikely that he can safely swallow food or liquid. These patients are usually examined clinically and are carefully followed, but not tested with radiologic imaging techniques until the tracheostomy cuff can be deflated. Patients who are on ventilators for assistance with breathing are usually in special ventilator units and their special needs are beyond the scope of this chapter.

We'll likely learn from the clinical records whether the patient has been losing weight, how the patient receives his nutrition (by mouth or by an alternative feeding method such as a nasogastric tube or gastrostomy tube), and laboratory values related to the patient's nutritional status. These laboratory values are usually interpreted by a physician or a dietitian. Three values most commonly used to ascertain nutritional status are serum albumin, total lymphocyte count, and prealbumin. An albumin of 3.5 or greater, a total lymphocyte count of 1,500 or greater, and a prealbumin ranging from 16–36 are generally considered normal. It is always wise to talk with the local dietitians and learn what laboratory tests and the ranges they use to indicate the various levels of severity of malnourishment. If the patient is taking his meals by mouth, the clinical records should state if he is on a regular or a special diet.

Patient/Family Interview

After the history has been obtained from the available documentation, we are now ready to interview the patient and family. In our context, the term "family" is used loosely; a family member may actually be a nonrelated caregiver or significant other. The questions asked of the patient and family are intended to help decide how to proceed with the proper method of evaluation and/or referral. Also, much of the information will be important when treatment options are considered.

> Some patients live in a nursing home or other care facility. Many of these institutions are short of staff, and that will have an influence on what your final recommendations can be for the patient.

As with any other history taking it is important to record who is providing the information. If the patient is unable to answer for himself, then it is important to know how close the informant is to the patient and the probable accuracy of the information that is provided.

Throughout this interview we observe the patient's speech and language status and look for any indications of impaired judgment or memory or signs of attention deficit. Obviously, any such problems will influence decisions about testing procedures and therapy techniques associated with the possible dysphagia. Also, we need to be alert to the need to follow up at another time with formal testing of speech, language, cognition, or hearing.

> Talk, listen, and observe your patient. Pay attention to speech, voice, language, and behavior.

History taking begins with open-ended questions such as asking the patient or informant to describe the swallowing problem and describe what makes swallowing better or worse. We want to know when the problem began and if there were any incidents that occurred at that time that could account for the onset. We also ask whether the onset was sudden or if the dysphagia developed gradually. Additionally, we need to know whether the problem has become progressively worse or has remained at the same level of severity for an extended period, and if the problem is always present or if it is intermittent and comes and goes with no particular pattern. Prognosis for the patient who has experienced a recent surgery or neurological insult resulting in dysphagia may be very different than for a patient whose dysphagia is of gradual onset and may be an early sign of degenerative neurological disease.

Once the preliminary questions have been asked, it is time to begin with more specific questions about whether there are any of the following symptoms during or after eating:

1. food/liquid from the nose (nasal regurgitation)
2. drooling

3. food residue found in the mouth after eating

4. dry mouth (xerostomia)

5. coughing/choking during or after eating or drinking

6. the sensation of a lump in the throat

7. a sticking sensation in the throat

8. pain or discomfort on swallowing (odynophagia)

9. voice changes

10. heartburn

11. frequent regurgitation or vomiting

12. frequent burping

13. taste problems

14. appetite changes

The most obvious cause of nasal regurgitation is failure to close the velopharyngeal port during swallowing. When a velopharyngeal disorder is so severe as to result in nasal regurgitation, it is likely that the patient's speech will be nasalized. Because that patient may be a candidate for management by dental prosthesis or possibly surgery, a referral to a special management team is needed. If the cause of the velopharyngeal disorder is not already known, a neurologic referral is certainly indicated to determine if the velopharyngeal disorder is symptomatic of a neurologic disease. Ideally, cancer patients who are to undergo a partial or total paletectomy should be seen by a prosthodontist preceeding the surgery.

Drooling or residue in the mouth after eating are often symptomatic of neurological impairment. These findings are common with patients who have had strokes and in children with certain neuromuscular disorders. Drooling does not necessarily mean that the individual cannot eat safely, but it is a "flag" that suggests that the patient may be at-risk for poor oral control of a liquid or food bolus. The "squirreling" of food in the cheeks because of decreased sensation or buccal muscle weakness can result in spillover into the unprotected airway, causing that person to choke on the residue some time after eating.

A dry mouth (xerostomia) can affect the oral stage of the swallow and decrease taste sensation. Xerostomia can occur from certain systemic diseases, radiation treatment to the mouth or neck, or any other cause that decreases salivary gland production such as various medications. Also, with advanced age, the amount of saliva that is produced is decreased. If there is decreased secretion of mucus in the pharynx, it can be difficult for a food bolus to travel smoothly into the esophagus and portions of the bolus may stick in the pharynx. There are "artificial saliva" products on the market that may be helpful. Depending on the patient's history, it may be appropriate to refer the patient to a dentist who is accustomed to treating xerostomia or it may be necessary to refer the patient to a physician for a medical examination.

Individuals who cough or choke during or after meals may describe the problem as a tickling in the throat or the sensation of something going down the wrong pipe or falling into the windpipe. Such a description cues the clinician that, when proceeding to a visual imaging examination (usually radiographic), which we will be discussing later in this chapter, the clinician should be on the lookout for penetration of food or liquid into the larynx. Just because a person coughs does not mean there is aspiration; rather, the cough may be a successful defense that prevents penetration into the trachea. Likewise, just because someone does not choke or cough does not mean that they do not aspirate; that person may have decreased sensation and be a "silent aspirator."

This is important because many dysphagic patients are silent aspirators.

The complaint of a sensation of a lump in the throat or of something sticking in the throat after swallowing can be difficult to diagnose. One cause for this complaint is the reflux of contents in the stomach or esophagus; that is, the contents "come up again." Of course, the complaint can be because food is indeed sticking in the patient's throat. Visual imaging techniques that are used for evaluation and will be discussed later, help to identify the cause for this sensation. If, on visual imaging, there is no food sticking in the throat, a consult with a gastroenterologist is generally warranted.

The report of voice changes needs to be followed up with additional questions. If the voice change occurs just after eating or drinking, it may be the result of food or liquid entering the laryngeal vestibule and either settling on or penetrating the vocal folds. The additional material on the vocal folds will change their vibratory pattern. On the other hand, a history of voice change may be indicative of a laryngological problem such as weakness or paralysis of a vocal fold or laryngeal cancer. Differential diagnosis is then performed with laryngoscopy by an otolaryngologist.

When patients report that they have experienced taste changes, appetite changes, odynophagia (pain on swallowing), heartburn, vomiting, or excessive stomach gas, it is important that a physician be consulted. These are not symptoms associated with oropharyngeal dysphagia — rather they are symptoms of a variety of possible medical problems that require a physician's attention.

Examination of the Patient

These discussions with the patient and family, provide the basis for an informal assessment of speech, language, and cognition. Although specific problems will not be discussed in this chapter, it is sufficient to suggest that, if the patient has significant cognitive or linguistic deficits, those problems can influence the decisions that will be made regarding task instructions, the type of diagnostic tests to perform, and recommendations for treatment.

The sensorimotor examination is performed to determine if there is any impairment of the face, mouth, pharynx, or larynx that can affect chewing or swallowing. The impairment can be sensory, motor, or structural. When a portion of the mouth, larynx, or pharynx has been altered (such as partial pharyngectomy or laryngectomy) or is malformed (such as Pierre Robin syndrome), the condition is considered structural. If the impairment is sensorimotor, the examiner then determines if the breakdown in function is in the peripheral or central nervous system. When assessing swallowing it is very important to assess sensory as well as motor function.

The oromotor examination and a complete discussion of the evaluation of swallowing is described elsewhere (Perlman et al., 1991). Nevertheless, it seems useful at this point to discuss certain observations that should be made during the examination.

Face

Sensory.   For a qualitative estimate of facial sensation, ask the patient to close his eyes and to touch the locations where you apply very light touch and then deep pressure, perhaps with a manicure stick or a feather. Test the upper and lower lips and the perioral region.

Motor.   Note the symmetry, strength, and tone of the muscles of the face. Assess the lower face at-rest, during conversation, on lip rounding, and when smiling. Most patients can swallow adequately even if the lips are weak; however, the complexity or severity of a patient's disease or disorder is more fully understood if the facial muscles are assessed. Although the upper face does not contribute to speech or swallowing, a complete cranial nerve examination would include observation of the muscles of eyes and forehead.

Mouth

Look at the oral mucosa for the presence or absence of oral secretions. Generally, the oral mucosa will glisten; but if a patient has xerostomia, the mucosa will appear dry. Excessive secretions suggests that the patient is unable to manage saliva satisfactorily. Too much saliva, particularly if it can be seen pooling in the oropharynx, is generally indicative of a serious swallowing problem.

Note the condition of the teeth and whether any are absent. If the molars are missing or if they are exceptionally worn down, the patient may not be able to chew solid foods satisfactorily.

Sensory.   As with the lips and perioral region, touch the tongue and the hard and soft palates lightly and ask the patient to indicate when he senses the touch. You can use a sketch of the lips, tongue, and palate and instruct the patient to point to the location you touched. A diagram adapted from that used by Silverman and Elfant (1979) may be a useful way for obtaining and recording this information.

Because the sensory innervation of the tongue comes from cranial nerves V, VII, and IX, taste and sensation may be affected along with the motor function to the face and muscles of mastication. If taste or sensation are found to be selectively impaired, you can use this information to the patient's advantage when performing radiographic examination and when making decisions regarding treatment. For example, if sensation is present only on the left side, be sure to place the food bolus on the left side of the tongue.

Also, look for the squirreling of food in the lateral sulci. This is suggestive of decreased sensation and can also indicate weakness of the cheek or tongue muscles.

Motor.   Observe the soft palate at-rest, during vowel prolongation, and during a gag. It is my policy to let the patient know that I am going to try to make him gag, because it generally builds trust and allows me to do other things in the patient's mouth without causing adverse reactions. Although on some occasions this can work against me, with the patient pulling away or overreacting. Although the absence of a gag can mean that the cranial nerve IX–X reflex is impaired, there are many people who just do not have a gag reflex but who have good palatal movement that can be seen when they produce the prolonged /a/.

The absence of a gag *may* be indicative of a swallowing problem. The presence of a gag does not tell you anything about the safety of the swallow.

Look at the tongue at-rest and on protrusion. Note if the tongue deviates on protrusion, if it is symmetrical, and if the size is within normal limits. Note also if there is a reasonable range of tongue motion adequate for touching the hard palate, retruding the tongue as is necessary for swallowing, and moving it to manipulate a food bolus as described earlier in this chapter. Look for fasciculations or tongue atrophy, particularly in dysarthric patients. Be attentive if there has been partial or total glossectomy, because these patients are at high risk for dysphagia.

Respiration, Speech, and Voice

We need to determine if the respiratory, phonatory, articulatory, or resonatory systems are impaired. Patients with respiratory problems may not be able to clear their lungs of foreign material as well as patients with normal lung function. Also, they may not be able to safely coordinate respiration and swallowing. Consequently, they need to be treated with caution when nutritional options are considered.

Problems with the articulatory system may be indicative of weakness or incoordination of the muscles that are used for chewing and swallowing as well as for speech; and, resonance problems may be suggestive of velopharyngeal incompetency or incoordination that can also impact on the efficiency of the swallow.

If the patient exhibits a wet, hoarse voice quality or if the voice is perceived as breathy or of weak intensity, it is important that a laryngoscopy be performed. Some individuals with paralysis or paresis of the vocal folds aspirate because an important valve protecting the airway has been compromised. When a laryngoscopy reveals excessive secretions in the hypopharynx or if a patient's voice is wet-sounding, it is likely that the patient is an aspirator. However, it is important to remember that a clear voice does not mean that the patient swallowed without aspiration.

Once the clinical examination is completed, the clinician decides how to proceed. It is possible that the speech-language pathologist will decide that the problem is not within his or her domain and that the patient should be referred to another specialist such as an otolaryngologist, gastroenterologist, or neurologist. For example, a referral to a gastroenterologist would be appropriate, if after a careful interview it becomes evident that the clinical signs suggest that the patient may be experiencing gastroesophageal reflux. Another example for the need to refer a patient would be if the patient's complaints of dysphagia are part of a cluster of symptoms such as hoarseness and/or odynophagia; in that case, the patient should be referred to an otolaryngologist. At times the patient needs to be seen by both the SLP and another specialist.

Reports indicate that only about 42% of the patients who aspirate are identified by clinical examination. This strongly reinforces the need for dynamic imaging of the swallow.

If the problem is in the domain of the SLP, then it is necessary to decide which instrumental procedures should be used for further diagnosis. Because the clinical examination neither reliably identifies patients who aspirate (Splaingard, Hutchins, Sulton, & Chaudhuri, 1988) nor provides adequate information for treatment planning, it's advisable to proceed with additional diagnostic procedures.

DIAGNOSTIC PROCEDURES

There are several objective diagnostic procedures available to the speech-language pathologist. Because the type of information obtained is not necessarily the same for each, you need to be able to decide which procedure will provide you with the most appropriate information, with the least risk or discomfort for your patient.

In many institutions, videofluoroscopy is the only diagnostic procedure for the assessment of swallowing, and in the majority of instances, it may be the only objective procedure that needs to be performed. There is more information available on the application and interpretation of videofluoroscopy than any of the other procedures. Nevertheless, it is important for you to know about the other techniques.

Videofluoroscopy

This procedure is also commonly referred to as the modified barium swallow (MBS) or the cookie swallow. In our institution, it is called the videofluoroscopic examination of oropharyngeal swallowing function (VFE/OPSF). Although the name is cumbersome, it describes what is tested and why. Other hospitals have used terms such as deglutition study or oropharyngeal motility study.

I choose to avoid use of the term modified barium swallow because the first word can easily get "lost in the shuffle," resulting in a patient inadvertently receiving a traditional barium swallow, a totally inappropriate test for evaluating oropharyngeal swallowing, and that, at times, can be dangerous for a dysphagic patient.

The problem with the term "cookie swallow" is that it does not provide any information as to the purpose of the examination; also the majority of patients at acute care hospitals never get far enough along in the examination to take a bite of cookie or other solid food, and so the term seems inappropriate in most instances.

VFE/OPSF is a moving picture X-ray examination of swallowing *function*. Although there are times when a portable fluoroscopy unit may be taken to a patient's bedside, generally patients are seen in radiology departments.

The patient is examined in the lateral (Figure 15-3a) and anterior-posterior (A-P) (Figure 15-3b) planes. Most of the information is obtained in the lateral plane, but the A-P view provides information relating to the symmetry of the swallow, the presence of a pocket that is called a diverticulum, and often permits gross observation of the movement of the vocal folds.

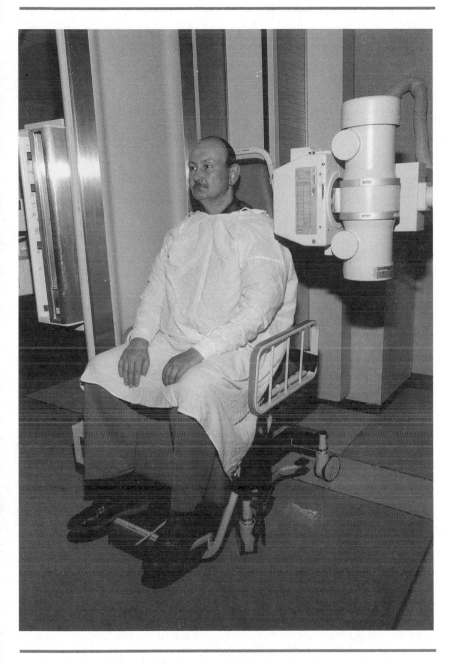

Figure 15-3a. Position of patient for videofluoroscopic examination in the lateral plane.

The patient is given radiopaque material (barium), and as the fluoroscopy camera images the patient during the oral and pharyngeal stages of swallowing, that image is recorded on videotape. This examination is not intended to identify lesions or structural abnormalities.

Figure 15-4 shows the lateral and A-P views of an individual with a normal swallow. As you can tell, there is very little barium remaining in the

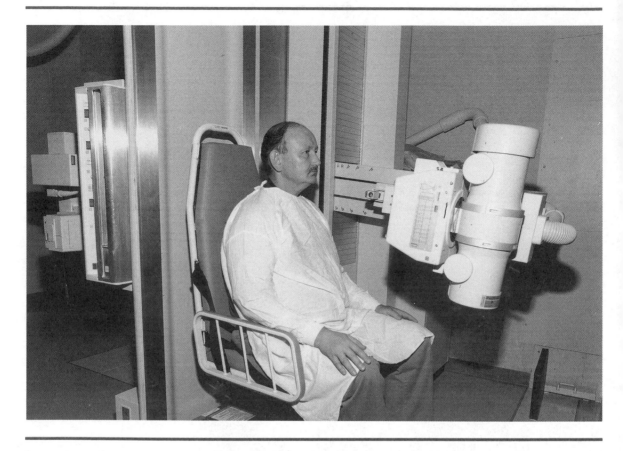

Figure 15-3b. Position for examination in the anterior–posterior plane.

mouth or pharynx. Figure 15–5 shows the residuals from the swallow of a dysphagic patient. On the lateral view there is significant barium residue in the pyriform sinuses and aspiration; note the barium on the vocal folds as well as in the trachea. The A–P view of another swallow from the same patient shows bilateral vallecular and pyriform sinus stasis; barium can be seen in the trachea.

Following the examination, the clinician can then look at the videotape of the swallow in slow motion or even frame-by-frame in an effort to identify oral, pharyngeal, or laryngeal events that may be contributing to the patient's dysphagia. The technique can assist in determining not only *if* the patient is aspirating, but *why* he is aspirating. Information on performing the VFE/OPSF is in Logemann (1983, 1993).

The videofluoroscopic procedure is an extremely informative examination technique, but the examiner needs to remember that this is an X-ray procedure and the patient is exposed to all the hazards of radiation. Therefore, the procedure should not be used indiscriminately. The procedure is generally contraindicated when no new or useful information will be obtained, if the patient has no swallow, or if a patient's level of alertness is

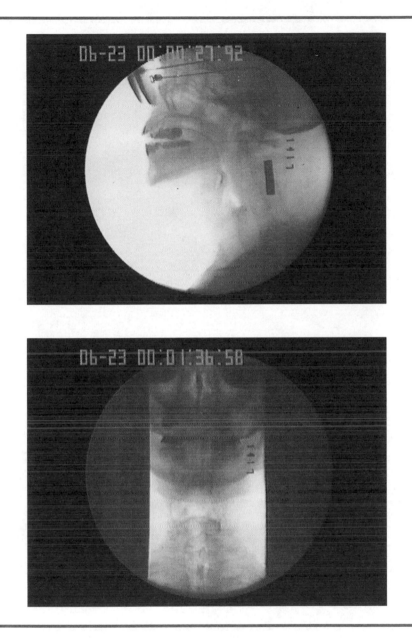

Figure 15-4. A fluoroscopic image in the lateral (top) and A–P (bottom) planes, showing no oropharyngeal dysphagia.

such that the individual cannot be safely nourished by mouth. If a patient is extremely ill, the decision to proceed with an examination needs to be considered very carefully; if the physician feels the evaluation is necessary, then either a nurse or physician, and possibly a respiratory therapist should be in attendance during the examination.

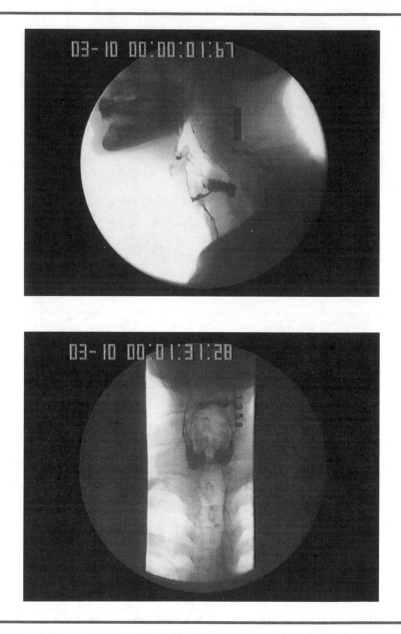

Figure 15–5. A fluoroscopic image in the lateral (top) and A–P (bottom) planes, showing significant barium residue and aspiration.

Videofiberoptic Endoscopy

Traditionally, fiberoptic endoscopy has been used by laryngologists and speech pathologists to assess laryngeal and velopharyngeal function during phonation and to determine if there is disease or disorder in the vocal tract. With the addition of a small camera onto the endoscope, these images can be videorecorded. The procedure can also be used to observe the swallowing process, although the information obtained from endoscopy is more restricted than that obtained from a videofluoroscopic examination.

During the examination, the endoscope is passed transnasally until the valleculae, epiglottis, hypopharynx, pyriform sinuses, and larynx can be viewed. The patient is given something to swallow such as milk, water, or applesauce, with a few drops of food coloring added and the examiner records the swallowing events on videotape. By coloring the food or liquid, it is easy to identify the test material and to determine if there is residue after the swallow. Avoid the use of yellow or red coloring; green is most frequently used.

The larynx, pyriform sinuses, epiglottis, and base of tongue are shown in Figure 15-6. This is the standard "starting point" when doing an endoscopic evaluation of swallowing.

This procedure permits visualization of the pharynx and larynx before and after the swallow; during the swallow the video image is obliterated. It is the best procedure for examining the larynx. By pulling the endoscope back until it is above the soft palate, the action of the velum can be observed throughout the swallow. Obviously, information is not obtained on the oral stage of the swallow with this procedure. The methodology for fiberoptic endoscopic examination of swallowing has been described by Langmore, Shatz, and Olson (1988).

Ultrasound

This imaging technique is used to track the movement of the tongue and the hyoid bone during swallowing and is, therefore, limited to assessing

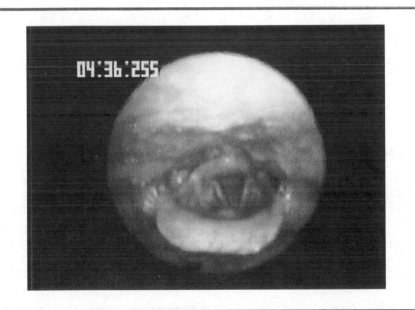

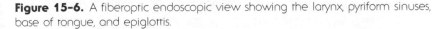

Figure 15-6. A fiberoptic endoscopic view showing the larynx, pyriform sinuses, base of tongue, and epiglottis.

oral function. The ultrasound transducer is held under the patient's chin; high frequency waves are transmitted and the reflected waves are received and transformed into a video image and then recorded on tape. Whereas the soft tissues of the tongue allow for passage of most of the ultrasound wave, the hyoid bone is so dense that it resists the passage of the waves and the reflected waves from the hyoid produce a shadow. Thus, the examiner can observe the movement of the tongue during the oral phases and can observe the movement of the shadow representing the motion of the hyoid bone during the pharyngeal stage of the swallow. Some investigators have used ultrasound to look at other aspects of the swallow, but that requires not only very special expertise but also highly sophisticated ultrasound equipment. Additional information about ultrasound can be obtained from Sonies (1991). Figure 15–7 shows the ultrasound machine and the transducer placed submentally.

Electromyography (EMG)

When a muscle fiber or group of fibers contract, the fibers generate a very small electrical signal; and, like a signal generated by a radio transmitter,

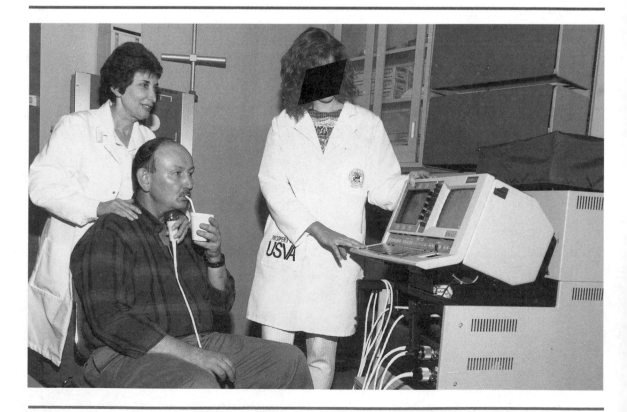

Figure 15-7. The ultrasound machine as it is used for obtaining information on the tongue and hyoid bone during swallow.

that signal can be picked up with the right type of antenna. In the case of EMG, the antenna is called an electrode. When fine wire electrodes are placed in a laryngeal, pharyngeal, or oral muscle and the individual performs a motor act that causes the muscle to contract, the small electrical signal emitted from the muscle is picked up by the electrodes, passed through an amplifier, and can be recorded. If the muscle is paralyzed, then no signal or an aberrant signal will be transmitted. An example of a rectified EMG signal from the superior pharyngeal constrictor muscle of a normal subject and from a patient with pharyngeal constrictor paralysis is shown in Figure 15-8.

Electromyography is not only used to determine if a muscle is paralyzed; neurologists also use EMG in the differential diagnosis of various neuromuscular diseases. For a more thorough discussion of EMG assessment of swallowing, refer to the article by Perlman (1993).

COMPLETION OF THE EVALUATION

At the completion of the swallowing evaluation, the clinician should be in a position to describe the severity of the patient's dysphagia and the symptoms that result in dysfunction. One method of describing severity is the Functional Assessment Scale developed by the Rehabilitation Institute of Chicago (RIC-FAS, 1992). This scale is used to rate swallowing function on a 7-point scale from normal to severe impairment.

When the clinician has carefully evaluated all findings, it is time to determine if the patient is a candidate for behavioral therapy under the direction of the speech language pathologist, or a candidate for dental prosthetic, medical, and/or surgical intervention. The final decision may be determined after consensus has been achieved, with input from various specialists who are part of a structured or unstructured, interdisciplinary, or multidisciplinary team. And so, it is extremely important that the speech-language pathologist be well-versed in the anatomy, physiology, and pathophysiology of oropharyngeal swallowing and to be able to interpret the results from those procedures used to assess swallowing function.

In most institutions, it is the speech-language pathologist who heads the dysphagia team or who serves as the key component in the diagnosis and management of patients when no formal team is in operation. Although the scope of this chapter does not include discussion of team management, there are certain responsibilities that a dysphagia clinical management team can assume that are worth mentioning. Some of the responsibilities include: (1) establishing protocols for identification of patients with dysphagia and for routing patients through the necessary clinics involved in assessment; (2) developing protocols for patient management and nourishment; (3) developing a method for chart entry and record keeping that is meaningful to all members of the team; and (4) providing patient and family education and ongoing staff training. Consequently, it is important that the speech-language pathologist be able to communicate effectively with the physician and other healthcare professionals, as well as families when interpreting examination results and recommending treatment options that have been determined as a result of the complete dysphagia evaluation.

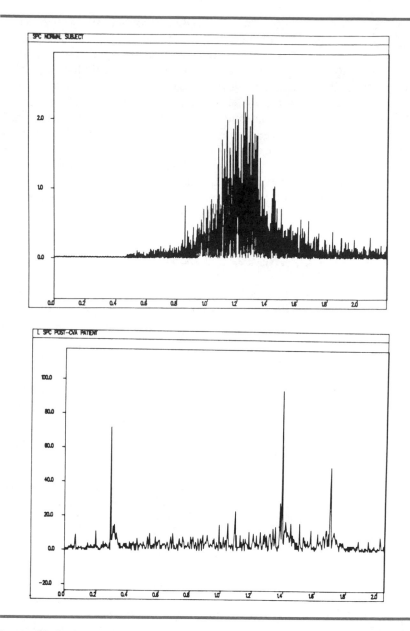

Figure 15-8. An example of rectified EMG signals from the superior pharyngeal constrictor muscle during swallow by a healthy individual, as well as an individual with paralysis of the pharyngeal constrictor muscle.

SUMMARY

The diagnosis and treatment of patients with oropharyngeal dysphagia has become a major portion of the caseload of many speech-language pathologists. Although the greater number of clinicians who work with this population are in hospitals, nursing homes, or rehabilitation centers, SLPs are frequently responsible for management of dysphagic children and adults in other environments as well.

Thorough examination begins with a review of the patient's history, an interview with the patient and/or significant others, clinical examination, and generally at least one objective technique. The clinical examination should consist of an informal assessment of speech, language, and cognition and an in-depth sensorimotor examination of those structures important to deglutition.

The most frequently used objective method for assessing swallowing is the videofluoroscopic examination of swallowing function. There are other techniques that are appropriate. The choice of technique depends on the question that is being asked about the patient.

At the completion of the swallowing evaluation, the clinician should be in a position to describe the severity of the patient's dysphagia, the causes of dysfunction, and make recommendations for treatment or for further evaluation. Diagnosis and management of dysphagia is generally most efficient and effective when there is team management. The configuration of the team is dependent on the type of institution and the patient population. It is often the SLP who heads the dysphagia clinical management team; and so, it is important that the speech-language pathologist be able to communicate effectively with physicians, other healthcare professionals, and families when interpreting examination results and recommending treatment options that have been determined as a result of the complete dysphagia evaluation.

REFERENCES

Arvedson, J. C., & Brodsky, L. (Eds.). (1993). *Pediatric swallowing and feeding.* San Diego: Singular Publishing Group.

Langmore, S. E., Shatz, M. A., & Olson, N. (1988). Fiberoptic endoscopic examination of swallowing safety: A new procedure. *Dysphagia, 2,* 216–219.

Logemann, J. A. (1983). *Evaluation and treatment of swallowing disorders.* San Diego: College-Hill Press.

Logemann, J. A. (1993). *Manual for the videofluorographic evaluation of swallowing* (2nd ed.). Austin, TX: Pro-Ed.

Perlman, A. L. (1991). The neurology of swallowing. *Seminars in Speech and Language, 12*(3), 171–183.

Perlman, A. L. (1993). Electromyography and the study of oropharyngeal swallowing. *Dysphagia, 8*(4), 351–355.

Perlman, A. L., Langmore, S., Milianti, F., Miller, R., Mills, R. H., & Zenner, P. (1991). Comprehensive clinical examination of oropharyngeal swallowing function: Veterans Administration Procedure. *Seminars in Speech and Language, 12*(3), 246–253.

RIC-FAS, Version 3. (1992). Rehabilitation Institute of Chicago (p. 71).

Silverman, E. H., & Elfant, I. L. (1979). Dysphagia: An evaluation and treatment program for the adult. *American Journal of Occupational Therapy, 33*(6), 382–392.

Sonies, B. C. (1991). Ultrasound imaging and swallowing. In M. Donner & B. Jones (Eds.), *Normal and abnormal swallowing: Imaging in diagnosis and therapy* (pp. 109–119). New York: Springer-Verlag.

Splaingard, M. L., Hutchins, B., Sulton, L. D., & Chaudhuri, G. (1988). Aspiration in rehabilitation patients: Videofluoroscopy vs. bedside clinical assessment. *Archives of Physical Medicine and Rehabilitation, 69,* 637–640.

RECOMMENDED READINGS

Beck, T. J., & Gaylor, B. W. (1990). Image quality and radiation levels in videofluo-roscopy for swallowing studies: A review. *Dysphagia, 5,* 118–128.

Bosma, J. F. (1957). Deglutition: Pharyngeal stage. *Physiological Reviews, 37,* 275–300.

Gritzmann, N., & Fruhwald, F. (1988). Sonographic anatomy of the tongue and floor of the mouth. *Dysphagia, 2,* 196–202.

Langmore, S. E. (1991). Managing the complications of aspiration in dysphagic adults. In B. Sonies (Ed.), *Seminars in Speech Language and Hearing, 12*(3), 198–208.

Miller, A. J. (1986). Neurophysiological basis of swallowing. *Dysphagia, 1,* 91–100.

Perlman, A. L., Booth, B. M., & Grayhack, J. P. (1994). Predictors of aspiration in oral-pharyngeal dysphagia. *Dysphagia, 9*(2), 90–95.

Selley, W. G., Flack, F. C., Ellis, R. E., Ellis, R. E., & Brooks, W. A. (1990). The Exeter dysphagia assessment technique. *Dysphagia, 4,* 227–235.

Veldeen M. S., & Peth, L. D. (1992). Can protein-calorie malnutrition cause dyspha-gia? *Dysphagia, 7,* 86–101.

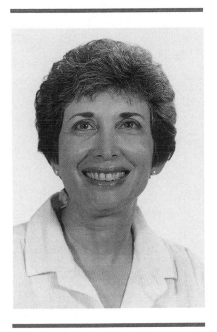

ADRIENNE L. PERLMAN, Ph.D.

Ph.D. 1985, The University of Iowa

Dr. Perlman is an Associate Professor in the Department of Speech and Hearing Science at the University of Illinois in Urbana-Champaign. Before receiving a Ph.D., she spent a number of years as a clinician, first in the public schools and eventually in a large community hospital. While working on her Ph.D. at the University of Iowa, she joined the staff at the VA Medical Center in Iowa City and served as Head of the Speech Pathology Section for 11 years. Her responsibilities at the University of Illinois are primarily research and teaching courses in swallowing and voice disorders. During the years, her research has been devoted to laryngeal physiology and the study of normal and disordered swallowing.

C H A P T E R

16

Adults with Mental Retardation

Louise Kent-Udolf, Ph.D.

This chapter will acquaint you with current trends in the assessment of communication for adults with mental retardation (MR). Specifically, my job is to tell you the attitudes, skills, and information that I want you to own before finishing a clinical practicum with adults with MR. I hope you will take these perspectives to heart when you serve individuals with MR and their families.

BACKGROUND

Unless you have a family member or a close friend or neighbor who has MR, you probably don't know much about it. All of my knowledge about the subject has been acquired since receiving my master's degree in speech-language pathology; none was acquired in formal courses. I learned about MR as a child from neighbors in Dallas, Texas and I learned more about it from children and parents in Stillwater, Oklahoma, where I first worked as a speech-language pathologist (SLP).

After I earned my doctorate, I continued to learn as I served in two large Michigan residential facilities for people with MR. At the same time, I taught psychology at Western Michigan University; and, not surprisingly, my teaching and academic interests became centered on MR, language acquisition, and learning.

The challenge to find and to integrate best practices for people with MR has led me through a fascinating and fulfilling career in speech-language pathology and behavior analysis. The point of this is to impress on you my belief that the field of mental retardation has a great deal to offer you as a specialty area. But, because this area lacks strong representation in academic and clinical programs in speech-language pathology, you will need to gain your expertise primarily through direct experiences with people with MR, their families, and clinicians who work with them.

Definitions

You and I need to agree on what we mean by **adult**, and I need to make you aware of the current definition of mental retardation. For our discussion here, adults with MR are 22 years of age or older and are no longer receiving services from public school special education programs.

The current definition of mental retardation, approved by the American Association on Mental Retardation in 1992 (Luckasson et al., 1992) is:

Further information about definitions of MR can be obtained from the AAMR, 17199 Kalorama Road NW, Washington, DC 20009.

> Mental retardation refers to substantial limitations in present functioning. It is characterized by significantly subaverage intellectual functioning, existing concurrently with related limitations in two or more of the following applicable adaptive skill areas: communication, self-care, home living, social skills, community use, self-direction, health and safety, functional academics, leisure, and work. Mental retardation manifests before age 18. (p. 1)

This definition is intended to influence how we think about people with mental retardation and the services we provide for them.

Perspectives on Mental Retardation

I want to share with you some perspectives that I and many other professionals in the field of MR embrace as standards for services. The overarching perspective is one of dignity in intervention. The goals for intervention are independence and inclusion. We want people with MR to have chances to become as independent as possible in every way. Where there are limitations, we want to remove them through instruction and through the use of **adaptations**. We want individuals with MR to have chances to be included in normal living environments; to be included in typical employment settings, as shown in Figure 16-1; to have access to all services and entertainment in our communities, as shown in Figure 16-2; and to have friends they are interested in interacting and communicating with and who are interested in interacting and communicating with them.

Adaptations are changes we make that allow people to do things that would otherwise be more difficult or impossible.

To help us achieve these goals, we apply certain standards. These standards can be applied to recommendations we make regarding intervention objectives, to specific activities we recommend, or to just about anything else that pertains to adults with MR, including, for example, the kinds

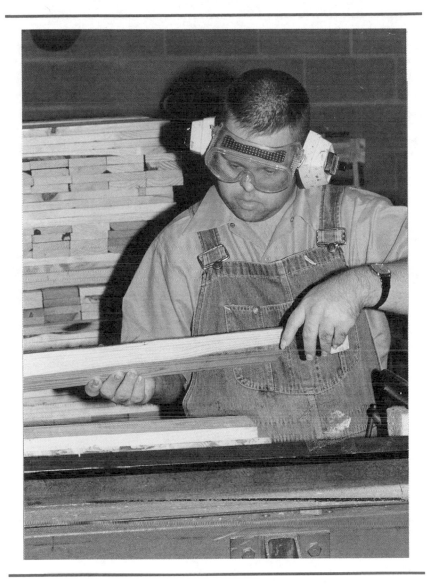

Figure 16-1. Robert Hirsch at work. People with MR deserve the opportunity to learn useful job skills for gainful employment. Courtesy of Bill Walker, Executive Director of the Center for the Retarded, Houston, TX, where Mr. Hirsch is a client.

of bedspreads we think are appropriate for adults with MR. I'm going to list some standards for service in the next sections, but it will be up to you to apply them in each context in which you work with people with MR.

Social Significance

People value some things more than others. We tend to prefer the things we perceive as valued in our society. For example, we value clean, well-fitted, stylish clothing.

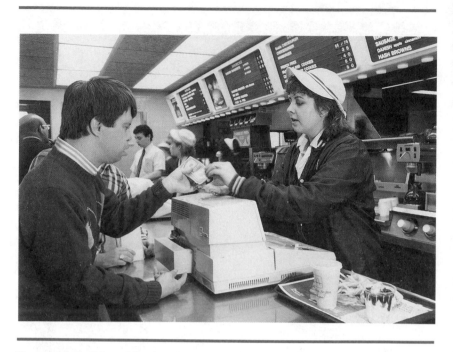

Figure 16-2. Wayne Crouse places his order: "Two all-beef patties, special sauce, lettuce, cheese, pickles, onions on a sesame seed bun." People with MR deserve the opportunity to learn useful interactive skills for everyday life, including visits to a fast food restaurant! Courtesy of Don Rabush, CEO of TARGET, Inc., Westminster, MD. From the brochure *Everyone Has to Live Somewhere*.

Functional

Functional is a term we use to describe activities that we consider essential in our society. In other words, if we think an activity must be performed, it's functional. Doing the laundry is an activity that most of us view as essential.

Social

Social refers to opportunities to interact and communicate with people of our own choosing. For individuals with MR, social interaction and communication with nondisabled people are viewed as essential for inclusion in the mainstream of society.

Age-appropriate

Treat adults with MR like adults.

This term describes what is appropriate for **typical** adults. For example, adults wear adult clothing even though they may be small in stature.

Durable

Durability, here, refers to skills; and durable skills are ones that have use and value over a long period of time. For example, telephone skills are useful indefinitely, provided there are telephones to use. Furthermore, using the phone is functional, age-appropriate for adults and of high social value.

Practical

Practical refers to just how many opportunities there will be to do or to use something. If there are opportunities everyday to engage in an activity, we say that learning to perform that activity is practical. For example, most of us eat at least three meals each day; so, table manners that are valued in our society can be practiced often. Laundry may need to be done only once a week, but doing the laundry is also viewed as practical, because there are relatively frequent opportunities for practice.

Preference

All of us want to express our preferences in the things we do and have. People with MR have preferences, too. High value is attached to opportunities to make choices in our society.

Everyone appreciates opportunities to make choices.

Culturally Correct

We are most comfortable in our own culture. Traditions and practices that are valued and accepted in a person's culture are considered culturally correct for that person. We live and work in a multicultural society today; and we should be sensitive to cultural differences.

In What Settings Are Services Available for Adults with MR?

People with MR are now in the mainstream of our society, receiving services in the same clinical settings as anyone else. For example, you can expect to serve adults with MR in community speech and hearing clinics, nursing homes, acute care hospitals, and rehabilitation hospitals. Speech-language pathologists in private practice serve adults with MR on contractual bases for state and local service agencies, and they also serve these individuals in their private caseloads. However, many SLPs are employed by private or state-operated institutions or by state and local service agencies, public and private.

Employment opportunities for SLPs serving adults with MR are expanding most rapidly in community service agencies and in private practices that serve them.

When Are Field-Based Services Appropriate?

Best practice says that the most effective way to teach adults with MR is to provide instruction in the environments in which the individuals are expected to function. Best practice also says that the most effective way to teach communication skills to adults with MR is to teach them in the con-

Best practice favors
ecological assessments.

text of activities in which they are embedded. Furthermore, best practice holds that the same is true for assessment.

Best practice says that assessments of communication skills should be conducted "in the field" in the environments in which individuals live, work, play, and transact the business of daily life. This means that assessments should be done in the home, on the job, on the bus, in the supermarket, at the pharmacy, at McDonald's, at the snack bar, at the post office, at the "Y," at K-Mart, at the bank, and so on. And we should be assessing the communication skills that are embedded in activities that typically occur in these environments, for example, buying bus tokens, buying donuts, ordering a pizza, cashing paychecks, playing cards with friends, getting haircuts, or going to church.

Ecological assessments of communication represent a departure from the usual methods in speech-language pathology, but I think this application of an ecological model is exciting and functional; and I think it's going to be important for SLPs serving people with MR to perform assessments and to deliver intervention in environments where their consumers are expected to function. This will require SLPs and other professionals to work together closely and to share "turf" to the extent that many traditional roles are "released" (Rainforth & York, 1987). Further, the adoption of an ecological model involves major shifts in philosophical and management paradigms on the part of administrators and such changes evolve slowly. For now, though, we need to concentrate on performing a **primary** assessment of communication, and this is done appropriately in a clinic environment. The ecological assessment is an important form of **secondary** assessment that you will frequently recommend.

THE ASSESSMENT PROCESS

The SLP as a Member of an Assessment Team

More often than not, the SLP assesses the communication skills of adults with MR as a member of an interdisciplinary team. Because the individual with MR presents a variety of needs, interdisciplinary teams are required to provide appropriate assessments and management. Minimally, a team includes a psychologist, a social worker, and a physician who may be represented by a nurse. Other service providers, such as SLPs, may also serve on such teams. My bias, of course, is that every team should include an SLP, as communication skills contribute heavily to a person's success in any environment. Team members conduct separate assessments and write separate reports after which they meet to discuss their findings and to draft a summary of their findings and recommendations. They then meet with the consumer and family members in an "assessment staffing" to discuss their findings and recommendations and to finalize the summary and recommendations.

Teams are expected to meet specific procedural standards as they perform their work. The purpose of these standards is to assure quality services. Only through adherence to standards do clinics and agencies qualify for eligibility to receive payment or services from insurance companies, Medicaid, and other funding sources.

The SLP's role in the assessment process varies as a function of how well and whether the team members function as a team. Assuming that the team functions well, the SLP can talk with and review the reports of other team members before the staffing. Access to the client's social history, psychological findings, educational history, the medical history, and current medical status makes it possible for the SLP to place the results of the primary communication assessment in ecological and functional contexts even though the assessment is performed in a clinic setting, rather than in natural environments. Without concurrent assessments from other professionals, it becomes more difficult for the SLP to provide a meaningful assessment.

How Do We Begin the Communication Assessment Process?

Obviously, you will need some information about the person before you meet him or her face-to-face. Put whatever identifying information you have into the format you plan to use for your written report. If you have no prior information on the person, use the information obtained at the time the appointment for the assessment was made. Highlight the information you lack as a reminder to yourself to fill in the gaps as you have the opportunity.

Review the Record

A review of whatever background information is available introduces you to the consumer. (I often use the term consumer, rather than patient or client, because it is preferred by the Texas Department of Mental Health and Mental Retardation.) From this review you will gain impressions that will help you conduct a useful assessment. You will gather information that will help you make meaningful interpretations of your observations and appropriate referrals for other kinds of professional services. Lastly, a careful review of existing information can help you form recommendations that will result in the person's becoming a more competent and independent communicator, immediately and in the near future.

To make efficient use of your preparation time, record your notes and questions in the appropriate sections of an outline of your written report. One important question is whether a reliable informant will accompany the consumer at the time of the assessment. Other questions will arise. Acronyms such as TRC (Texas Rehabilitation Commission) will appear in the text of reports without clarification. Diagnostic codes that are foreign to you may be used. You may have questions about the purposes of medications that the consumer is receiving. And you may find discrepancies between reports on anything from date of birth to social quotient. In every instance, you will want to know what opportunities the individual has to interact with nondisabled people outside the family. You will want to know how consumers spend their weekends and what they do during a typical day.

You may need to gather background information about the consumer. You need school records, a reliable developmental history, a medical history, a current physical, and a social history including a description of the

You need a reliable informant to obtain the needed information.

present living arrangement and programming during the day. You may be able to get some of this information from informants. To obtain copies of documents, however, you will need to obtain permissions for their release and to request them.

When you finish your review of the background information, organize what you have learned into the relevant sections of your report. Be sure to highlight any specific questions to be asked of the informant(s) during the assessment in the sections where the information will be reported.

Plan Your Interaction With Informants

The outline for your written report can serve as a guide for how you will spend your assessment time with the consumer. Right away, however, you will encounter a challenging problem: How are you, a stranger, going to engage an adult with MR in a conversation that will allow you to gather the kind of information you need? And, what if the person doesn't talk at all?

You will need one or more informants who know the consumer well. Identify your informants and make an appointment to talk with them on the same day and at the same place where you will assess the consumer. Plan to interview the informants **before** you interview the consumer. Parents and family members or direct-care staff who have known the consumer for at least 6 months can provide you with reliable information about how the consumer communicates.

When you talk with informants, ask them to tell you about the consumer as a person: What makes the person laugh? What makes her angry or cross? How does the consumer tell others what she wants? How does she handle frustration? Does she have a job? If so, what does she like about it and how does she get there? Does the consumer have a best friend? Does she wear makeup? Is she interested in the opposite sex? Does the individual take an interest in decorating her bedroom? Does she like to go shopping? Does she like to eat out? How does she spend her weekends? Does she independently wash and dry her hair? Does the person do her own laundry? Does she cook or help prepare meals? Does she like to play card games? Does she belong to the "Y" or to a health club? Is exercise a regular part of the person's weekly routine? Does she have friends without disabilities? If so, what do they do together? Does the consumer have adult brothers and sisters? If so, are they active in the consumer's life? Does she use the telephone and how often does she receive calls?

You don't need to address all of these questions, and don't just ask questions. Listen. If the informants are talkative, let them talk as long as they stay on topic. Informants can help prepare you for your consumers. Plan to spend 30–45 minutes with informants before you interview consumers.

Listen to informants. Practice your interviewing skills.

Plan a Functional Communication Interview

Based on what you learn from reviewing the available information, plan how you will interview the consumer. You probably will have a fairly accurate picture of how the person communicates. If the person talks at all, you will be able to informally assess articulation, voice, rate, fluency, pitch, loudness, pragmatics, expressive vocabulary, language, and suprasegmental aspects of speech such as melody, stress, and inflectional patterns.

You will need to include an oral examination, which is covered in some detail in Chapter 4. This is a very important part of the assessment and is always expected. The consumer will be more likely to cooperate if you perform the exam midway through the interview, rather than at the beginning or at the end. Treat the person with the same respect you would accord any other adult and expect the same in return. Demonstrate what you want the consumers to do. Let them look in your mouth. And let them examine any instruments or props you use. Be aware that as you conduct the oral examination it is possible to assess language at the same time: "Let me see your teeth." "Show me how you chew." You are performing an oral examination, but you are also communicating with the consumer.

In some instances, consumers may have difficulties swallowing or chewing. When this is the case, teams often depend on the SLP for assessments, referrals, and recommendations regarding adaptive equipment and management techniques. Additional material about these aspects is presented in Chapter 15. When you need this kind of expertise on the job, you can turn to more experienced SLPs and other professionals for advice. It is your professional responsibility, however, to seek continuing education in this area, if you find that you continue to need expert help.

Whether the consumer talks or not, you need to record the interview. Even though you are doing all the talking, listening to tape will remind you of what you did and said, and how the consumer responded.

If the person doesn't talk, you will still be able to assess social routines, the communication of personal ID information, receptive vocabulary, receptive language, language-related concepts such as time, and language-related cognitive skills such as visual memory and sequencing. There may be an art to talking with people who don't talk. If it is an art, I'm confident that it's one you can master. I'll give you some tips to get you started later on. For now, let's focus on how to set an adult tone for the interview and how to make it interesting, informative, and fun.

The substance of communication assessments for adults with MR is quite different from speech and language examinations for children or for adults with other types of histories and diagnoses. As you begin the interview, you will need to introduce yourself and make some small talk to help the consumer feel relaxed and at ease with you. Plan this. Rehearse it. It's part of the assessment. You are interested in how the consumer responds to these social approaches.

Next, assume a more formal attitude toward the consumer. Tell the person that you are now going to be asking some questions that will help you assess how he communicates. Under the pretext of completing a form, ask basic information such as full name, address, telephone number, birthdate, age, marital status, employment, and so on. Ask the consumer to print his name. Show the consumer a calendar and ask him to show you his birthday. Ask him to guess how old you are. Locate the current date on the calendar and ask how long it will be until Christmas or his birthday.

After gathering the basic data, compliment the consumer on something: shoes, purse, eyes, hair — anything that catches your attention as nice.

> The oral examination is a must. Don't forget it.

> Communication doesn't require speech.

Observe closely how the consumer responds to this sort of social gesture. Just as you might ask any new acquaintance, ask about what the consumer does during the day.

Be sure to assess denial, an important form of negation. For example, even though you may know that the consumer has never been married, ask. Why? Many times professionals working with adults with MR are asked if an individual is capable of giving informed consent or, less often, whether an individual is competent to stand trial. People dealing with such issues may look to you for help. Documentation showing that a person can reliably deny the truth value of statements, ranging from concrete to abstract, can be helpful in this regard. Don't confuse denial with other forms of negation such as rejection or nonexistence. Denial requires the person to indicate that a statement about an object, person, place, and so on is false.

Give the consumer generous amounts of time to respond. Rephrase your comments or questions to give the consumer the benefit of every doubt. Supply prompts and encouragers including starters such as "Your first name is Charlie and your last name is . . . ?" Pause. Be prepared to keep the interview going on your own. Even though consumers may never say a word, they usually will participate. Typically, adults with MR appreciate the respect and attention you give them; and when family members are present, they appreciate it, too.

Most adults with MR work at jobs in the community or in workshops run by agencies. Ask questions about the work station that you can confirm or that require explanations and demonstrations. For example, "How do you get to work in the morning?" "Do you drive?" "What day of the week do you get paid?" Ask questions that reveal the consumer's memory, language, and language-related concepts such as money, measurement, time, health, and safety. "What do you do when you get tired?" "What do you do when you run out of work?" "What time do you usually get to work in the morning?" "What do you do on your break?" "Show me here on the map where you live."

Point to the emergency numbers in the front of the telephone directory and ask what they are for. Before you put the telephone book aside, wonder out loud how much it weighs. Ask how we could weigh it. Ask the consumer to guess how much you weigh. You are interested in how the consumer responds and if she seems to understand you and the situation.

Switch the conversation to leisure activities. Looking at a *TV Guide*, ask the consumer to tell you about a favorite show. Ask about shopping. "Where did you buy those shoes?" "What size are they?" Compare your shoe size with hers. Wonder which size is larger. Wonder about the price of shoes generally. "I have some money here." Put $.75 in change on the table. "Do you think this is enough money for a pair of shoes?" "How about a Coke? Could we buy a Coke with it?" "Show me how you could use this money to get a Coke out of a machine." Ask which coin is largest, which one is worth most. Ask which is the larger of two identical coins. Ask whether the consumer can count and then ask him to count the coins. Find out if he knows the names of the coins. "This is a quarter and this one is a . . . ." Or, "Give me the nickel. You can keep the quarter."

Most adults with MR can tolerate at least 45 minutes of this kind of interview. When the consumer begins to show signs of tiring, tell him that

How would you assess a person's ability to give informed consent for surgery?

People who don't speak can still communicate.

you are almost finished. Ask him to estimate how long you've been talking. Give him a pad of paper and a pencil and say something like, "Up 'til now I've been asking all the questions. Now, it's your turn. Ask me something." Give several prompts as needed. Whisper, "Ask me what my favorite color is." "Ask me my middle name." "Ask me where I'm going when we finish here." Thank the consumer for participating in the interview. Pay him another compliment. Observe what he does when you announce that the interview is finished.

Tips on Talking With a Person Who Doesn't Speak

Just because someone doesn't talk, we cannot safely assume that the person doesn't hear, isn't listening, or doesn't comprehend what is being said. Communication doesn't require speech. When a consumer doesn't talk back to you, continue to try to establish eye contact as you work to engage the person in some sort of give-and-take of communication. Pause frequently, sometimes with a questioning intonation and sometimes not. Do things as you talk. For example, take out your billfold and open it. "I have my billfold right here." Silently look at some of your own family snapshots or photos of pets or friends. Then start to talk about the photos. "This is my dog. His name is Manfred. He was stolen out of my car one time when we went hunting. He was a good dog." Then look up, "Do you have a dog?" Pause. "Maybe you have some pictures."

People who don't speak aren't necessarily without language.

Move on to something else. Take out your driver's license and show it to the person. "This is my driver's license." Pause. "That's me. Look at that. What a face." Pause. "I use this for ID when people ask to see my ID." Pause. "Do you have any ID?" When you pause, you are giving the person an opportunity to "jump in" and you are watching for any reaction. Does she look up, look away, smile, show interest in any perceptible way? Does she seem to understand what is expected during a conversation? Pursue other directions. Take out some folding money or change. Talk about what you can do with it, count it, name it. Ask her which coin she wants, which one is worth most.

Think receptive. Don't ask the person to talk. Ask him to hand you objects that you name. Ask him to show you what one does with things and how they work. Ask him to do things that will reflect his language comprehension skills. For example, "Would you reach over there and get the phone book for me?" No response. "Look over here." Pause. "Show me the phone book." Pause. "Give it to me, please." "Thank you." Drop it on the floor. "Wow! It's heavy!" Pick it up. "How much do you think it weighs?"

Use things you wear and carry on your person as props: your car keys, a ballpoint pen, billfold, change, family pictures, handkerchief, rings, watch, glasses, earring, shoes, socks. If you carry a briefcase, stock it with pens, pencils, highlighters, paper, small spiral notebooks, a small magnifying glass, napkins, city map, *TV Guide*, a package of chips, and other things that might serve as interesting conversational referents.

Think memory. "Where did I put my keys?" "Could you show me where the water fountain is?" Think visual. "Let's see, here. I'm all turned around. Can you show me how to put this piece of paper in this binder?"

Interview Protocols

I got the idea for interviewing adults with MR from Audrey Holland's *Communicative Abilities for Daily Living* (CADL) (1980), a test she authored for adults with aphasia. She included a small group of adults with hearing impairments and adults with MR in the norming sample. Interestingly, the performance of the adults with MR was similar to that of her group with anomic aphasia. You probably have access to this test and the manual, if you aren't already familiar with them.

Although the CADL is suitable, as is, for some people with MR, my experience has been that it is very difficult for the majority of the group. It's impossible for some. I want you to take a look at it, however, because it captures the essence of what we want to do in an interview with adults with MR. It's functional, it covers a range of communicative functions, it's fun, it's socially interactive, it has interesting props, and it poses interesting everyday situations. It will stimulate your creativity.

Based on my awareness of the CADL and with the help of another SLP (Penny Pennington), I included an interview protocol for people with MR in *Shop Talk* (Kent-Udolf & Sherman, 1983). It won't rescue a hopeless situation, but if you have access to it, you may find it useful. You have the publisher's permission to copy it, and you don't need anyone's permission to adapt it for your personal use.

The truth is that we aren't going to find or create an interview protocol that will suit all adults with MR. The abilities, modes of communication, interests, cultures, and life histories of these individuals vary drastically. It's more reasonable for us to individualize the interview protocol than to expect the consumer to accommodate us.

THE WRITTEN REPORT

After you have interviewed the consumer, you have your notes and a tape of what transpired. How are you going to organize the information you have into a useful report?

What you want to achieve is a neat report that includes several elements divided into three parts. Part I is an overview that can be presented in tabular or sentence outline form. Part II presents the results of the interview organized into five sections: social routines, identifying information, basic language skills, language related concepts, and cognitive concepts.

Part III includes your prognosis for improvement in communication and your recommendations. Given Part I and Part II, in Part III you predict the future, barring unforeseen events and with the assumption that your recommendations will be followed.

Part I

This section should include identifying information about the consumer, a summary of the most relevant aspects of the history, a description of communication modes used and their attributes, and the diagnosis. You should also identify your informants and other sources of information. If your referral source states a specific reason for referral, this reason should be included here. Summarize the findings of the oral examination and what you think are the consumer's current communicative needs for now and the immediate future.

Provide a description of communicative modes used by the consumer and characterize their primary attributes. If it is relevant, this is where you address intelligibility, rate, loudness, voice, and so on, as you would for a person without MR. In addition, include information about other communicative modes such as body language, gestures, sign, and written language and describe how each contributes to communication.

Speech is only one mode of communication.

End with a diagnosis. This is usually, but not always, developmental language delay (secondary to MR). There may be, of course, more than one diagnosis. For example, there may also be a voice disorder. Be aware that you are not being asked to diagnose mental retardation or level of cognitive development. Your focus should be on communication, speech, language, hearing, voice, and the oral mechanism.

Part II

In this part, I organize the information obtained from the interview around five categories. Any set of categories is going to be somewhat arbitrary and there will be overlap among them. I caution you not to pursue perfection in this regard. Do try to avoid reporting the same information in more than one category.

Social Routines

Describe how the consumer performs in the contexts of social routines. Describe his use of polite forms and social skills in speech and nonspeech modes such as gestures, smiling, and eye contact. We are interested in all the ways that the consumer initiates and responds to events that for you and me would occasion social responses. For example, how does he acknowledge your introduction? How does he acknowledge your compliments? Is eye contact appropriate and comfortable? Does he return your smile? Does he laugh at your jokes?

Review your notes and the tape. You will be surprised at how much information you have in this category.

Personal Identification

Describe what the consumer knows about himself and how he communicates it. Intelligibility is critical here whether the consumer talks, prints, points, or fingerspells. The world has a low tolerance for errors having to do with identification information. If the consumer doesn't talk, does he accurately communicate his address in some other language mode when you ask where he lives? Does he have identification with him?

Everybody should carry ID.

Basic Language Skills

In this category, describe receptive and expressive attributes of vocabulary, basic semantic relations such as possession, attributes, and negation (especially, denial), morphology, syntax, and pragmatics. If speech is not the primary communicative mode, describe the content of what was communicated and how. Report your observations of vocal imitation in this category.

Language Related Concepts

Describe how the consumer communicates with respect to time concepts (minutes on watches, days on calendars, seasons of the year, and words and phrases such as past, later, after a while, never, soon, and a long time). It's important to know how and whether people can sequence events in time. For example, to call home using a pay telephone, I must pick up the receiver, put a quarter in the slot, wait for the tone, and then punch in the numbers 8 4 9 9 7 8 7 **in order**, starting with 8.

Number concepts include any meaningful uses of numbers from money to weights and measures. Make note of the client's use or understanding of words such as first, last, pounds, sizes, inches — in fact, any words that suggest an awareness of amounts of anything.

Spatial concepts range from an awareness of one's body in space to the abstract use of space in a game of chess. Describe the consumer's awareness of space as revealed through its use. For example, how does she enter the room? How does she leave? Does she remember the way back to the waiting area? If uncertain or confused, does she ask for directions? If she prints her name on a Consumer Information Form, how does she use the space? If she carries a billfold with her, how are the contents arranged?

Concepts of safety and health require us to recognize what is dangerous in the here and now and what might be bad for us in the future. For example, I try to handle sharp knives carefully to avoid what I know to be a clear and present danger, but I avoid eating foods with high fat content to avoid a less certain future risk. Does the consumer express awareness of these kinds of causes and effects? Is he able to communicate physical complaints? What is the consumer's level of awareness of the relationship between cleanliness and disease? How does he respond when you ask why we should turn away from others when we sneeze?

Concepts of change include the changes that come about as a function of the seasons, aging, normal growth and development, decay, changes in temperature, changes due to wear or to exposure to the sun. Does the consumer express or seem to understand references to these sorts of relationships?

Cognitive Concepts

This is a category that includes memory for any and everything from spatial patterns to tunes and words of songs. Of special importance is the kind of visual memory that allows us to reassemble things, for example, to glue the handle back on a cup, we must remember how the cup looked before it was broken. This category also includes the ability to group things by category and to cite examples from categories. Reading and writing are cognitive skills, as is drawing a picture from memory. Describe anything that you observe during the interview that fits in this category.

Part III

Part III includes your prognosis for improvement in communication and your recommendations. When stating a prognosis, it is critical that you state "prognosis for what." People expect you to tell them whether you think **communication** will improve. If you say no more than "Prognosis is good," your audience won't be certain what you are talking about; and they may think you are saying something different from what you intend. **Prognosis for improvement in communication** is quite different from prognosis for improvement in level of intellectual functioning.

Prognosis for what?

I base my judgment of prognosis for communication on the existing level of communication, on apparent eagerness to communicate, persistence, variety of modes used, willingness to try novel modes, humor, and opportunity for interaction with nondisabled people in a variety of environments. I often qualify the prognosis with the recommendations. In other words, the prognosis for improved communication may be **good** only if the recommendations are followed.

Sometimes it is important to state a prognosis for intelligibility of speech or for voice or for speech itself. When it's appropriate or requested, I don't let the diagnosis of MR unduly influence my judgment. I know that people with MR can learn and change and I respect their abilities and the breadth of their accumulated life experiences. I am alert to instances, however, when years of therapy have not produced appreciable changes. When intelligibility of speech is an issue, I often qualify the prognosis with a recommendation for instruction in the use of backup systems, such as key word signing or a billfold communication system.

When writing your recommendations, go back to the beginning of your report. State your recommendations in the order in which you have addressed the information on which they are based. For example, if you were unable to obtain reports of prior diagnostics or therapy, recommend that these documents be obtained early in your list of recommendations. If you have questions about hearing, recommend an audiological assessment. If you have questions about dentition or voice or if you have any medical concerns, you will need to formulate appropriate recommendations and referrals.

If you have indicated a positive prognosis for communication, conclude with recommendations for intervention that are consistent with your prognosis and refer the consumer to suitable sources for service delivery. To target communication skill deficits that are embedded in high priority activities, I often recommend ecological assessments of communication. Before making specific recommendations for intervention, I hope that you review the standards for service discussed earlier in this chapter.

Recommend ecological assessments to refine objectives: Assess performance in the environments in which it is expected to occur.

DESCRIPTION OF REFERENCES

I have kept my list of references short, hoping that you will take advantage of each of them. Three of them are referred to in the text; the other three are equally useful. Each is included for special reasons. The Snell (1987) book is, to me, the best text ever published in the field of special education. I particularly recommend that you read the chapters on assessment (pp. 64–109) and on domestic and community skills (pp. 390–434). Be prepared for a challenging read! It's not easy, but it says it all.

The article by Mirenda (1993) expresses current trends in service delivery and reveals some of the passion of those who serve people with severe disabilities. This is required reading.

The article by Rainforth and York (1987), in my opinion, is the clearest statement of what is meant by "role release," a concept that is crucial to effective interdisciplinary teamwork.

I have included the Wilcox and Bellamy (1987) catalog because it is unique and it explains by example what we mean by "age-appropriate" and "functional." It will give you valuable ideas for assessment and for programming.

Holland's *CADL* (1980) and my own book, *Shop Talk* (1983) are included because they provide examples of functional communication interviews.

SUMMARY

I'm not going to try to summarize this chapter for you. I've thought about it and it's too much for me. I do want to take this opportunity to preach, however.

When you serve an adult with mental retardation, it's true that you are serving that individual; but you are also serving that person's family and everyone else who serves that person. You have the opportunity to make differences that matter to many people.

As you interact with adults with MR, be aware that you have the power to influence the attitudes and actions of others. Let your performance demonstrate how to show respect and how to evoke participation and humor.

One way to show respect is to "give credit for life experiences." What I mean is that age equivalents for test scores don't tell the whole story. Even though a person may be described as having a mental age of 4 years, that person isn't 4 years old and shouldn't be treated like a 4-year-old child. Make an effort to model the standard of chronological age-appropriateness whenever possible. You might be surprised at the effects.

REFERENCES

Holland, A. L. (1980). *Communicative abilities in daily living: A test of functional communication for aphasic adults.* Austin, TX: Pro-Ed.

Kent-Udolf, L., & Sherman, E. R. (1983). *Shop talk: A prevocational language program for retarded students.* Champaign, IL: Research Press.

Luckasson, R., Coulter, D. L., Polloway, E. A., Reiss, S., Schalock, R. L., Snell, M. E., Spitalnik, D. M., & Stark, J. A. (1992). *Mental Retardation: Definition, classification, and systems of supports.* Washington, DC: American Association on Mental Retardation.

Mirenda, P. (1993). AAC: Bonding the uncertain mosaic. *AAC Augmentative and Alternative Communication, 9,* 3–9.

Rainforth, B., & York, J. (1987). Integrating related services in community instruction. *Journal of the Association for Persons with Severe Handicaps (JASH), 12,* 190–198.

Snell, M. E. (1987). *Systematic instruction of persons with severe handicaps.* Columbus, OH: Charles E. Merrill.

Wilcox, B., & Bellamy, G. T. (1987). *The activities catalog.* Baltimore: Paul H. Brookes.

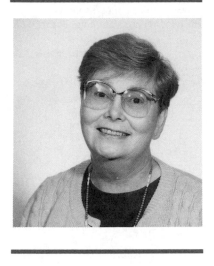

LOUISE KENT-UDOLF, Ph.D.

M.A. 1957, Indiana University
Ph.D. 1966, The University of Iowa

Dr. Kent-Udolf is a principal in a private practice of speech/language pathology and behavior analysis in Houston, Texas. Prior to entering private practice she held positions as professor, clinician, and administrator. Most recently, she served as an administrator at The Mental Health and Mental Retardation Authority of Harris County and at The University of Texas Health Science Center Speech and Hearing Institute, both in Houston, Texas. Her special interests throughout her career have been in the fields of mental retardation and behavior analysis.

CHAPTER

17

Children Who Are Hard of Hearing

Jill L. Elfenbein, Ph.D.

In this book, discussion of children who have hearing losses is divided into two categories. Children who are deaf are described in Chapter 18. In this chapter, we consider children who are hard of hearing. These are the children who have hearing losses that fall in the mild to severe hearing loss range. You will discover that even a mild hearing loss can have a marked effect on communication skill development.

Figure 17-1 provides an example of how degree of hearing loss is determined. There are some differences among audiologists about the cutoff points between categories. For example, some use 80 dB HL as the cutoff for profound hearing loss/deaf; others use 90 dB HL. The actual cutoff points are of limited importance. We base our assessment protocol, prognosis, and treatment plan on the child's abilities, not on the label of hard of hearing or deaf.

DEFINING THE TERM "HARD OF HEARING"

The term "hard of hearing" covers a large and heterogeneous population. Ross (1990) reports an estimate that 16/1000 school-age children have average thresholds between 26 and 70 dB HL. He notes that, if we add chil-

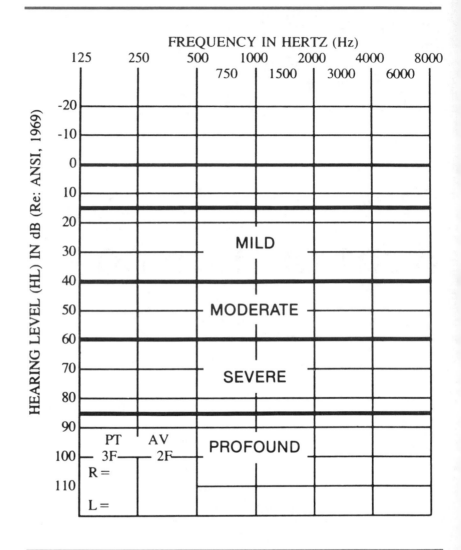

Figure 17-1. Examples of cutoff points used by clinicians to describe degree of hearing loss for children.

dren with milder but educationally significant hearing losses, the number of children considered to be hard of hearing would be nearer 30/1000.

Figure 17-2 provides a representation of conversational level speech plotted on an audiogram. The most intense speech sounds are the vowels. Consonant sounds are less intense than vowels. Some consonants, such as /s, f, t, tʃ, ʃ/ are characterized by energy focused in the high frequencies.

Individuals who are hard of hearing demonstrate a broad range of speech perception abilities. Figure 17-3 shows audiograms for two 18-month-old children whose hearing losses are newly identified. These children have had vastly different exposure to speech and other sounds in their environments and thus will present different patterns of communi-

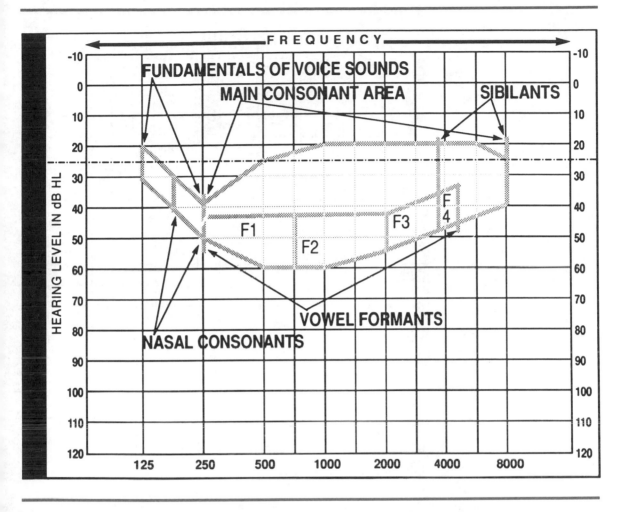

Figure 17-2. Acoustic spectrum of the speech signal plotted on an audiogram. From *Assessment and Management of Hearing-Impaired Children* (p. 183) by M. Ross, D. Brackett, and A. B. Maxon, 1991. Austin, TX: Pro-Ed. Copyright 1991 by Pro-Ed. Reprinted by permission.

cation skill acquisition. Child A has a mild, high-frequency, sensorineural hearing loss. Her responses to environmental sounds and her level of communication skill acquisition may not differ enough from those of her normally hearing peers to raise the red flags that lead to referral for evaluation. However, she is missing valuable acoustic input. This is particularly a problem when she is in a poor listening environment, such as playing with her brother on the kitchen floor while the dishwasher is running. Child B has a bilateral, flat, moderate, sensorineural hearing loss. He hears only intense environmental sounds and receives little information from conversational speech. It is likely that his communication skills are significantly delayed relative to those of age peers with normal hearing. Both Child A and Child B are hard of hearing.

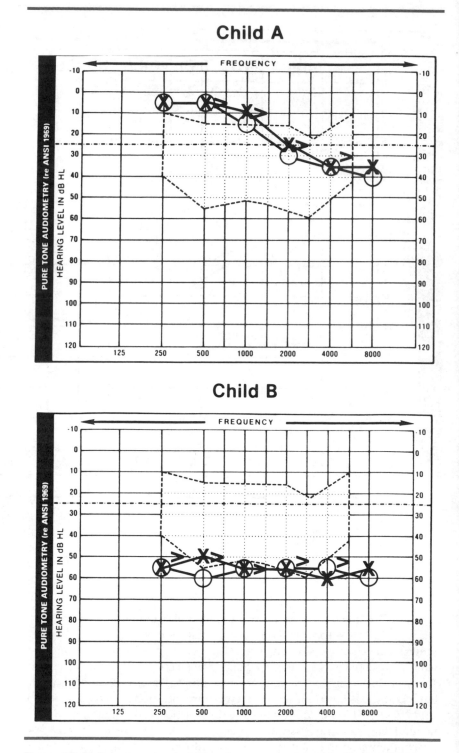

Figure 17-3. Pure-tone threshold data for example cases described as Child A and Child B. Audiogram form reprinted from "Audiological Evaluation of the Mainstreamed Hearing-Impaired Child" by J. R. Madell, 1990, *Hearing-Impaired Children in the Mainstream* edited by M. Ross, 1990. Copyright 1990 by York Press, Inc. Reprinted by permission.

Figure 17-4 shows aided audiograms for Child A and Child B; that is, thresholds obtained in sound field while they are wearing their hearing aids. Amplification of the speech signal makes more of the speech signal audible; however, it does not give the children normal or even near normal hearing. Threshold data such as these indicate neither the distortion that may be present nor the difficulty that children will have in coping with background noise.

Distortion or absence of low intensity, high-frequency speech sounds has a marked effect on the information an individual can extract from conversation. The listener may be unable to discriminate among words that have similar phonemic structure, such as *mass, match,* and *mash.* It is difficult for young language learners to know whether they are hearing one word with multiple meanings or three separate words.

High-frequency speech sounds also carry significant amounts of information about the morphological markers used in English. Consider the problems that children will have if they don't hear the /t/ in contractions such as "can't," the /s/ that signals plural in "books," and the /s/ or /t/ that changes the verb "walk" to the third person singular "walks" or the past tense "walked."

The listening environment is another factor that has a strong impact on the speech perception abilities of individuals who have hearing losses. Finitzo-Hieber and Tillman (1978) demonstrated that the speech recognition abilities of children with hearing losses drop much more sharply than do those of children with normal hearing under two conditions: an increase in background noise or an increase in the reverberation time of the room (the time it takes the sound that echoes off of hard surfaces to decay). When both background noise and reverberation time are high, the ability to recognize speech is severely limited. Hawkins (1988) concluded that, for a child who is hard of hearing to function adequately, a listening environment should have a reverberation time of 0.5 seconds or less and a signal-to-noise ratio of +15 or greater. That is, the signal level should be at least 15 dB above the noise level and echoes should decay rapidly. Data gathered from typical classroom settings indicate that few classrooms meet either standard.

The term "hard of hearing" encompasses children who have permanent conductive hearing losses, such as hearing loss associated with ossicular chain malformation, and children who have mixed hearing losses as well as children with sensorineural hearing losses. In addition, there is mounting evidence that children who have normal hearing in only one ear (those with unilateral losses) and children who have normal hearing only some of the time (those with fluctuating conductive hearing losses resulting from otitis media) are at a disadvantage in auditory learning situations such as the average classroom. They, too, may be described as hard of hearing.

Hearing loss is not the only disability we find in children who are hard of hearing. Estimates are that approximately 30% of children with hearing losses have at least one other disability (Gallaudet University Center for Assessment and Demographic Studies, 1992). Additional disabilities may include problems that affect communication skill development in predictable ways, such as cerebral palsy, craniofacial anomalies, and mental retar-

Ask your audiology professor about alternatives to aided audiograms.

Noise is unwanted sound — it can be anything from a conversation in the hallway outside your door to the hum of a heating unit.

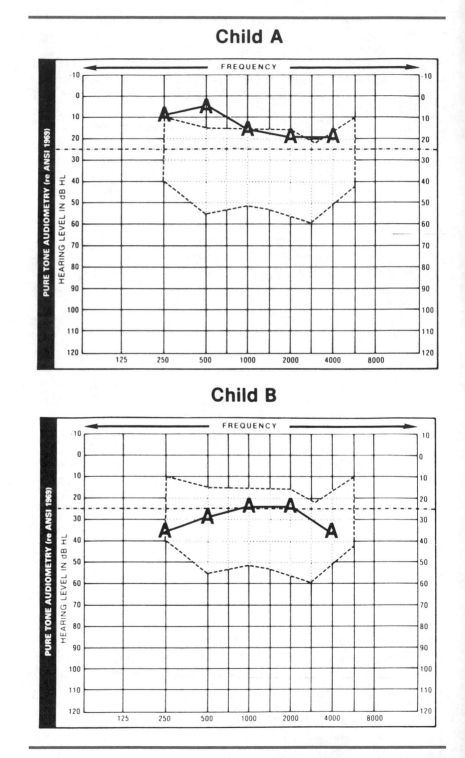

Figure 17-4. Aided audiograms for example cases described as Child A and Child B. Audiogram form reprinted from "Audiological Evaluation of the Mainstreamed Hearing-Impaired Child" by J. R. Madell, 1990, *Hearing-Impaired Children in the Mainstream* edited by M. Ross, 1990. Copyright 1990 by York Press, Inc. Reprinted by permission.

dation. They may also include problems such as cardiac irregularities that result in prolonged hospitalization and/or may be life-threatening. In such instances, we sometimes see an indirect affect on communication skill. We may also see a direct effect on parents' perceptions of the importance of communication skill deficits.

REASONS FOR SPEECH AND LANGUAGE ASSESSMENT

As is true for the other groups of children that you are studying, it is common for parents to request evaluation because of concerns that a child's communication skills are different from those of other children. This is often the reason that a child's hearing loss is first identified.

Another common reason for assessment is to determine the direction of treatment and/or to monitor progress. For the child who is hard of hearing, treatment may take many forms, including one-on-one sessions focusing on the development of speech articulation or language skills, group discussion of strategies used to cope with communication breakdown, and provision of assistive listening devices for the classroom. In many instances, the breadth of the questions posed will require that a team of teachers and clinicians gather data and consider solutions.

PLANNING THE ASSESSMENT PROTOCOL

Children who are hard of hearing often demonstrate communication skills like those of younger children who have normal hearing. Thus, we can use many of the same strategies for both groups. Indeed, the questions that we need to answer and the instruments that we use will often be identical. The primary purpose of this part of the chapter is to identify the ways that protocols must be modified to meet the special needs of children who are hard of hearing.

Team Approach

Children who have hearing losses are often followed by a team of professionals with special skills in the areas of hearing loss and/or education. Members typically include speech-language pathologists, audiologists, teachers specializing in hearing impairment, otologists, psychologists, and classroom teachers. Other support personnel such as reading specialists may also be involved. As you begin to outline an assessment battery, you need to consider what information will be available from the other members of the team and which pieces of the puzzle the team will be expecting you to add.

Environment

When selecting and arranging the room in which you will work, it is important to provide for good transmission of acoustic information. Noise levels must be low. Something as simple as the fan used to cool the room on a hot June day can have a tremendous impact on a child's ability to communicate.

Lighting must be appropriate for transmission of visual cues. The light should be on your face. Avoid sitting in front of a window. If the light source is behind you, your face will be in shadow, making it difficult for the child to speechread. Be sure that the chairs are positioned so that the child does not have to twist or turn to get a good view of your face.

Hearing Aids and Other Assistive Listening Devices

Many children who have hearing losses wear hearing aids. If they do, it is essential to check the hearing aids before beginning an evaluation. Do not assume that, because parents and teachers believe that the evaluation is important, they will ensure that the hearing aids are functioning properly. Equipment does not always cooperate. For example, Elfenbein, Bentler, Davis, and Niebuhr (1988) discovered that 10% of children who were aided monaurally and 52% of children who were aided binaurally arrived for a day-long psychoeducational and communication skill evaluation with a malfunctioning hearing aid.

Options for dealing with hearing aid malfunction will vary, depending on the setting in which you work. If you work with an audiologist, you may be able to obtain a loaner hearing aid of the same make and model that the child wears. If you are doing end-of-the-year assessment in a school system, you may be able to juggle your schedule and work with a child whose hearing aids are functioning. In some instances, you may decide to proceed under less-than-ideal conditions such as having a child who uses two hearing aids wear only one. Be sure to document such situations in your report.

Children often use FM amplification systems, sometimes called "auditory trainers," in their classrooms. Such devices are used to combat the problems created by noise, reverberation, and distance between the student and teacher. When using these devices, the teacher wears a microphone and transmitter that sends her voice via radio waves to a receiver worn on the student's belt. The signal is then routed from the receiver to the child's ear using one of a variety of available schemes. Although it is important to know if such equipment is used in the classroom, it is not necessary to use this equipment during an evaluation conducted in the type of environment described earlier. An exception to this would be a child who uses an FM system rather than a hearing aid as primary amplification.

Communication Modality

Although most children described as hard of hearing use speech as their primary means of communication, there are other possibilities. A girl who has a moderate hearing loss and lives with parents who are deaf may use American Sign Language (ASL) as her first language. A boy who has a moderate hearing loss and severe dysarthria may use speech for receptive communication and some type of language board to express himself.

Multicultural Factors

As noted elsewhere in this book, especially in Chapter 2, clinicians must be sensitive to cultural differences among the families with whom they work. Members of different cultural groups may have markedly different views about the causes of disabilities and the nature of appropriate treatment procedures. These must be understood before we can help the family make plans for diagnosis and treatment.

Children who are hard of hearing may have a strong link to Deaf culture if their parents identify themselves as Deaf. Although the Hearing culture and many of the parents with whom we work view hearing loss as a pathology, some parents, especially those who are Deaf, do not.

Many clinicians are familiar with manually coded English (MCE) systems such as Signed English (Bornstein, Saulnier, & Hamilton, 1983) and Signing Exact English (Gustason, Pfetzing, & Zawolkow, 1980). When working with families who communicate using ASL, it is important to remember that ASL and English are different languages. Although it is possible to adapt MCE skills for some social interactions, an interpreter is needed for information exchange.

> The capitalized term Deaf refers to individuals who belong to a cultural group that shares a signed language (Humphries, 1993).

Test Administration Procedures

A child who is hard of hearing presents a unique combination of communication needs and experiences that will likely require some adaptation of test administration. First, the child needs time to scan the pictures or other materials before auditory stimuli are presented. You do not want the child's attention divided between your face and the table top. Second, the child who has a hearing loss may be more alert to visual cues than a child who has normal hearing. Be careful not to provide subtle cues such as glancing at the correct response after stimulus presentation. Third, children who are hard of hearing often misunderstand or are misunderstood. If you request repetition, the child may interpret this as a need to change the response. Be prepared to score the child's first response. Fourth, hearing loss can affect the child's perception of test stimuli. When possible, you will probably want to select instruments that permit repetition. You may also elect to modify standard administration procedures. If you choose the latter option, be sure to document the modification and weigh its impact as you interpret the data.

Assessment Battery

Much of the information covered in the previous chapters of this book is directly applicable to work with a child who is hard of hearing. You need to devise a combination of formal and informal evaluation strategies that will provide data to answer the specific diagnostic questions that you delineate for each child.

Parent Interview

The approach that you use for other parent interviews can serve as the basic framework for this interview, too. Questions such as those about the types of treatment/communication approaches that have been used, types of classroom placement, names of clinicians and teachers, and progress seen by the parents all provide important information. You may find that the school and the parents employ different approaches to communication. Perhaps a child is in a preschool program that focuses on audition without speechreading, but uses audition plus speechreading at home. A child whose family has moved often may have been exposed to a wide range of approaches.

You will need to add questions that provide you with information about the hearing loss, such as etiology (if known), age at identification, any changes in the loss, names of the physician and audiologist who are following the child, and the date and results of the last audiologic evaluation. Information is also needed about any amplification used. For example, what was/is the age aided, type of amplification used at home, type of amplification used at school, name of the audiologist or hearing aid dealer who fit the device(s)? These data will help you determine what sort of speech signal the child has received in the past and is currently receiving.

Child Interview

Children are often excellent sources of information about their communication skills and deficits. Not only can they pinpoint specific problem areas, they can also identify those that they would most like to change. When we work with young children, it is possible to motivate change with praise or tangible reinforcement. As ages increases, it becomes more and more important that the children work to make changes because they value the change.

Depending on your relationship with the child, you may choose to begin the assessment with a formal interview or elect to wait until you have gained rapport through play or other activities. One of the best approaches is simply to ask the child questions about whether she has problems being understood or understanding others, when these situations occur, how she feels in these situations, what she feels the causal factors are, and what she does when she encounters communication breakdown. Children who are hard of hearing are usually quite candid about the impact of communication skill deficits on classroom, family, and social interactions.

An example of a guidesheet for assessing students' understanding of classroom interactions is shown in Figure 17-5. Similar sorts of questions can be asked about a child's interactions at the dinner table or a scout troop meeting.

Auditory Perception

Audiologists are often responsible for determining what information a child can obtain from a speech signal presented without visual cues. How-

---

A Guidesheet to Assess Student's Knowledge of Classroom Interaction

---

Instructions: You know all about our class by now, but a new student might need some help. Please answer the following questions. We will use your answers to help new students learn about our class.

---

1. Write down exactly what happens in this class on most days. Be sure to explain what happens first, second, next, and so on.

2. Write down the important rules in this class and explain WHY we have each rule.

3. Describe your teacher. Tell what your teacher is like so the new student will get to know this person.

4. Tell WHERE the teacher usually stands when he or she wants everyone to pay attention. Tell WHAT the teacher usually says or does first to get the students' attention.

5. Tell what makes the teacher mad so the new student will not get into trouble with the teacher.

6. Explain the homework system. This will be helpful to the new student:
   (a) How do you find out what the homework is?
   (b) How do you remember what books or papers to take home?
   (c) How do you remember to bring your homework back to school?

7. Tell what is hardest for you in this class. (It might be hard for the new student also.)

8. Tell what YOU do when you do not understand something in this class.

9. How is reading group different from whole class discussion? Tell as many differences as you can.

10. Can you think of anything else the new student should know about this class?

Figure 17-5. A guidesheet for assessing students' knowledge of classroom interaction. From "Assessment Issues for Three Aspects of School Communication" by S. Tattershall, and L. Kretschmer, 1988. *Journal of the Academy of Rehabilitative Audiology (JARA)* Monograph XXI. Copyright 1988 by *JARA.* Reprinted with permission.

ever, speech-language pathologists may consult regarding test selection and/or administer some tests.

When these tests are conducted in sound booths, the level of the test signal can be closely monitored and it is an easy matter to eliminate visual cues. However, when auditory perception is assessed via live voice in a treatment room, a different approach must be taken. If you ask the child to turn away from you, the microphone on the hearing aid will also move, thus creating a shadow effect that will reduce the intensity of the speech signal. The solution is to cover your face. This is best done with a speaker mesh screen of the type shown in Figure 17-6. Using a book or a piece of card-

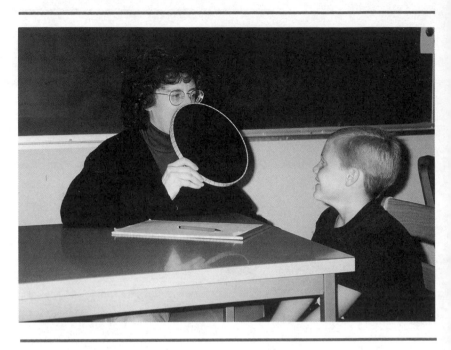

Figure 17-6. Assessment of auditory perception using a speaker mesh screen to mask speechreading cues.

board will likely reduce the high-frequency components of your speech and confound your data (Niday & Elfenbein, 1991).

When selecting instruments to assess auditory perception, it is important to keep other aspects of the child's communication skills in mind. If the vocabulary and syntax levels of test items are too difficult for the child, it will not be possible to determine whether errors reflect deficits in perceptual abilities, language skills or some combination of the two. The child's speech skills also need to be considered. Some auditory perceptual tasks require that the child repeat stimulus items. If the child is not able to say the test items, you will not know if they were heard correctly. For example, if a child often deletes /t/ in word final position and the stimulus item is "beet," does the response "bee" indicate that he didn't hear the final /t/?

A good example of an instrument that can provide you with data about a wide range of auditory perceptual skills is the *Test of Auditory Comprehension* (TAC) (Trammell, Farrar, Francis, Owens, Shepard, Thies, Witlin, & Faist, 1976). Its 10 subtests, outlined in Figure 17-7, provide tasks as basic as discrimination of speech from environmental sounds and tasks as complex as comprehending a story told in background noise. Because normative data are provided by age and degree of hearing loss, it is possible not only to determine a child's strengths and weaknesses, but also to compare the child to age peers with the same degree of loss.

Subtests of the Test of Auditory Comprehension	
Subtest	Description
One	Discriminates between linguistic and nonlinguistic sounds
Two	Discriminates between linguistic, human nonlinguistic, and environmental sounds
Three	Discriminates between stereotypic messages
Four	Discriminates between single-element core-noun vocabulary presented in a sentence
Five	Recalls two critical elements from a sentence
Six	Recalls four critical elements from a sentence
Seven	Sequences three events from a story
Eight	Recalls five details from a story
Nine	Sequences three events from a story presented with a competing message
Ten	Recalls five details from a story presented with a competing message

Figure 17-7. Subtests from the *Test of Auditory Comprehension*. Adapted from *The Test of Auditory Comprehension* by J. Trammell et al., 1976. North Hollywood, CA. Foreworks.

Oral Mechanism

It is easy for clinicians to see a child with a hearing loss as a set of ears and attribute all of the child's communication problems to the hearing loss. Be sure to consider all possibilities. The child could have mild craniofacial anomalies that have not yet been detected or may be in need of referral for dental care.

Speech Production

Most children who are hard of hearing demonstrate speech articulation skills that reflect the acoustic signal they receive. Table 17-1 shows data by manner of production for three groups of children ages 5–18 years who have different degrees of bilateral sensorineural hearing loss. Beyond the normal developmental patterns of speech sound acquisition, these children demonstrate the greatest problem with fricatives and affricates. This is consistent with the nature of the speech signal that they hear. Substitutions and oral distortions are the most common errors with the numbers of omissions increasing as hearing loss increases. Errors in the production of vowels are not expected.

Children who are hard of hearing may present with some hoarseness, pharyngeal resonance, and hyper- or hyponasality. They typically do not

Table 17-1. Articulation test performance (percent correct) of three groups of children who are hard of hearing.[a]

Group[b]	Nasals		Stops		Glides		Affricates		Fricatives	
	X̄	SD	X̄	SD	X̄	SD	X̄	SD	X̄	SD
<45 dB HL	98.07	6.93	93.58	12.59	96.15	9.38	91.02	8.64	77.92	17.61
45–60 dB HL	96.87	7.21	96.52	7.28	89.84	14.59	73.95	27.86	73.09	20.33
61–88 dB HL	98.86	3.76	96.96	5.75	82.62	14.24	68.18	26.30	73.27	13.38

[a] *Note:* Adapted from "Oral Communication Skills of Hard of Hearing Children" by J. Elfenbein, M. Hardin-Jones, and J. Davis, 1994. *Journal of Speech and Hearing Research, 37.* Copyright 1994 by Journal of Speech and Hearing Research. Adapted by permission.
[b] Pure-tone-average for the better ear.

demonstrate the severe problems with phonation, speech rate, intelligibility, pitch control, and vocal quality demonstrated by children who are deaf.

Speech production is usually assessed with the same speech articulation tests used with children who have normal hearing. However, some sets of target words and elicitation phrases may contain vocabulary items or syntactic structures that are too difficult for some children. One common solution is to attempt to elicit the target through imitation. This may be effective in some instances, but there is also a possibility that children will have difficulty hearing the phonemes that you are asking them to imitate. An alternative is to substitute a word or elicitation phrase that is appropriate to the child's language skill level.

As is often the case with children who are normally hearing, a child's speech skills at the word level may be quite different from those in conversational speech. If the formal test used includes only word or sentence level tasks, it is important to obtain a conversational sample for comparison.

Sit in on a class discussion or an indoor recess period to obtain a sample of typical speech production patterns.

Language Skills

The language skills of children who are hard of hearing also reflect the deficits that exist in the acoustic input they receive (Davis, Elfenbein, Schum, & Bentler, 1986; Elfenbein, Hardin-Jones, & Davis, 1994). For example, children who have bilateral mild, moderate or severe sensorineural hearing losses often demonstrate vocabulary skills that lag behind those of their normally hearing peers. Words that have multiple meanings and idioms are particularly difficult. These children also have difficulty learning the use of morphological endings and complex syntax structures — tasks that require information coded in high-frequency and/or unstressed components of the English language. They do not, however, typically demonstrate the severe receptive and expressive language skill deficits often demonstrated by children who are deaf.

As with the assessment of speech skills, instruments used with normally hearing children are also used with children who are hard of hearing.

In most cases these are appropriate. However, you need to consider how the type of task can affect the child's performance. As was noted during the discussion of auditory perception, imitation tasks combine perception and production. You may want to combine the two or you may not. If you want to evaluate production without the influence of perception, select a different approach.

As you develop your own cache of assessment tools, you may want to borrow from other disciplines. For example, the *KeyMath Diagnostic Arithmetic Test* (Connolly, Nachtman, & Pritchett, 1971) is useful in evaluating a child's ability to apply language skills to an academic task. The same basic math concepts are evaluated in simple computation problems and in word problems. Data from tasks such as these can be helpful in explaining the impact of language skill deficits to educators, parents, and the children, themselves.

Language is the key to academic success.

Speechreading

For the child who is hard of hearing, speechreading is considered to be a supplement to audition, not a substitute. Traditional speechreading tests for children were not developed from this perspective. In light of this, clinicians who gather information about speechreading often design their own bisensory evaluations. For example, some compare message comprehension when both auditory and visual cues are available to message comprehension when only auditory cues are available. Others vary environmental factors such as background noise to simulate different real-world listening situations.

If you choose to design your own task, you will need to use the child's language skills as a guide for devising test messages. Language skills are a key factor in the top-down processing required to speechread. As you analyze your data, do not focus simply on the number of words the child can correctly identify. Determining whether the child can gather the gist of the message and what types of strategies she employs when she does not understand may provide a better idea of how speechreading affects the child's daily interaction. For example, does she ask for repetition, change position to improve angle for speechreading, or turn down background noise?

INTERPRETING FINDINGS

Data From Other Team Members

Data from other specialists may be shared in many ways. If weeks elapse between evaluations, you may receive formal written reports. When a child is evaluated by several individuals on the same day, information may be exchanged informally as it is gathered or at a formal staffing. Whatever the format of the discussion, speech-language pathologists need to be familiar with the terminology and procedures used by their colleagues.

Take advantage of the resources around you. Ask other professionals about the work they do.

Remember that each team member holds pieces of the puzzle that you are trying to solve together. Otologists can provide information about the medical status of the auditory system and any medical treatment planned. Psychologists and teachers can provide information about cognitive abilities, learning patterns, academic achievement, and psychosocial skills. With the addition of data from the speech-language pathologist and the audiologist, the big picture will begin to form.

Analyzing Your Data

In most instances, you will be using instruments that provide normative data only for normally hearing children. This is certainly a relevant comparison group, because children who are hard of hearing must function in classroom and social situations geared to the skill levels of their normally hearing peers. For example, a child whose vocabulary is 2 years behind that of his classmates is going to be at a marked disadvantage in a class discussion.

Be wary of normative samples of children with hearing loss that include children with a broad range of degree of hearing loss and little or no information about the presence of additional disabilities. There is little to be gained by comparing a child's performance to data from such a heterogeneous group.

When you do use instruments that provide normative data delineated by age and degree of hearing loss, take advantage of the opportunity to put a child's performance in perspective. For example, the data may show that although the child's skills are poorer than those of children with normal hearing, his skills are average relative to children with the same degree of hearing loss.

There may be situations in which you choose not to focus on comparison to normative data. When a child is known to be performing far behind his normally hearing peers, it may be more helpful both to you and the parents to analyze the child's performance in terms of developmental patterns seen in his skills rather than as a percentile rank relative to his age group.

It is also helpful to compare a child's communication skills to performance on academic achievement measures. Communication skill strengths and weaknesses often explain patterns of strength and weakness in academic performance. For example, data that show differences in a child's auditory perception in quiet and in noise can be used to explain differences between a child's ability to communicate one-on-one at the teacher's desk and participate in group discussions while seated next to a cage full of gerbils racing their exercise wheels. In much the same way, patterns of academic performance may provide indications for the direction of treatment.

Parent Conference

The primary focus of a parent conference is to discuss how the information you have gathered answers the questions that led to the evaluation. Our role is to sort through the data and develop a description of the problem. This must then be presented to the parents, along with treatment options. The goal is to provide them with the foundation they need to make informed decisions.

When assessment is for the purpose of diagnosing hearing loss and associated communication skill problems, it is important to remember that such situations trigger a variety of emotions in family members. Anxiety is common. It is not enough to be able to identify the emotions. Clinicians need to develop strategies for helping clients deal with them. For example, if parents are anxious about their abilities to meet the challenges of raising a child who is hard of hearing, we can reassure them that we are there to help and that we have suggestions for how to begin (Schum, 1986).

Monograph No. 9, in the NSSLHA series (Schum, 1986), is an excellent resource for information about counseling.

When counseling families about a child's progress in treatment, it is easy to slip into a pattern of reporting a series of percentile ranks and age-equivalents that indicate that the child who is hard of hearing is behind age peers. If the question was "Is continued treatment necessary?" such data may support the answer. However, if the gap between what is expected and what the child is doing persists, it will be more productive to focus on progress made, indicators of the next step to be taken, and the relationships that exist between communication skills, psychosocial development, and academic achievement.

Child Conference

Whether the child participates in the discussion of assessment findings generally depends on age. School-age children should receive direct feedback about the session. Although parents may discuss your findings with their child, the child also needs the opportunity to discuss the results directly with you.

One of the topics often discussed by parents and clinicians is the need to foster independence in children with hearing losses. A clinician-child conference makes the child an active participant in the treatment process. It also provides for information transfer through a neutral party. A child may view parents' concerns about her communication skills in the same way she views their concerns about her bedroom cleaning habits.

In some instances you will find a need to meet with the parents and the child separately. In others, the entire conference can be conducted with the family as a whole, or you can meet with the parents first and then invite the child to join you. The information that you gather during the evaluation process will help you determine the need for private meetings.

OTHER RESOURCES

Student clinicians interested in working with children who have hearing losses will find that information on this topic is available from a wide variety of sources. The additional readings section at the end of this chapter provides a list of selected books, journals, and organizations that will be useful as you explore rehabilitative audiology. Although many of the titles include only the word "deaf," you will find that they also have information to offer about the child who is hard of hearing.

SUMMARY

Most children who are hard of hearing develop communication skills more like those of peers who are normally hearing than who are deaf. As a result, the approach taken to assessment of communication skill development is much like that used with children who have normal hearing. This chapter provided general guidelines for making decisions about the types of skills to assess and ways to modify standard evaluation procedures to limit the impact of hearing loss on the evaluation process. Clinicians will need to adapt these guidelines to the needs of individual children. For each child, factors such as age of onset of the hearing loss, degree of the hearing loss, history of (re)habilitative services, the presence of additional disabilities, and family support will combine to affect the development of communication skills.

REFERENCES

Bornstein, H., Saulnier, K., & Hamilton, L. (1983). *The comprehensive signed English dictionary.* Washington, DC: Gallaudet University Press.

Connolly, A., Nachtman, W., & Pritchett, E. (1971). *KeyMath Diagnostic Arithmetic Test.* Circle Pines, MN: American Guidance Service.

Davis, J., Elfenbein, J., Schum, R., & Bentler, R. (1986). Effects of mild and moderate hearing impairments on language educational, and psycho-social behavior of children. *Journal of Speech and Hearing Disorders, 51*(1), 53–62.

Elfenbein, J., Bentler, R., Davis, J., & Niebuhr, D. (1988). Status of school children's hearing aids relative to monitoring practices. *Ear and Hearing, 9*, 212–217.

Elfenbein, J., Hardin-Jones, M., & Davis, J. (1994). Oral communication skills of hard of hearing children. *Journal of Speech and Hearing Research, 37*, 216–226.

Finitzo-Hieber, T., & Tillman, T. (1978). Room acoustics effects on monosyllabic word discrimination ability for normal and hearing-impaired children. *Journal of Speech and Hearing Research, 21*, 440–458.

Gallaudet University Center for Assessment and Demographic Studies (1992). *1991–1992 Annual Survey of Hearing-Impaired Children and Youth.* Washington, DC: Gallaudet University.

Gustason, G., Pfetzing, D., & Zawolkow, E. (1980). *Signing exact English.* Los Alamitos, CA: Modern Sign Press.

Hawkins, D. (1988). Options in classroom amplification. In F. Bess (Ed.), *Hearing impairment in children* (pp. 253–265). Parkton, MD: York Press.

Humphries, T. (1993). Deaf cultures and culture. In K. Christensen & G. Delgado (Eds.), *Multicultural issues in deafness.* White Plains, NY: Longman.

Madell, J. R. (1990). Audiological evaluation of the mainstreamed hearing-impaired child. In M. Ross (Ed.), *Hearing-impaired children in the mainstream* (pp. 27–44). Parkton, MD: York Press.

Niday, K., & Elfenbein, J. (1991). The effects of visual barriers used during auditory training on sound transmission. *Journal of Speech and Hearing Research, 34*, 694–696.

Ross, M. (1990). Definitions and descriptions. In J. Davis (Ed.), *Our forgotten children: Hard of hearing pupils in the schools.* Washington, DC: Self Help for Hard of Hearing People, Inc.

Ross, M., Brackett, D., & Maxon, A. (1991). *Assessment and management of mainstreamed hearing-impaired children.* Austin, TX: Pro-Ed.

Schum, R. (1986). *Counseling in speech and hearing practice* (Clinical series 9). Rockville, MD: National Student Speech, Language, and Hearing Association.

Tattershall, S., Kretschmer, L., & Kretschmer, R. (1988). Assessment issues for three aspects of school communication. In R. Kretschmer & L. Kretschmer (Eds.), Communication assessment of hearing impaired children from conversation to classroom. *Journal of the Academy of Rehabilitative Audiology, 21*(Monograph Suppl.), 173–197.

Trammell, J., Farrar, C., Francis, J., Owens, S., Shepard, D., Thies, T., Witlin, R., & L. Faist. (1976). *Test of Auditory Comprehension.* North Hollywood, CA: Foreworks.

RECOMMENDED READINGS

Books/Monographs

Bradley-Johnson, S., & Evans, L. (1991). Psychoeducational assessment of hearing-impaired students. Austin, TX: Pro-Ed.

Butler, K. G. (Ed.). (1989). Communicative competence of hearing impaired students: Implications for assessment and learning. *Topics in Language Disorders, 9*(4).

Christensen, K. M., & Delgado, G. L. (1993). *Multicultural issues in deafness.* White Plains, NY: Longman.

Davis, J. (1990). *Our forgotten children: Hard-of-hearing pupils in the schools.* Washington, DC: Self Help for Hard of Hearing People, Inc.

Krestchmer, R. R., & Krestchmer, L. W. (1988). Communication assessment of hearing-impaired children: From conversation to classroom. *Academy of Rehabilitative Audiology, 21*(Monograph, Suppl.).

Ross, M., Brackett, D., & Maxon, A. B (1991). *Assessment and management of mainstreamed hearing-impaired children: Principles and practices.* Austin, TX: Pro-Ed.

Thompson, M., Biro, P., Vethivelu, S., Pious, C., & Hatfield, N. (1987). *Language assessment of hearing impaired school age children.* Seattle, WA: University of Washington Press.

Journals

American Annals of the Deaf
American Journal of Audiology
Ear and Hearing
Journal of the American Academy of Audiology
Journal of the Academy of Rehabilitative Audiology
Journal of Communication Disorders
Journal of Speech and Hearing Disorders
Journal of Speech and Hearing Research
Language Speech and Hearing Services in the Schools
Seminars in Hearing
Seminars in Speech and Language
Topics in Language Disorders
Volta Review

ORGANIZATIONS

Academy of Rehabilitative Audiology
c/o Judy Abrahamson
Olin E. Teague Veterans' Center
Audiology/Speech Pathology
Temple, TX 76504

Alexander Graham Bell Association for the Deaf
34117 Volta Place, NW
Washington, D.C. 20007

American Speech-Language-Hearing Association
10801 Rockville Pike
Rockville, MD 20852

Educational Audiology Association
c/o Peggy Von Almen
Utah State University
Department of Communicative Disorders
Logan, UT 84322-1000

National Center for Information on Deafness
Gallaudet University
800 Florida Avenue, NE
Washington, DC 20002

Self Help for Hard of Hearing People, Inc.
7800 Wisconsin Avenue
Bethesda, MD 20814

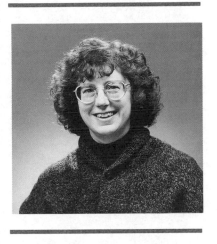

JILL L. ELFENBEIN, Ph.D.

M.A. 1975, University of Iowa
Ph.D. 1986, University of Iowa

Dr. Elfenbein is an Assistant Professor in the Department of Speech
Pathology and Audiology, The University of Iowa, with clinical
teaching and research emphasis in rehabilitative audiology. She holds
the ASHA Certificate of Clinical Competence in both Audiology and
Speech-Language Pathology. Her work experience also includes school
and hospital positions.

CHAPTER

18

The Child
Who Is Deaf

Nancy Tye-Murray, Ph.D.

Parents react in many different ways when an audiologist tells them that their baby has a severe or profound hearing impairment. One common reaction is for parents to say, "O.K., we'll get hearing aids for her, and she can learn to lipread us." They assume hearing aids and lipreading lessons can make the hearing loss inconsequential. Unless the parents know some-one who has had a significant hearing impairment from birth, they may not realize initially that their child's speech development, language acquisition, conversational skills, and academic and social achievement will likely differ from what is common for children with normal hearing. Parents may become aware of these consequences only gradually, as they receive counseling from speech and hearing professionals and as they acquire many months and even years of firsthand experience in watching their child grow. They will also learn to appreciate the long-term commitments that will be required of them, the child, other members of their family, and the child's school system for the child to realize her full potential.

At this stage of your training, you too may be unfamiliar with how a hearing impairment affects children's speech and language development. The purpose of this chapter is to introduce you to these and related issues. The first section describes children's hearing capabilities and then reviews some of their speech and language problems. In the second section, we

Hearing impairment affects almost every aspect of a child's cognitive and social development.

consider your role as a speech-language pathologist. The third section focuses on procedures for assessing speech and language skills, with the final section focusing on procedures for assessing auditory and speechreading training needs.

Before we begin, a few terms must be defined. A child who has a *severe* hearing impairment cannot hear sounds presented at a level softer than 70 dB HL. A child with a *profound* hearing impairment cannot hear sounds presented at a level softer than 90 dB HL. Persons who are *prelingually* hearing-impaired had their hearing impairment when they were learning language and speech. They may have been born with a hearing impairment (in which case they have a *congenital* hearing impairment) or they may have lost their hearing early in life, perhaps as a result of meningitis, high fever, or head trauma. As we will learn, these persons often require assistance from a speech-language pathologist. Persons who have *postlingual* hearing loss had normal or nearly normal hearing when they were learning language and speech. They then lost their hearing in late childhood or adulthood. Typically, these people speak intelligibly and have normal language patterns, especially if they incurred their hearing loss as adults. Most persons with postlingual hearing losses will not seek your services. In this chapter, we are concerned only with prelingual hearing losses.

DESCRIPTION OF CHILDREN WHO HAVE SEVERE AND PROFOUND HEARING IMPAIRMENTS

The next order of business is to consider the hearing capabilities of children who have severe and profound hearing impairments and then to consider some of their common speech and language problems.

Hearing and Speech Recognition Skills

By understanding what is heard by a child with a severe and profound hearing impairment, you can better select appropriate therapy objectives and teaching methods. For example, if you know a child cannot hear you or himself speak, you will probably rely more on visual and tactile aids to teach articulation and less on auditory modeling.

As Figure 18-1 illustrates, many different audiometric configurations fall under the rubric of severe and profound hearing impairments. For instance, the child denoted by the letter "A" in Figure 18-1 has a severe hearing loss. He has some hearing across a wide range of frequencies (250 Hz to 8000 Hz). With appropriate amplification, Child A may recognize some speech auditorily and may be able to speechread (i.e., recognize speech when using hearing and vision simultaneously) very well. This child may also hear many of his own speech sounds while talking, such as the vowel segments (which tend to be louder than consonants) and consonants that have high amplitude, such as the nasals /m/ and /n/. He will likely hear the rhythm and prosody of his own speech.

Child B, also represented in Figure 18-1, has a profound hearing impairment. Like many people with profound impairments, she is not com-

Children who have severe and profound hearing impairments are a heterogeneous group: They vary widely in their receptive and expressive communication skills.

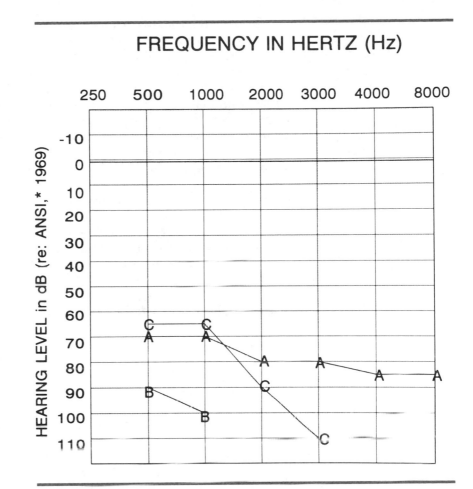

FREQUENCY IN HERTZ (Hz)

Figure 18-1. Audiometric configurations for three different types of hearing impairments. Letters indicate the level at which a threshold was obtained. Child A has a severe hearing impairment, Child B has a profound hearing impairment, and Child C has a severe-to-profound hearing impairment.

pletely deaf. She has some measurable hearing in the low frequencies (250 and 500 Hz). This child will probably not recognize any speech auditorily. She may or may not be a good speechreader. Her speechreading skill will depend on a number of factors. For example, visual speech recognition is determined in part by innate talent, and she may be either a naturally good or a naturally poor speechreader. Using residual hearing, she might listen to prosodic cues and recognize when one word ends and the next word begins. (When speechreading, a little bit of residual hearing can provide a great deal of benefit.) Finally, if she has ample vocabulary and knowledge of grammar, she will be able to "fill in" words she cannot speechread. For instance, if she speechreads the sentence, "The salt and _____ are on the table," she might be able to guess the word, "pepper." Child B will hear little if any of her own speech; she may only hear some rhythmic cues.

Many children have a combined severe and profound hearing impairment. Their hearing typically is better in the low frequencies than the high frequencies. For example, Child C in Figure 18-1 has a "sloping" hearing impairment. This child will hear some words auditorily. His listening skills will appear to be more inconsistent than those of Child A or B. Because he has some hearing in the low frequencies, he will often detect the presence of speech and recognize some words. However, because much of the acoustic information that distinguishes one word from another is contained in the mid and high frequencies, he often will not discriminate the words even though he seems to hear them. Thus, his family and teachers (and even you) may sometimes accuse him of "not listening" or "not paying attention." Child C may have reasonably good speechreading skills and he probably will hear the rhythm and prosody of his voice while speaking. He will not hear many of his own consonant productions, particularly sounds that have high frequency information, such as /s, t/. He may hear his own vowel productions but they may all sound similar to him.

Speech Characteristics

When describing the speech of children with severe and profound hearing impairments, we usually talk about overall intelligibility, segmental errors (errors in the sounds of speech), and suprasegmental errors (errors in speech rhythm and prosody). As a general rule, children with more residual hearing will speak better and produce fewer segmental and suprasegmental errors than children with less residual hearing. However, how well a child speaks also depends on numerous other factors, including the speech therapy received, motivation to speak, the consistency of appropriate amplification use, the age of first receiving hearing aids, and the child's speech environment. For example, is speech heard often? Do those around the youngster provide a good speech model? Is reinforcement provided when the child tries to speak?

Overall Intelligibility

Most children with profound hearing impairments are difficult to understand. On average, you will rarely identify more than 20% of the words they say. Intelligibility deficits are a recalcitrant problem. You will have as much difficulty understanding the speech of an adult with a profound hearing impairment as a 7-year-old child, even if the adult has received many years of speech therapy.

Segmental Errors

Children with hearing impairments produce many segmental errors, both when speaking vowels and diphthongs and when speaking consonants. Children most commonly neutralize vowels, so the phrase *see you* might sound like "sa ya." They also substitute one vowel for another. Other vowel errors include diphthongization (the word *pot* may sound like "poat"), prolongation, and nasalization. Diphthongs may sound distorted or sound like a single vowel.

Consonantal errors include voiced/voiceless confusions, substitutions, omissions, distortions, and errors in consonant clusters. For example, a child with a hearing impairment might intend to speak the word *boat*, but actually say "poe." In this production, the youngster has substituted the voiceless /p/ for the voiced /b/ and omitted the final /t/ sound. As you acquire experience in working with children who are hearing impaired, you will realize that many children produce consonants that are visible on the face more accurately than consonants that are not visible. For instance, a child is more likely to produce the word *pat* correctly than the word *cat*. The /p/ entails visible lip closure, whereas the tongue dorsum closing gesture for /k/ cannot be seen. Apparently, a child with a significant hearing impairment relies heavily on visual information for acquiring speech.

Suprasegmental Errors

You may find that the speech of your clients with hearing impairments sounds *breathy, labored, staccato,* and *arhythmic.* Many such children place equal stress on all syllables or stress words inappropriately. They speak very slowly, pausing often. They may not coarticulate sounds in the same way as normally hearing talkers. For instance, a child might say the word *basket* as "ba-a-sa-ka-a-ta." In this production, the child has articulated each sound as if it were an isolated unit.

You may rate your children's voice quality as unpleasant. Their pitch may sound excessively high or variable. Pitch breaks, with pitch abruptly changing from high to low, are common. Children may speak too softly or too loudly and often their intensity will fluctuate inappropriately.

In light of the many segmented and suprasegmental errors, it is not surprising that so many children with severe hearing impairments have extremely poor intelligibility. When these speech problems coexist with language problems, communication becomes difficult indeed.

Language

The majority of persons with profound hearing impairments use one of three modes to communicate: American Sign Language (ASL), manually coded English, and spoken language. Before we consider problems of language, let us consider the three communication modes.

ASL is a manual system of communication. A person does not use ASL and speak at the same time. ASL has a different grammar than spoken English. One ASL sign might represent a concept that would require many English words to express. Facial expressions and body language can impart a variety of meanings to the signs.

As the name implies, manually coded English is comprised of manual signs corresponding to the words of English. It also has the same syntactic structures. Typically, the person who uses manually coded English speaks

Currently, there is a strong "Deaf Culture" movement. Persons who are a part of this movement advocate that children who have significant hearing impairments use ASL as their primary language and learn English as a second language.

simultaneously while signing. For instance, as a boy says, "The cat is inside," he will sign the article "the," and then one sign each for "cat," "is," and "inside." The combined use of sign and speech as an educational philosophy is referred to as *total communication*. The child will use every available means to receive a message, including sign, residual hearing, and lipreading.

Aural/oral language is the same language used by persons with normal hearing. The child with a hearing impairment who uses aural/oral language will speak messages and use speechreading to receive messages.

Regardless of which communication mode they use most frequently, most children who are profoundly hearing impaired do not learn the English language very well. One way to appreciate how hearing impairment affects language development is to compare normally hearing and hearing impaired groups. Beginning speech-language pathologists often become disheartened when they learn that 8-year-old normally hearing children have a better knowledge of grammar than do adults with profound hearing impairments. Moreover, most adults with hearing impairments never acquire a vocabulary better than that of a normally hearing fourth grader. Speech-language pathologists often categorize language difficulties as either problems of form (syntax and morphology), content (semantics and vocabulary), or pragmatics (use).

Form

The list comprising problems of form is extensive. Children with hearing impairments may overuse nouns and verbs and rarely use adverbs, prepositions, or pronouns. They may omit function words. Most of their sentences have a simple subject-verb-object structure, and their sentences have few words compared to those produced by normally hearing children. Compound or complex sentences are rare, as are morphemes that mark plurality or past tense. In telling a story about her cat, one child said, "Socks jump. Cup fall over. Mess big. Mom mad about Socks." In this narrative, the child omitted function words such as *was* and tense markers such as *-ed*. Her syntactic structures were very simple. Although the listener could probably follow her story, the sentences sound telegraphic.

Sometimes children order their words incorrectly. A child may say, "Saw cat big," meaning she saw a big cat.

Not only do they rarely speak compound or complex sentences, children with hearing impairments usually cannot interpret them when they speechread or read. For example, they often interpret sentences in the passive voice (*The cat was chased by the dog*) as though in the active tense (*The cat chased the dog*). They might interpret a nominal sentence (*The ending of the school year saddened the teacher*) objectively (*The school year saddened the teacher*).

Content

Perhaps one of the most pervasive language problems among children with hearing impairments is a restricted vocabulary. Children often learn only common everyday words. They may have gaps in their vocabularies, wherein they do not know words relating to an entire concept, such as outer space. Hence, words such as *planet, Martian, star, spaceman,* and *rocket* may all be unfamiliar. They often use words in limited ways. For instance, a child with a hearing impairment may use a word such as *happy* as a predicate (e.g., *The boy is happy*) but not as a modifier (e.g., *The happy boy is here*). Most children cannot identify synonyms and antonyms or understand idioms such as *She was mad as a hornet.*

Pragmatics

As you interact with a child with a hearing impairment, you might note that the child uses questions inappropriately. (For instance, one child's first question to a new acquaintance was, "How much does your husband make?") The child may not know how to initiate or maintain a conversation or know how to repair breakdowns in communication. In some circumstances, the child might nod and bluff, pretending to understand something. A child also may not know many of the social graces of conversation. For example, he may not know how to take turns while conversing, how to acknowledge that he has heard the message, and how to change the topic of conversation. Overall, the child probably will not use language functionally as well as his normally hearing peers.

There are at least three reasons why some children do not learn conversational pragmatics very well. First, they do not receive extensive practice in using language. Their unfamiliarity with many language structures and reduced vocabulary limit their ability to converse. Moreover, they have fewer conversational partners to interact with because few normally hearing persons know manually coded English or ASL. Another reason is children with hearing impairments cannot overhear their parents or other people talking. Thus, they do not receive the everyday, incidental models of how to use language. Finally, children with hearing impairments do not receive the same formal instruction as normally hearing children. For instance, a parent may carefully explain the rules of politeness to a child with normal hearing (do not interrupt; say "thank you"; let someone else say something). The parent may not explain the rules to her child with a hearing impairment, either because of the child's limited language or because of the parent's limited skill in using manually coded English or ASL.

Can you think of reasons why children who have hearing impairments may not use language very well?

Interim Summary

Children with severe and profound hearing impairments will present an array of speech and language problems. Their speech will be marred by segmental and suprasegmental errors. Few people will understand their speech. Their language will exhibit errors of form, content, and pragmatics. The children will use a reduced range of syntactic structures, they will omit or misuse morphemes, and they will have a restricted vocabulary. They may have difficulty in using language and participating in conversations.

THE ROLE OF THE SPEECH-LANGUAGE PATHOLOGIST

As a speech-language pathologist, you may play three important roles in the habilitation program of the child with a hearing impairment. These roles include: speech and language evaluation, speech-language and speech perception training, and consultation.

Evaluation

You will probably evaluate the child's speech production and language skills at the beginning and the end of his academic school year and perhaps on other occasions. You may also evaluate the child's need for auditory and speechreading training. The initial evaluation allows you to identify the child's specific strengths and weaknesses. This information can help you formulate therapy objectives and can also be used by the child's educational planning team. For instance, the test results may help the team decide whether the child should be placed in a mainstream classroom with a sign interpreter or a self-contained classroom with other children who are hearing impaired.

Your evaluation at the end of the school year will indicate if therapy objectives were achieved and if the child has progressed in speech and language skills. The test results might also help the educational planning team decide if the child should go to summer school.

Historically, most children with hearing impairments attended residential schools. Since the 1970s, more children remain in their home communities for their education.

Therapy

One of your roles will be to provide speech and language therapy to the child with a hearing impairment. Typically, school-aged children receive speech-language therapy two or more times per week, for about 30 minutes at each session.

Children usually receive formal auditory and speechreading training from a speech-language pathologist, although the child's classroom teacher or an audiologist occasionally provides this training, instead. *Auditory training* develops the child's ability to recognize speech using only audition. *Speechreading training* develops the child's ability to recognize speech by simultaneously listening and watching.

Consultation

You will frequently consult with a child's parents, teachers, audiologist, and other members of the child's educational planning team. One of your responsibilities is to provide general information. You can familiarize parents and teachers with a child's speech and language skills, and how the child's skills compare to those of other children. You can also describe how speech and language skills typically progress in normally hearing children and children with hearing impairments and factors that may accelerate progress. This information will help those who know the child to develop appropriate expectations. It also may provide them with ideas about how best to nurture their child's development.

You might recommend that parents and teachers view commercially available sign language video cassettes, participate in a weekly "sign group," and attend sign language classes.

You can help parents and teachers learn to speak and sign complete sentences. Many parents and teachers do not match their words to their signs when they use a total communication approach. A mother might say, "John, get in the car" and simultaneously sign the word "John" and then "car," without signing the verb and connecting words. This presents a poor language model. The child may only receive the message, "John car."

You will also suggest ways for helping the child to generalize what she has learned in therapy to more real-world settings by informing the parents and teachers about the child's current therapy objectives and suggesting practice materials. For example, you might send a list of vocabulary words home. A parent can practice the words with the child, perhaps in a flashcard game format. You can also observe the child in the classroom and then suggest ways in which the classroom teacher can integrate speech and language practice into the daily routine.

Finally, the audiologist might use your information about the child's language skills to help him select appropriate audiological tests. For instance, if your test results indicate the child has an extremely limited vocabulary, the audiologist will not evaluate the child's speech perception skills with recorded sentence lists.

Interim Summary

You will play three roles in providing services to a child with a hearing impairment. First, you will assess the child's speech and language skills and her need for auditory and speechreading training. Second, you will provide speech-language therapy and, often, auditory and speechreading training. Finally, you are an important resource for the classroom teacher, audiologist, the parents, and other members of the child's educational planning team. You provide information about the child's progress and suggest ways to nurture the youngster's development.

SPEECH AND LANGUAGE ASSESSMENT

In this section, we first review general principles to remember when assessing a child's speech and language. We then consider specific procedures.

General Principles

There are five general principles to keep in mind when assessing speech and language. First, children often use speech and language differently in one setting than another and they perform differently on varying tasks. For example, children are more likely to produce a sound correctly when they are imitating their speech-language pathologist than when they are telling a story to their classmates. For this reason, you should construct a profile of the child's speech and language proficiency from numerous formal and informal measures. In assessing speech, you might formally obtain an imitated speech sample consisting of isolated words and sentences, a citation speech sample ("Tell me the name of this picture") and a spontaneous sample of continuous speech. You might informally observe the child in therapy, in the classroom, and on the playground while he speaks to other children. By using a variety of speech tasks, you can determine how robust certain skills are and whether or not they have generalized to real-world settings. This information will help you plan therapy objectives and evaluate progress.

The second principle to remember is that the speech-language evaluation should be performed with the child's preferred mode of communication, such as manually coded English. If you do not know the child's sign system, get an interpreter. The child must understand the tasks and the test items if you are to obtain a true reflection of his speech and language skills.

Third, before formally evaluating a child, establish a rapport. You will find many children with hearing impairments are shy about using their voices, especially around strangers. If the child does not feel comfortable in your presence, he will not provide speech or language samples that represent his skills. (In fact, you may not receive samples at all!)

Fourth, select specific test procedures that are appropriate for the child's age and language. For example, if an articulation test has picture cards, the child must have the vocabulary necessary to name the pictures.

Finally, try to use at least some tests that have been developed for children with hearing impairments (although this may not always be possible, because few tests are available). Other tests have not been designed to be administered with sign. Moreover, norms of many tests reflect the performance of normally hearing children and not children with hearing impairments.

Assessing Speech Skills: Intelligibility, Segmentals, and Suprasegmentals

You have several options available for obtaining a speech sample for intelligibility assessment. You can audio- or videorecord a spontaneous conversation with the child and/or you can engage the child in a story retelling activity, in which the child retells a story you have just told. Alternatively, the child can read a list of sentences or a paragraph. The intelligibility of a sample can be evaluated in two different ways. First, the recordings can be played to a group of listeners, who can assign each sample a value from a rating scale (Johnson, 1975). (Also see Chapter 8.) For example, "1" on a 5-point scale might correspond to "I understood none of the child's message," and "5" correspond to "I understood all of the child's message." The listeners also might estimate how much of the child's speech they understood, such as 10% of the words, 20%, and so forth. The second way to evaluate a speech sample is to transcribe the spoken message (and the signed message when the sample is spontaneous speech) and reference the spoken transcription to the printed text or signed transcription. You then can determine what percentage of the words or sounds were correctly spoken.

Measures of speech intelligibility vary as a function of several different variables. For instance, a child will be more intelligible when reading a paragraph than speaking a list of unrelated sentences. Her listeners will understand more of her speech if they have heard the speech of other children with hearing impairments before. Listeners will also recognize more speech if they can hear and see the child rather than only hear her. When recording intelligibility scores, you will be wise to comment on these variables, especially if you want to monitor the child's progress over time. If you do not, the child's intelligibility score might improve because of a change in an extraneous variable. You may misinterpret the change as denoting an improvement in the child's speaking proficiency.

Segmental speech testing determines which sounds the child can articulate and which sounds she cannot. Variables that you will consider when selecting test procedures include the context and the methods for eliciting sound productions. You might evaluate segmental speech production by using a choice of contexts, including nonsense syllables, isolated words, sentences, and spontaneous speech. Methodologically, the child may imitate you or might produce the sounds by naming picture cards or reading printed words aloud or by speaking spontaneously. You might use conventional articulation tests to assess segmental speech skills, such as the *Goldman-Fristoe Test of Articulation* (Goldman & Fristoe, 1969) and the *Test of Minimal Articulation Competence* (T-MAC) (Secord, 1981). Some speech-language pathologists modify the tests by eliminating test words that are not in the child's vocabulary. If modifications are made, you must record them alongside the child's scores.

Suprasegmental speech skills can be evaluated by rating the child's spontaneous speech as described by Subtelny, Orlando, and Whitehead (1981) or by asking the child to perform specific speech tasks. For instance, you might determine whether or not the child can sustain the vowel /a/ for 5 seconds (to assess breath management) or whether he can speak two-syllable phrases with correct stress and pitch variation (to assess his ability to imitate stress patterns) (Levitt, 1987).

Assessing Language Skills

Figure 18-2 presents examples of language tests sometimes used with children who are hearing impaired. They are organized according to whether they primarily assess form, content, or pragmatics.

Assessment procedures can generally be classified as checklists (e.g., Moog & Geers, 1975), tests (e.g., Quigley, Monranelli, & Wilbur, 1976) or language sample analyses (e.g., Kretschmer & Kretschmer, 1978). In compiling a checklist, you check whether or not a particular behavior is present. For example, you might check yes or no for the statement, The child recognizes the meaning of subject-verb-object sentences. Tests contain items that formally assess a child's ability to use language structures. If negation is assessed, the child might be asked to change the sentence, *He will go* to *He will not go*. Language sample analyses are usually performed on samples of both the child's receptive and expressive language. You might describe the semantic classes the child uses and recognizes, her complex sentence productions, and her communication competence.

> Allow plenty of time for language testing. You may need to extend testing over several days. It can be exhausting for both you and the child.

Interim Summary

You will use a variety of tasks to evaluate speech and language skills of children with hearing impairment. It is important that you use a child's

Form

Rhode Island Test of Language Structure (RITLS) (Engen & Engen, 1983)

Grammatical Analysis of Elicited Language (GAEL) (Moog & Geers, 1979)

Grammatical Analysis of Elicited Language (pre-sentence level (GAEL-p)
(Moog, Kozak, & Geers, 1983)

Test of Syntactic Ability (TSA) (Quigley, Montanelli, & Wilbur, 1976)

Written Language Syntax Test (WLST) (Berry, 1981)

Berko Morphology Test (Berko, 1984)

Test for Auditory Comprehension of Language (TACL) (Carrow, 1973)

Developmental Sentence Analysis (DSS) (Lee, 1974)

Content

Semantic content analysis (Kretschmer & Kretschmer, 1978)

Peabody Picture Vocabulary Test — Revised form (PPVT-R) (Dunn & Dunn, 1981)

Reynell Developmental Language Scales (Reynell, 1977)

Function

Pragmatic content analysis (Kretschmer & Kretschmer, 1978)

Performative content analysis (Hasenstab & Tobey, 1991, see their Table 1)

Figure 18-2. Examples of language tests that assess form, content, and pragmatics. Assessments that were designed specifically for hearing-impaired children and teenagers are denoted with an asterisk (*).

preferred mode of communication when testing and that you establish a rapport with the child before testing begins. When possible, include some tests developed specifically for persons who are hearing impaired.

In assessing speech skills, you will evaluate speech intelligibility, segmental speech production, and suprasegmental speech production. Your assessment procedures may include rating scales, transcriptions, and standard tests.

In assessing language skills, you will evaluate form, content, and pragmatics. Your assessment procedures may include checklists, standard tests, and language sample analyses.

ASSESSING SPEECH PERCEPTION SKILLS

If you provide auditory and/or speechreading training, the audiologist can tell you what speech information a child's hearing aid or cochlear implant provides. However, you will probably need to gather additional information to determine what *level* of speech perception training the child should receive. Some methods are offered by Erber (1982), Stout and Windle (1986), and Tramwell and Owens (1977).

Assessing Auditory Training Needs

Auditory testing involves assessing four hierarchical task levels: awareness (level 1), discrimination (level 2), identification (level 3), and comprehension (level 4) (Erber, 1982). Training activities are also structured around these four task levels.

During *awareness testing,* the child must detect the presence or absence of sound. For instance, she may raise her hand every time you speak her name. In the second level, *discrimination testing,* she must make gross discriminations between two items. You might ask her to distinguish a loud versus a soft sound or a 1-syllable word versus a 2-syllable word. During *identification testing,* the child must label a word or phrase after you speak it. She might be given a closed set of choices from which to choose (Figure 18-3). In the final level, *comprehension testing,* the child must comprehend speech. She might listen to a 1-paragraph story and then answer questions about it.

Once you have finished your assessment, you will select auditory training objectives to advance the child from her current skill level (e.g., she currently can identify monosyllabic words when her choices are limited to four) toward the next (she will practice identifying words when her choices are limited to six).

Auditory-verbal educational programs strongly emphasize auditory training in their curricula. In auditory-verbal programs, children are taught to rely on their residual hearing; sign language is usually not permitted.

Assessing Speechreading Training Needs

The goals of speechreading training are twofold: (a) to teach the child how to distinguish sounds that look alike on the face (sounds that look alike are called *visemes*) and (b) to develop the child's ability to understand the gist of a sentence. This first goal defines *analytic* speechreading training, whereas the second goal defines *synthetic* speechreading training.

You can use nonsense syllables (such as pa, ba, ma) and rhyming words to assess the child's need for analytic speechreading training. Figure 18-4 presents an example of a test that evaluates syllable recognition. For this test, you say one of the test items and the child points to the picture corresponding to what she heard. In scoring the responses, you determine how many items the child correctly identified and also look at her error patterns. Which phonemes did the child tend to confuse? Do the phonemes that were confused belong to the same viseme group or different viseme groups? (See Figure 18-5.) The test results will indicate if training should begin with teaching the child to discriminate between sounds belonging to different viseme groups (*mat* versus *cat*) or the same viseme group (*mat* versus *bat*).

You also assess the child's needs for synthetic training. Figure 18-6 presents an example of a sentence recognition assessment activity. For this

Children usually receive less speechreading training in school than auditory training. Children who use a total communication approach are more likely to receive it than children who use oral communication (because oral children receive primarily auditory training).

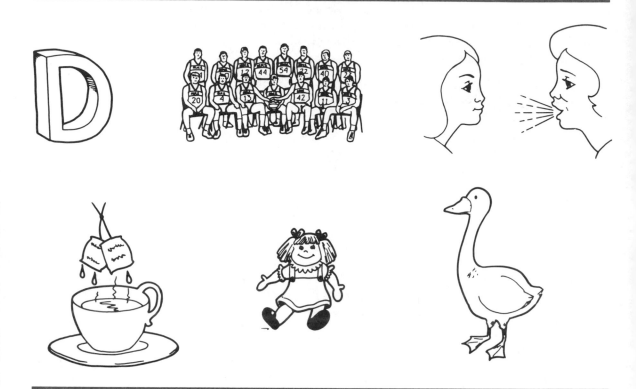

Figure 18-3. Example of a response set that can be used during identification testing. The target sounds in this exercise are /t/ and /d/. The speech-language pathologist might say "Show me the team" or "Show me the *D*." The child then must point to the corresponding picture. From *Communication Training for Hearing-Impaired Children* (p. 48) by N. Tye-Murray, 1992, Austin, TX: Pro-Ed. Copyright 1992 by Pro-Ed. Reprinted by permission.

activity, you speak a sentence and the child points to the picture that illustrates it. The child need not recognize every word to perform the task correctly. If she performs well on this task, you may then assess if the child can paraphrase sentences and then repeat them verbatim, without the assistance of picture cues. The test results will help you to design training objectives to advance the child along this continuum of tasks.

Auditory and speechreading training will develop the ability of a child with a hearing impairment to recognize speech. One reason you assess auditory skills is to determine which level of auditory training is appropriate: awareness, discrimination, identification, or comprehension. A reason you assess speechreading skills is to determine therapy objectives for analytic and synthetic speechreading training.

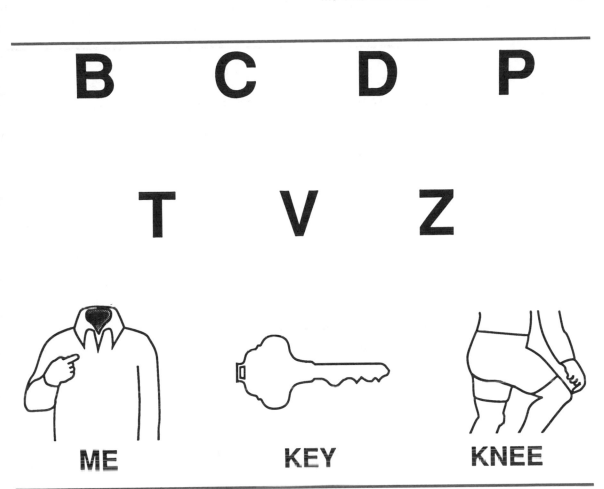

Figure 18-4. Example of a test that can be used during analysis of speechreading. The syllables rhyme, so the child must hear the first sound of a word in order to identify it correctly. From *Audiovisual Feature Test for Young Children* by R. S. Tyler, H. Fryauf-Bertschy, and D. Kelsay, 1991. Iowa City: The University of Iowa. Copyright 1991 by the University of Iowa. Reprinted by permission.

FINAL REMARKS

This is an exciting time to be working with children who are severely and profoundly hearing impaired for at least two reasons. First, new hearing devices, such as digital hearing aids and cochlear implants, allow these children to hear better than ever before. Children who use the new hearing devices demonstrate unprecedented progress in their speech and language development and their speech perception learning.

Secondly, many computerized teaching aids have recently become available. These aids include the IBM Speechviewer for teaching segmental and suprasegmental speech production (Allen, 1992; Rosenberg, 1988) and laser videodisc programs for teaching speechreading (Tye-Murray, Tyler, Bong, & Nares, 1988). Computerized teaching aids can increase the

Consonant Viseme Groups

1. /p, b, m/
2. /f, v/
3. /ð, θ/
4. /ʃ, ʒ, tʃ, dʒ/
5. /t, d, s, z, j, k, n, g, l/

Vowel and Diphthong Viseme Groups

1. /u, ʊ, o/
2. /aʊ/
3. /ɔ, ɔɪ/
4. /i, ɪ, e, ʌ, ɛ, æ, aɪ/

Figure 18-5. Consonant viseme groups and vowel viseme groups. Members of a viseme group appear the same on the face.

quality of your therapy and allow you to monitor children's performance on a daily or weekly basis (because the computer usually keeps an ongoing record of the child's performance during therapy). Not least important, computerized teaching aids can make therapy more fun for you and your clients.

SUMMARY

Children who have severe and profound hearing impairments typically develop deviant speech and language patterns. Your role as a speech-language pathologist is to assess their speech and language skills, provide speech and language therapy, and consult with their parents and other professionals who work with them. You probably will provide speechreading and auditory training to the children as well. In this chapter, we consider the hearing capabilities of children who have severe and profound hearing impairments and their characteristic speech and language problems. We then consider ways that you can assess their speech and language, and their speech perception training needs.

ACKNOWLEDGMENT

Preparation of this chapter was supported by research grants DC00242 and DC00976-01 from the National Institutes of Health/NIDCD.

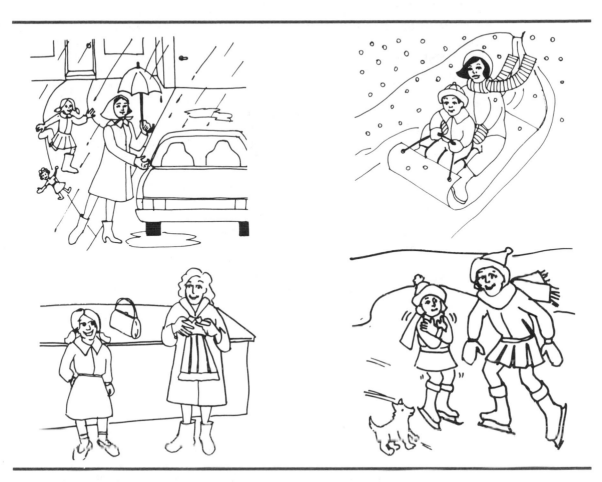

Figure 18-6. Example of a response set that can be used during synthetic speechreading testing. The speech-language pathologist might recite the sentence, *The woman holds the new dress.* The child then must point to the corresponding picture. From *Communication Training for Hearing-Impaired Children* (p. 50) by N. Tye-Murray, 1992. Austin, TX: Pro-Ed. Copyright 1992 by Pro-Ed. Reprinted by permission.

REFERENCES

Allen, B. (Ed.). (1992). IBM announces Speech Viewer II. *Speech Viewer Times, 1,* 2.

Berko, J. (1958). The child's learning of English morphology. *Word, 14,* 150–177.

Berry, S. (1981). *Written Language Syntax Test.* Washington, DC: Gallaudet College Press.

Carrow, E. (1973). *Test for Auditory Comprehension of Language.* Lamar, TX: Learning Concepts.

Dunn, L., & Dunn, L. (1981). *Peabody Picture Vocabulary Test—Revised.* Circle Pines, MN: American Guidance Service.

Engen, E., & Engen, T. (1983). *Rhode Island Test of Language Structure Manual.* Baltimore, MD: University Park Press.

Erber, N. P. (1982). *Auditory training.* Washington, DC: Alexander Graham Bell Association for the Deaf.

Goldman, R., & Fristoe, M. (1969). *Test of Articulation.* Circle Pines, MN: American Guidance Service.

Hasenstab, M.S., & Tobey, E. A. (1991). Language development in children receiving Nucleus multichannel cochlear implants. *Ear and Hearing, 12(4),* 55S–65S.

Johnson, D. D. (1975). Communication characteristics of NTID students. *Journal of the Academy of Rehabilitative Audiology, 8*(1), 17–32.

Kretschmer, R., & Kretschmer, L. (1978). *Language development and intervention with the hearing impaired.* Baltimore, MD: University Park Press.

Lee, L. (1974). *Developmental sentence analysis.* Evanston, IL: Northwestern University Press.

Levitt, H. (1987). *Fundamental Speech Skills Test.* New York: City University of New York.

Ling, D. (1976). *Speech and the hearing-impaired child: Theory and practice.* Washington, DC: Alexander Graham Bell Association for the Deaf.

Moog, J. S., & Geers, A. E. (1975). *Scales of early communication skills for hearing impaired children.* St. Louis: Central Institute for the Deaf.

Moog, J. S., Kozak, V. J., & Geers, A. (1983). *Grammatical Analysis of Elicited Language (GAEL-p).* St. Louis: Central Institute for the Deaf Press.

Quigley, S. P., Monranelli, D. S., & Wilbur, R. B. (1976). Some aspects of the verb system in the language of deaf students. *Journal of Speech and Hearing Research, 19,* 536–550.

Reynell, J. K. (1977). *Reynell Development Language Scale.* Windsor, Ontario, Canada: NFER Publishing.

Rosenberg, R. (1988, November 3). New IBM system helps deaf, hearing-impaired. *The Boston Globe.*

Secord, W. (1981). T-MAC: Test of Minimal Articulation Competence. Columbus, OH: Charles E. Merrill.

Stout, C. G., & Windle, J. V. E. (1986). *The developmental approach to successful listening (DASL).* Houston: Stout & Windle.

Subtelny, J. D., Orlando, N. A., & Whitehead, R. L. (1981). *Speech and voice characteristics of the deaf.* Washington, DC: Alexander Graham Bell Association for the Deaf.

Tramwell, J., & Owens, S. (1977, November). *The Test of Auditory Comprehension (TAC).* Paper presented at the annual convention of the American Speech-Language-Hearing Association, Chicago.

Tye-Murray, N. (1992). *Communication training for hearing-impaired children and teenagers: Speechreading, listening, and using repair strategies.* Austin, TX: Pro-Ed.

Tye-Murray, N., Tyler, R. S., Bong, B., & Nares, T. (1988). Using laser videodisc technology to train speechreading and assertive listening skills. *Journal of the Academy of Rehabilitative Audiology, 21,* 143–152.

Tyler, R. S., Fryauf-Bertschy, H., & Kelsay, D. (1991). *Audiovisual Feature Test for Young Children.* Iowa City: The University of Iowa.

RECOMMENDED READINGS

Erber, N. P. (1982). *Auditory training.* Washington, DC: The Alexander Graham Bell Association for the Deaf.

Ling, D. (1976). *Speech and the hearing-impaired child: Theory and practice.* Washington, DC: The Alexander Graham Bell Association for the Deaf.

Quigley, S. P., & Paul, P. V. (1984). *Language and deafness.* San Diego: College-Hill Press.

Tye-Murray, N. (1992). *Cochlear implants and children: A handbook for parents, teachers and speech and hearing professionals.* Washington, DC: The Alexander Graham Bell Association for the Deaf.

Tye-Murray, N. (1992). *Communication training for hearing-impaired children and teenagers: Speechreading, listening, and using repair strategies.* Austin, TX: Pro-Ed.

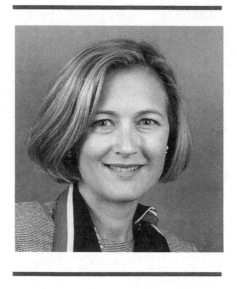

NANCY TYE-MURRAY, Ph.D.

Ph.D. 1984, The University of Iowa

Dr. Tye-Murray is a senior research scientist in the Department of Otolaryngology — Head and Neck Surgery, The University of Iowa. She directs the aural rehabilitation and speech production program for children and adults with cochlear implants. Her special research interests are the use of conversational strategies by individuals with hearing impairments and their families, speechreading training, the role of auditory information in acquiring and maintaining speech production, and performance of adult cochlear implant users over time.

INDEX